Essential Quick Review
PROSTHODONTICS

Essential Quick Review
PROSTHODONTICS

Editor-in-Chief

Priya Verma Gupta MDS FPFA
Professor
Department of Paedodontics and Preventive Dentistry
Divya Jyoti College of Dental Sciences and Research
Ghaziabad, Uttar Pradesh, India

Co-Author

Dr Suraj R Suvarna MDS
Professor
Department of Prosthodontics
Shree Bankey Bihari Dental College and Research Centre
Masuri, Uttar Pradesh, India

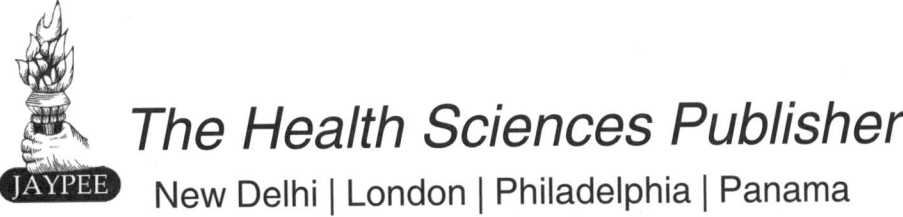

The Health Sciences Publisher
New Delhi | London | Philadelphia | Panama

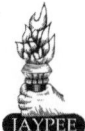 **Jaypee Brothers Medical Publishers (P) Ltd**

Headquarters
Jaypee Brothers Medical Publishers (P) Ltd
4838/24, Ansari Road, Daryaganj
New Delhi 110 002, India
Phone: +91-11-43574357
Fax: +91-11-43574314
Email: jaypee@jaypeebrothers.com

Overseas Offices

J.P. Medical Ltd
83 Victoria Street, London
SW1H 0HW (UK)
Phone: +44 20 3170 8910
Fax: +44 (0)20 3008 6180
Email: info@jpmedpub.com

Jaypee-Highlights Medical Publishers Inc.
City of Knowledge, Bld. 235, 2nd Floor, Clayton
Panama City, Panama
Phone: +1 507-301-0496
Fax: +1 507-301-0499
Email: cservice@jphmedical.com

Jaypee Medical Inc.
325 Chestnut Street
Suite 412, Philadelphia, PA 19106, USA
Phone: +1 267-519-9789
Email: support@jpmedus.com

Jaypee Brothers Medical Publishers (P) Ltd
17/1-B Babar Road, Block-B, Shaymali
Mohammadpur, Dhaka-1207
Bangladesh
Mobile: +08801912003485
Email: jaypeedhaka@gmail.com

Jaypee Brothers Medical Publishers (P) Ltd
Bhotahity, Kathmandu, Nepal
Phone: +977-9741283608
Email: kathmandu@jaypeebrothers.com

Website: www.jaypeebrothers.com
Website: www.jaypeedigital.com

© 2017, Jaypee Brothers Medical Publishers

The views and opinions expressed in this book are solely those of the original contributor(s)/author(s) and do not necessarily represent those of editor(s) of the book.

All rights reserved. No part of this publication may be reproduced, stored or transmitted in any form or by any means, electronic, mechanical, photocopying, recording or otherwise, without the prior permission in writing of the publishers.

All brand names and product names used in this book are trade names, service marks, trademarks or registered trademarks of their respective owners. The publisher is not associated with any product or vendor mentioned in this book.

Medical knowledge and practice change constantly. This book is designed to provide accurate, authoritative information about the subject matter in question. However, readers are advised to check the most current information available on procedures included and check information from the manufacturer of each product to be administered, to verify the recommended dose, formula, method and duration of administration, adverse effects and contraindications. It is the responsibility of the practitioner to take all appropriate safety precautions. Neither the publisher nor the author(s)/editor(s) assume any liability for any injury and/or damage to persons or property arising from or related to use of material in this book.

This book is sold on the understanding that the publisher is not engaged in providing professional medical services. If such advice or services are required, the services of a competent medical professional should be sought.

Every effort has been made where necessary to contact holders of copyright to obtain permission to reproduce copyright material. If any have been inadvertently overlooked, the publisher will be pleased to make the necessary arrangements at the first opportunity.

Inquiries for bulk sales may be solicited at: jaypee@jaypeebrothers.com

Essential Quick Review: Prosthodontics

First Edition: **2017**

ISBN: 978-93-86056-21-4

Printed at Rajkamal Electric Press, Plot No. 2, Phase-IV, Kundli, Haryana.

Editorial Board

Priya Verma Gupta MDS FPFA
Professor,
Department of Paedodontics and Preventive Dentistry
Divya Jyoti College of Dental Sciences and Research
Ghaziabad, Uttar Pradesh, India

Gunjan Gupta MDS
Assistant Professor
Department of Periodontics
Shree Bankey Bihari Dental College and Research Centre
Ghaziabad, Uttar Pradesh, India

Nishant Gupta MDS
Assistant Professor
Department of Orthodontics and Dentofacial Orthopedics
Shree Bankey Bihari Dental College and Research Centre
Ghaziabad, Uttar Pradesh, India

Rishab Malhotra MDS
Assistant Professor
Department of Paedodontics and Preventive Dentistry
Jaipur Dental College
Jaipur, Rajasthan, India

Preface

I am very pleased to introduce you to the first edition of Essential Quick Review; A series for final year undergraduate students.

The series will be available in eight subjects, i.e., Periodontics, Operative Dentistry and Endodontics, Paedodontics, Prosthodontics, Oral Surgery, Oral Medicine and Radiology, Orthodontics and Public Health Dentistry covering essential parts of each subject. This book will not only help the student to attain the knowledge, but will also give an idea how to attempt a question during the examination, covering entire syllabus in a limited period of time.

The book gives a complete outline for writing an essay type, a short answer type or a viva-voce type of question. The language used is very simple enabling a better understanding with well-illustrated diagrams wherever possible. Each book also carries a section that contains recently asked questions covering majority of the universities in India.

What makes it different from other books is, that it is supported with a supplementary booklet for each subject that contains three sections, i.e., definitions, classifications and viva-voce covering the entire syllabus enabling the student to undergo a quick revision.

The study material provided in this book is an attempt to provide an additional help to students for easy retention and reproduction of subject in the examination. This book is in no way a replacement to standard text books.

I thank all my subject matter experts for their valued suggestions and contributions. A very special word of thanks to my family for being the source of constant encouragement. I profusely thank Shri Jitendar P Vij (CEO), Mr Ankit Vij (Group President), and production team of M/S Jaypee Brothers Medical Publishers (P) Ltd, New Delhi for their enthusiasm and constant efforts in bringing out this book.

Dr Priya Verma Gupta

Contents

Section 1 Complete Dentures

1. Introduction to Complete Dentures 3-5
2. Diagnosis and Treatment Planning 6-15
3. Impression and Mouth Preparation 16-20
4. Primary Impression and Laboratory Procedures 21-36
5. Secondary Impression and Laboratory Procedures 37-42
6. Maxillomandibular Relations 43-48
7. Laboratory Procedures Prior to Try-In 49-56
8. Laboratory Procedures for Insertion 57-64
9. Relining and Rebasing 65-69
10. Special Complete Dentures 70-74

Section 2 Removable Partial Dentures

11. Introduction to Removable Partial Dentures 77-82
12. Diagnosis, Treatment Planning and Mouth Preparation 83-87
13. Major and Minor Connectors 88-96
14. Rests and Rest Seats 97-101
15. Direct and Indirect Retainers 102-107
16. Surveying 108-113
17. Principles of Removable Partial Denture Design 114-119
18. Secondary Impressions for Removable Partial Denture 120-122
19. Laboratory Procedures for Removable Partial Denture Design 123-125
20. Types of Removable Partial Denture and its, Correction and Repair 126-130

Section 3 Fixed Partial Dentures and Implants

21. Introduction to Fixed Partial Dentures 133-136
22. Treatment Planning and Mouth Preparation 137-141
23. Occlusion 142-146
24. Abutments 147-150
25. Tooth Preparations 151-159
26. Types of Fixed Partial Dentures 160-165
27. Impression Making 166-170

28. Provisional Restorations and Laboratory Procedures 171-175
29. Cementation 176-181
30. Maxillofacial Prosthetics and Implant 182-186

Section 4 Recently Asked Questions

31. Recently Asked Questions 189-220

SECTION 1

COMPLETE DENTURES

CHAPTER 1

Introduction to Complete Dentures

LONG ESSAY

Question 1

Define prosthesis and write in detail about branches of prosthodontics?

Answer

- Prosthesis may be defined as an appliance which replaces the lost or congenitally missing tissue restoring both function and the appearance of the tissue. Prosthesis, denture, denture prosthesis and restoration may be used synonymously
- Prosthetics is an art and science of designing and fitting artificial substitutes to replace lost or missing tissues
- Prosthodontics/prosthetic dentistry/dental prosthetics is the branch of dentistry pertaining to the restoration and maintenance of oral function, comfort, appearance and health of the patient by the restoration of the natural teeth and/or the replacement of missing teeth and contiguous oral and maxillofacial tissues with artificial substitutes.

Branches of Prosthodontics

Prosthodontics has several branches as follows:
- Removable prosthodontics.
  - Complete denture prosthodontics
  - Partial denture prosthodontics.
- Fixed prosthodontics
- Maxillofacial prosthodontics
- Implant prosthodontics.

Removable Prosthodontics

The branch of prosthodontics concerned with the replacement of teeth and contiguous structures for edentulous or partially edentulous patients by artificial substitutes that are removable from the mouth.

Fixed Prosthodontics

The branch of prosthodontics concerned with the replacement and/or restoration of teeth or both by artificial substitutes that are not readily removable from the mouth.

Maxillofacial Prosthodontics

The branch of prosthodontics concerned with the restoration and/or replacement of the stomatognathic and associated facial structures with prosthesis that may or may not be removed on a regular or elective basis.

Implant Prosthodontics

The phase of prosthodontics concerning the replacement of missing teeth and/or associated structures by restorations that are attached to dental implants.

Complete Denture Prosthodontics

The replacement of the natural teeth in the arch and their associated parts by artificial substitutes.

Removable Partial Denture Prosthodontics

The science and techniques of designing and constructing partial denture.

Types of Prosthesis

Denture

An artificial substitute for missing natural teeth and adjacent tissues. A denture may be partial or complete.

Partial Denture

A dental prosthesis that restores one or more but not all of the natural teeth and/ or associated parts and that is supported in part by natural teeth, dental implant supported crowns, abutments, or other fixed partial dentures and/or the mucosa.

Based on patient's capability to remove or not to remove the prosthesis, a partial denture may be fixed or removable.

Fixed partial denture

A partial denture that is luted or otherwise securely retained to natural teeth, tooth roots and/or dental implant abutments that furnish the primary support for the prosthesis.

They are of two types:
1. Screw retained fixed partial denture
2. Cement retained fixed partial denture.

Removable partial denture

Any prosthesis that replaces some teeth in a partially dentate arch. It can be removed from the mouth and replaced at will.

Complete Denture

A removable dental prosthesis that replaces the entire dentition and associated structures of maxillae and mandible.

Objectives

The desired objectives in complete denture prosthesis are as follows:
- Aesthetics: The restoration of the facial dimension and lost contour with normal appearance
- Mastication: The restoration of the function of mastication for adequate nutrition
- Phonetics: The restoration of speech due to loss of teeth. The complete dentures help the patient to speak as distinctly as breathing factors will permit
- The complete dentures will provide the patient with oral comfort and improve the sense of wellbeing
- Preservation of oral structures: The patient should be informed about the changes to be expected in the supporting tissues and convinced him of the need for regular check-ups and further treatment.

Aesthetics

- The main part of the face to suffer change by the loss of the teeth and consequent resorption of the alveolar process is the lower third
- The lips lose their normal pose and exhibit an unnatural expression
- The wrinkle of face and aged appearance sets in
- The prosthodontics should correct and as far as possible restore the normal appearance
- It requires an artistic sense to develop the correct facial contour in order to restore harmony in each individual type of expression
- The colour of artificial teeth must be harmonious with the colour of the eyes, hair and patient's complexion
- The form, size and arrangement of the teeth and their treatment by grinding to simulate wear appropriate to the age of the patient must also be done.

Mastication

- When the function of mastication is impaired, the digestive organs fail to properly digest the food which results in poor health and a curtailment of the span of life
- The substitutes for the natural teeth should be provided that function as far as practicable
- The achievement of these objectives will, of course, be limited by the physiologic and psychologic condition of the patient.

Phonetics

- The third objective is the correction of speech defects resulted from absence of natural teeth or from improper arrangements of teeth
- The best result is most often obtained by placing the teeth as nearly as possible in position occupied by the natural teeth
- These can be done by using the proper form of teeth selection and adjusting the bulk of base material as well as the reproduction of the rugae of the palate.

SHORT ESSAY

Question 1

Write about indications and contraindications of complete dentures.

Answer

Indications

- Presence of acceptable edentulous ridge or ridges with sufficient vertical space to accommodate the dentures or dentures without affecting any major change in the patient's vertical dimension after the post-extraction tissue changes occurred
- Serious loss of masticatory function or impairment of aesthetics, speech and psychologic wellbeing
- Treatment of patients where remaining teeth cannot be retained owing to extensive carious destruction or periodontal bone loss.

Contraindications

The fabrication of complete denture is difficult in the following situations:
- An edentulous patient who has not worn dentures in many years

Chapter 1 Introduction to Complete Dentures

- Unmanageable mechanical problems associated with major lack of vertical inter-arch space
- Patient with no salivary function as a result of radiation or drug therapy
- Altered systemic health, e.g. uncontrolled diabetes, Parkinson's disease, epilepsy, etc.
- Allergy to acrylic resin
- Patient with severe or total paralysis of motor nerves of tongue, cheeks, lips or floor of the mouth
- Excessive loss of maxilla or mandible as a result of radical surgery
- Large maxillary or mandibular tori.

SHORT NOTES

Question 1
Write a short note on treatment options for edentulous patients.

Answer
- Edentulous in one or both arches with no prior denture experience
    - Complete dentures
    - Implant-supported overdentures
    - Implant-supported fixed prosthesis.
- Edentulous in both arches with an adaptive complete denture experience
    - Complete dentures
    - Implant-supported overdentures
    - Implant-supported fixed prosthesis.
- Edentulous in one or both arches with current maladaptive denture experience
    - Implant-supported overdentures
    - Implant-supported fixed prosthesis.

Question 2
Write a short note on clinical and laboratory procedures of complete denture prosthesis.

Answer
- First appointment
    - History, examination, diagnosis, treatment planning, prognosis and patient education
    - Preliminary impressions corrected and tested.
- Laboratory preparations for the second appointment
    - Pouring diagnostic casts, custom tray fabrication.
- Second appointment
    - Final impressions.
- Laboratory preparations for the third appointment
    - Boxing, cast pouring, occlusal rims on base plate.
- Third appointment
    - Recording of jaw relations
    - Selection and arrangement of artificial teeth.
- Fourth appointment
    - Tryin.
- Laboratory preparation for the fifth appointment
    - Waxing, flasking, curing, polishing and finishing.
- Fifth appointment
    - Insertion and instructions to the patient.
- Sixth appointment
    - Twenty-four hours post-insertion check for adjustments.
- Recall for check-up periodically.

Chapter 2: Diagnosis and Treatment Planning

LONG ESSAY

Question 1

Discuss in detail the clinical significance of diagnosis and treatment for ensuring success of complete denture treatment.

Answer

- Diagnosis is the examination of the physical state, evaluation of the mental or psychological make-up and understanding the needs of each patient to ensure a predictable result
- Diagnosis in complete denture is a continuing process and is not accomplished in a short time. In many patients, the most important finding escapes the operator until the planned treatment is near to completion
- The diagnostic record for complete denture treatment can best be complied by using a systematic diagnostic form
- From this information a treatment plan and prognosis can be developed. The dentist must consider each patient as an individual. It is possible to categorise patients and anticipate certain problems but always remember that not all patients will fit a predetermined group.

According to difficulty faced, patients can be categorised in the following types:

- Group 1: Relatively easy, compromises can be made during the treatment (70%)
- Group 2: Somewhat difficult, they make about 20% of all patients
- Group 3: Difficult, about 10% of the patients who have anatomical and psychological problems.

Treatment Planning

- Developing a course of action that encompasses the ramification and sequelae of treatment to serve the patient's needs
- Treatment planning is a consideration of all of the diagnostic findings, systemic and local, which influence the surgical preparations of the mouth, impression making, maxillomandibular relation records, occlusion to be developed, form and material of the teeth, denture base material and instructions in the use and care of dentures
- In evaluating a patient, a decision should be reached whether or not successful therapy can be instituted for that patient
- This decision should be based upon the result of the examination
- It should be based upon a physical examination; the patient's attitude may negate the construction of successful complete denture
- The success of complete denture treatment depends on so many physical and mental variables. It is advisable to use a complete checklist to ensure that all the influencing conditions have been examined.

Diagnostic Form

Patient Data

Name _____
Tel. Ph.: (Home) _____ (Business) _____
Age _____ Sex _____
Occupation and social position _____
Tooth shade _____ Mucosa shade _____
Cosmetic index: Class I (high), Class II (medium), Class III (low).
Personality: Philosophic, exacting, hysterical and indifferent

Medical History

- General health
- Major ailments (if any)
- Whether under any medication:

Dental History

1. Chief complaint _____
2. Period of edentulousness _____
   Maxilla _____
   Mandible _____
3. Reason for extraction _____
   Caries _____
   Periodontal diseases _____
   Others _____
4. Previous denture history-number _____
   Satisfactory/Unsatisfactory _____
   If unsatisfactory, state the reasons _____

Existing dentures experience

- ❏ Retention
- ❏ Stability
- ❏ Extension
- ❏ Aesthetics
- ❏ Phonetics
- ❏ Occlusion.

Extra-oral Clinical Examination

1. Face form: Ovoid _____
   Square _____ Tapering _____
2. Profile _____ Straight _____
   Convex _____ Concave _____
   (Class I) (Class II) (Class III)
3. Complexion: Fair _____
   Medium _____ Dark _____
4. Lips: Active _____ Flaccid _____
   Normal _____ Long _____
   Medium _____ Short _____
   Thick _____ Thin _____
   Normal _____
5. Muscle tone: Class I (Normal) _____
   Class II (Slightly impaired) _____
   Class III (Greatly impaired) _____
6. Temporomandibular joint:
   Normal _____ Crepitus _____
   Clicking _____ Deviation _____
7. Neuromuscular coordination:
   Class I: (Excellent)
   Class II: (Fair)
   Class III: (Poor)

Intra-oral Clinical Examination

Arch size

- ❏ Class I: Large
- ❏ Class II: Medium
- ❏ Class III: Small.

Arch form

- ❏ Class I: Square
- ❏ Class II: Ovoid
- ❏ Class III: Tapering.

Shape of the ridge

- ❏ Class I: U-shaped or square
- ❏ Class II: V-shaped
- ❏ Class III: Flat
- ❏ Class IV: Knife edge.

Inter-arch space

- ❏ Class I: Ideal inter-arch space to accommodate the artificial teeth
- ❏ Class II: Excessive inter-arch distance
- ❏ Class III: Insufficient inter-arch distance.

Ridge parallelism

- ❏ Class I
- ❏ Class II
- ❏ Class III.

Ridge relationship (Angle classification)

- ❏ Class I: Normal
- ❏ Class II: Retrognathic
- ❏ Class III: Prognathic.

Bony undercuts

- ❏ Maxilla: Class I (None), Class II (Slight), Class III (More)—require removal
- ❏ Mandible: Class I (None), Class II (Slight), Class III (More)—require removal.

Tori

- ❏ Class I (Absent)
- ❏ Class II (Mild): Surgery optional
- ❏ Class III (Large): Require surgical removal.

Palatal throat form

- ❏ Class I: Gentle (large and normal in form with a relative immovable band of resilient tissue 5–12 mm distal to a line drawn across the distal end of the tuberosities)

- Class II: Medium (sized normal in form with immovable tissue 3–5 mm distal to a line drawn across the distal end of the tuberosities)
- Class III: Abrupt (drop of soft tissue 3–5 mm anterior to a line drawn across the palate at the distal end of the tuberosities).

Lateral throat form

- Class I: Large
- Class II: Medium
- Class III: Small.

Mucosa condition

- Class I: Healthy: Uniform thickness and firm
- Class II: Irritated and thin
- Class III: Pathological thick and flabby.

Border and frenum attachments

- Class I: High
- Class II: Medium
- Class III: Low.

Saliva

- Class I: Normal quality and quantity
- Class II: Excessive saliva with much mucin
- Class III: Scanty with mucin.

Tongue size

- Class I: Normal
- Class II: Large
- Class III: Small.

Tongue position

- Class I: Normal
- Class II: Retracted
- Class III: Retracted.

Gag reflex

Radiographic Examination

Pre-extraction records.

Treatment Plan and Prognosis

- Tissue conditioning
- Pre-prosthetic surgery
- Tooth selection shade mould and material.
  - Maxillary anterior
  - Mandibular anterior
  - Maxillary posterior
  - Mandibular posterior.

Prognosis

- Mandibular denture criteria for retention
  - Factors: Good prognosis, bad prognosis.
- Criteria for stability
  - Factors: Good prognosis, bad prognosis.
- Maxillary denture criteria for retention and stability
  - Factors: Good prognosis, bad prognosis.
- From this checklist, a accurate treatment plan and prognosis is formulated by collecting and interpreting diagnostic data
- The problems should be identified early and explained clearly to the patient prior to the treatment
- Problems that are explained after they occur, may delay treatment, will be considered by the patient as excuses for poor dental skill
- It will have an adverse effect on doctor-patient relation.
- A logical approach to diagnosis begins with a patient interview, which may also include a dental and medical history, followed by radiographic and oral examinations
- So, a proper emphasis should be given in collecting, interpreting and transferring the diagnostic information into a treatment plan.

Explanation of Diagnostic Form

The information required to interpret the diagnostic data properly is given above. The discussion is followed to fully correlate the diagnostic findings and clinical practice.

Patient Data

Name

It is necessary for the purpose of identification and record.

Age

The age of the patient gives an indication of his ability to wear and use dentures efficiently. Young patients are generally in good health, and this is reflected in the oral tissues.

- In young patient, resorption of ridges is rare and all the anatomical and physiological factors are more favourable than in older patients
- The young people possess more powers of accommodation or adaptability, and learn to use artificial dentures with little apparent effort
- Patients over 40 have tissues that do not heal as quickly and have a mental attitude not to adapt to new situation
- Many patients over the age of 60 years find it difficult to adapt to new situations
- Tissue repair is often slow and in many cases there was extensive destruction of denture supporting tissues
- Age is also important in the selection and arrangement of artificial teeth.

Sex

- In general, women are more difficult to please with appearance of their denture than men
- They are more aware of their face and lips than men
- Any change in this part of body is readily apparent to them
- Women during menopause can be difficult to treat due to psychological problems, dry mouth, burning sensation in the mouth and general vague pain
- Men tend to be more occupied with their work and less concerned with their dentures. They are move inclined towards comfort and function.

Occupational and social position

- Knowing the patient's occupation and social position helps the dentist in determining what the patient expects from his dentures. In general:
  - Higher the social position, more demanding the patient is about aesthetics
  - A patient who speaks before group of people would be concerned about speech patterns more than one who paints for living
  - Tooth position for a musician who plays a wind instrument would be more critical than for person who does not use the mouth in making a living
  - Person who works in cafeteria is in high risk for frequent eating.
- At this time dentist should also identify discrepancy between expectations and reality before the start of treatment otherwise success will elude both dentist and patient.

Tooth shade

- The preliminary shade selection should be made in the first visit without the patient participation as most patients have a wrong concept about the size and colour of teeth
- These require some patient education
- The final selection of tooth shade and mould is usually done at third visit and patient's participation should be needed at that time.

Mucosal shade

- The colour of the denture base material should match with the colour of the mucosa
- For proper selection of shade manufacturers, supplied colour tabs may be used at chair side.

Cosmetic index

- It is the aesthetic expectations of the patient
- The patients are classified as high, medium and low cosmetic indices
  - Class I: High cosmetic index. Patients with high cosmetic indices are often exacting, appreciative and cooperative
  - Class II: Moderate cosmetic index. The patients are of moderate expectations
  - Class III: Low cosmetic index. The patients with low cosmetic indices are often indifferent and uncooperative.

Patient personality

- Meeting the mind of the patient is essential before institution of treatment. To understand a patient, the psychological assessment is required. House (1937) classified the patient as philosophical, exacting, indifferent and hysterical.
  - Philosophical patients:
    - These patients are with best mental attitude
    - These patients are rational, sensible, calm and well-adjusted in difficult situation
    - Their motivation is generalised as they desire denture for the maintenance of health and appearance and feel that having teeth replaced is a normal, acceptable procedure. Prognosis is excellent.
  - Exacting/Critical patients:
    - These patients are methodical, precise, accurate, and immaculate in dress and appearance, at times makes severe demands
    - They are dissatisfied, distrust and want guarantee or remake at no additional charge
    - A firm control of these patients is essential.
  - Indifferent patients:
    - These patients have questionable or unfavourable prognosis. These patients have little concern for their teeth or health
    - They have little appreciation for the efforts of their dentist
    - Often seek treatment because of insistence of their family
    - They will give up early, if problems are encountered in new teeth
    - Their attitude can be discouraging to the dentists who treat them
    - Education programme in dental condition is recommended treatment plan.
  - Hysterical/Sceptical patients:
    - They are those patients who have bad results with previous treatment and therefore, are doubtful that anybody can help them

- They often have a recent series of personal tragedies such as loss of spouse, business problems
- Sometimes they demand unrealistic expectation, i.e. patients demand aesthetic and function equal or greater than natural teeth. They have poor prognosis.

Medical History

General health

- Generally, a patient who possesses a good general health will be able to accept and adapt to a complete denture better than those in poor health
- So, the dentist must know about the systemic diseases that may affect complete denture therapy, e.g. AIDS, anaemia, arthritis, Bell's palsy, carcinomas, tuberculosis, diabetes, lupus erythematosus, nicotinic stomatitis, Parkinson's diseases, Pemphigus vulgaris, Paget's diseases, Plummer Vinson syndrome and scleroderma
- The medical history questions are to alert the dentist:
  - A positive answer indicates the necessity of further investigation
  - The dentist should know what medicines the patient is taking
  - Some medicines have direct effect on the oral cavity
  - Tranquillizers and antidepressants may cause dry mouth
  - Hormone therapies often cause extreme sore mouth for edentulous patients.

Debilitating diseases

- Patients having debilitating diseases should be under medical control
- Diabetes, tuberculosis and blood dyscrasia require extra instructions in oral hygiene, eating habits and rest of tissues.

Diseases of joint

- Osteoarthritis of the temporomandibular joint (TMJ) presents a problem in complete denture construction as mandibular movements are painful
- This causes jaw relation and impression procedures difficult.

Cardiovascular diseases

In presence of cardiovascular diseases, the patient's physician should be consulted as denture appointments may be contraindicated or shortened and along with premedication.

Neurological diseases

Parkinson's diseases and Bell's palsy involve nerve and patients may be treated but the problems of denture retention and jaw relation records should be encountered with special attention.

Malignancies

- The diagnosis of oral lesions should be done by biopsy, and treatment with surgery, and radiotherapy should be followed by denture construction only after proper healing
- The clinical examination of the tissues after post-insertion of denture is essential.

Menopause

- The hormonal changes cause bone changes, generalised osteoporosis
- The mental changes may cause burning mouth, gagging and vague pain in the patients
- Medical or psychiatric treatment may be required before dentures are constructed.

Diet

- The patient should be questioned about his diet
- Dentist must remember that a patient who has been edentulous may have unconsciously changed his diet due to his inability to masticate properly and if the nutritional intake of patient is found to be lacking, an adequate diet should be prescribed.

Dental History

Chief complaint

- It is the patient's reasons for seeking dental treatment or new dentures
- The exact words of patient should be noted.

Dates of extraction of the teeth

- This helps to ascertain the rate of resorption and gives an idea of stability of the denture bearing tissues
- The longer the patient been edentulous, the more bone resorption usually is noted
- More resorption in one area than in other is difficult to treat with a complete denture
- The patients who have been edentulous for a long time and did not wear artificial dentures are difficult to treat.

Reasons for extraction of the teeth

- The reasons for loss of natural teeth help to ascertain the rate of resorption of ridges

- The rate is more expected in tooth loss due to periodontal disease. Extraction due to caries usually produces less resorbed ridges.

Previous denture history

- The denture history is very important in evaluation of the prognosis of complete denture treatment
- The number of dentures that the patient has had and the length of time each has been worn help in evaluating the anticipated prognosis
- A patient with a successful denture treatment will probably be having good prognosis again.

Existing or present dentures

- The reasons for dissatisfaction with the present dentures may also affect the type of replacement to the patient
- The following should be checked:
    - Occlusion
    - Retention
    - Stability
    - Aesthetics
    - Phonetics
    - Extension.

Extra-oral Clinical Examination

Face form

- There are four basic shapes of a person.
    1. Square.
    2. Square tapering.
    3. Tapering.
    4. Ovoid.
- The shape of the maxillary central incisor should be similar to that of face when placed upside down
- This method is known as geometric theory.

Facial profile

- The incisogingival and mesiodistal curvatures of incisor teeth are similar to the profile curvature of face
- So, facial profile is helpful for selection of anterior tooth.

Complexion

- It is important guide in the shade selection. The shade should have harmony with complexion
- The relationship of colour of hair or eye is questionable in shade selection.

Lips

- Short lips show more tooth structure
- The opposite is true for long lips
- Thin lips are difficult to treat because the slight over support may greatly affect facial expression.

Temporomandibular joint

- The TMJ should be examined digitally by placing the fingers on the joints when the patient opens and closes the mouth
- Any pain, clicking and crepitus or abnormal movements should be noted
- Discomfort or pain has been associated with excessive increase or decrease of vertical dimension and arthritis.

Neuromuscular coordination

- The mandibular movements should be coordinated
- Uncontrolled movements cause difficulty in determining correct centric relation and protrusive records and forbid the use of a balanced occlusion with anatomic tooth.

Intra-oral Clinical Examination

Arch size

- Class I (large): Best for retention and stability
- Class II (medium): Good for retention and stability
- Class III (small): Poor for retention and stability
- Denture stability will be hampered, if there is a great discrepancy between the upper and lower arch
- The choice of cuspless posterior teeth will lessen the problem.

Arch form

- Generally arch form is classified as:
    - Class I (square): The square arch is best form to prevent rotational movements and provides stability to the dentures
    - Class II (tapering): The tapering arch prevents rotational movements to a lesser degree
    - Class III (oval): The oval arch is round in shape and gives little or no resistance to rotational movements.
- If the arch form is not same in the maxilla and mandible, there will be problem with tooth arrangement and stability.

Shape of the ridge

- The contour of the residual ridge determines the amount of vertical and horizontal denture basis
    - Class I (square): The square and U-shaped ridges are best for denture stability and retention
    - Class II (V-shaped): The V-shaped ridges are less favourable as slight pressure on the denture base

causes displacement of the denture from the underlying soft tissues
- Class III (flat): The flat ridges offer the poorest resistance to horizontal forces
- Class IV (knife edge): The knife edged ridges also can offer little resistance to vertical forces.

- The pressure on the ridges traumatises the mucosa covering the top of the ridge and sufficient relief should be provided on it.

Inter-arch space

- The inter-arch distance between the ridges are approximately parallel. In case of normal interspace, the arrangement of teeth is easy and stability of the denture is good
- Excessive inter-arch space is usually accompanied by severe resorption and produces leverages on the denture base and decreases stability
- Insufficient inter-arch space creates difficulty to accommodate the artificial teeth.

Ridge parallelism

- Class I: When both the ridges are parallel, no sliding movement of the denture occurs during function
- Class II: When the mandibular ridge is divergent from the occlusal plane anteriorly one denture will slide forward
- Class III: When the maxillary ridge is divergent from the occlusal plane anteriorly or both the ridges are divergent anteriorly both the dentures will slide forward.

Ridge relationship

- Class I (normal):
  - The maxillary ridge crest is directly above the mandibular ridge
  - This is most favourable ridge relation for complete dentures and balanced occlusion is possible.
- Class II (retrognathic):
  - The mandibular ridge is narrower and shorter than the maxillary ridge that makes the setting of posterior teeth difficult
  - These patients often have wide range of mandibular movement that makes the balance occlusion necessary
  - They frequently show habitual closure position anterior to centric relation.
- Class III (prognathic):
  - The mandible is larger and wider than maxillae
  - These patients show no excursive movement but only open and close hinge jaw movement
  - This makes balance occlusion unnecessary
  - These patients show a posterior, and sometimes, an anterior cross-bite.

Bony undercuts

- Bony undercuts are found on both the maxillary and mandibular ridges
- On maxilla, undercuts are usually present in anterior ridge and lateral to the tuberosities. Undercuts do not help in retention but cause loss of border seal.

Tori

- Small mandibular or maxillary tori usually present no problem in denture fabrication
- If undercuts are present in tori, they should be removed surgically
- If very thin mucosa overlies, the tori relief in denture should be provided.

Mucosa condition

- Class I: Healthy
- Class II: Irritated
- Class III: Pathologic, e.g. papillomatous.

Border and frenum attachments

- Class I (low): The border or frenum attachments close to the vestibule (less than 6 mm)
- Class II (intermediate): The border or frenum attachments close to the ridge crest (between 6–12 mm)
- Class III (high): The border or frenum attachments high up the ridge crest (more than 12 mm).

Saliva

- Class I: Amount and consistency of saliva is normal
- Class II: Excessive thin saliva containing water or thick saliva contains much mucus. Excessive saliva may cause gagging and interface with impression making
- Class III: (Xerostomia) Saliva is scanty and mucinous may reduce retention of denture.

Tongue size

- Class I: normal in size
- Class II: Large in size
- Class III: Excessive large.

Tongue position

- Wright (1949) classified tongue position as follows:
  - Class I
    - The tongue completely fills the floor of the mouth
    - The lateral borders of the tongue rest on or against the residual ridges

- The tip of the tongue rests just lingual to anterior mandibular ridges
- This is the normal position of tongue and is the most favourable for denture border seal.
- Class II
  - The tongue is flattened and broad with its apex in normal position.
- Class III
  - Retracted tongue: The apex is curled upward or downward and depressed in the floor of the mouth. The retracted tongue fails to provide a seal and also unseat the mandibular denture.

Gag reflex

- Gagging is due to psychological and somatogenic causes
- The gag reflex is assessed by gently touching the palate with a mouth mirror
- The patient may gag during impression making
- To prevent that sedatives may be employed, but the medicines should be avoided
- The patient should be kept in an upright position and his attention is distracted
- The use of fast setting impression material and quick manipulation is essential.

Radiographic Examination

- The panoramic radiographs are valuable to examine the osseous structures that support the denture
- The nature of the supporting bony structure has been classified by Wical and Swoope as follows:
  - Class I: Approximately two-thirds of mandibular alveolar bone remains
  - Class II: Approximately two-thirds to two-ninth mandibular alveolar bone remains
  - Class III: Approximately one-thirds or less mandibular alveolar bone remains.
- This classification is based on the measurement of the distance from the inferior border of mandible to the lower edge of the mental foramen divided by three
- Approximately 25% of edentulous mouths show the presence of some types of retained pathology like roots, unerupted teeth, cysts, etc.
- A pantographic X-ray is valuable in estimating the bone quantity but it has little value in evaluating bone quality
- An image of retained root or unerupted tooth in a pantographic X-ray should be viewed in a periapical X-ray
- If the retained root or tooth is present for many years symptomless and shows no pathology, removal may not be necessary. Of course, a regular yearly check-up is necessary.

Pre-extraction Records

- All types of pre-extraction record are helpful
- Study casts and close up photographs are most useful, but radiographs and patient's recollection can also be used.

Treatment Plan and Prognosis

- After all the relevant information has been gathered in the form of a chart, prognosis and treatment plan should be formulated
- Treatment plan is the sequence of procedures planned for the treatment of a patient after diagnosis
- A treatment plan includes necessary pre-prosthetic surgery and tissue conditioning
- It should include the procedures to be followed, materials to be used and time schedule required for treatment
- It should be presented to the patient along with the prognosis and the fee to the patient for approval.

SHORT ESSAY

Question 1

Write about ridge relationship.

Answer

Antero-posterior

- Class I (Angle's classification) jaw relation
- Class II (Angle's classification) jaw relation
- Class III (Angle's classification) jaw relation.

In case of class II and III, the dentist has to encounter great difficulties during placement and arrangement of tooth for balanced occlusion. On the contrary, in class I jaw relation, the problem of arrangement of teeth is comparatively simple procedure.

Ridge Relationship (Lateral)

- Mandibular ridge is much wider than maxillary ridge
- Maxillary ridge is much wider than mandibular ridge
- Maxillary and mandibular ridges are almost of same width.

In the first two cases, difficulties will be encountered in setting up the teeth. In the first case, it may be necessary to arrange the teeth in cross-bite relation. In the second case, the occlusion may be limited to the second premolars and molars only.

Inter-arch Distance

- An ideal inter-arch distance at vertical dimension of occlusion is 16–18 mm
  - Normal: When there is a normal distance between the ridges, the conditions are favourable for arrangement of anterior and posterior teeth
  - Excessive: When there is an excessive distance between the ridges, it is very difficult to get stability of the dentures during mastication because of the large distance between the occlusal surfaces of the upper and lower teeth to their respective ridges
  - Inadequate: When there is very limited space between the ridges, setting of teeth may have to be mutilated to arrange them in proper position.

Nature of Denture-bearing Tissue

- The denture bearing mucosa and submucosa overlying the bone are not of uniform thickness
- Thick and compressible mucosa because of their extreme resiliency returns to their original position when compressed
- They may loosen the dentures after the pressure is released
- An extensive papillary hyperplasia due to traumatic ill-fitting denture should require surgery
- A new denture should be constructed then
- Thin incompressible mucosa never allows the dentures to bring into intimate contact with soft tissues lessening retention
- Average thick mucosa allows the dentures to bring into intimate contact with the soft tissues and good retention and prognosis is obtained.

Maxillary Ridge Prognosis

- The prognosis for the maxillary complete denture can be divided into factors that can affect retention and stability
- The factors are as follows:
  - Size of ridge
  - Shape of palatal vault
  - Bilateral tuberosity undercuts
  - Size of tuberosity
  - Maxillary torus.

SHORT NOTES

Question 1

Write a short note on surgical mouth preparation?

Answer

The prosthodontic should be aware of the situation before the extraction of teeth and perform the preparation accordingly following the list of staging of the surgical procedures.

Surgical Preparation During Extraction of Teeth

- Removal of sharp bony spicules and tips of interdental septum using the rongeur forceps
- Application of sharp pressure between thumb and index finger after, all extraction of teeth to even contouring the ridge.

Surgical Preparation of Edentulous Mouth

- Removal of retained roots or unerupted teeth, and dental cysts
- Reduction of sharp bony mass, e.g. mylohyoid ridges, sharp ridges, enlarged tuberosities, and torus
- Removal of soft hyperplastic tissues caused by denture hyperplasia or flabby anterior ridges
- Removal of high frenum attachments
- Deepening of shallow sulcus to increase denture bearing area
- Orthognathic surgery to improve ridge relation
- Important denture procedures
- Surgery of congenital defects.

Question 2

Write a short note on nutritional counselling.

Answer

- Nutritional counselling is a very important step in treatment planning of a complete denture patient
- The quality of diet for such patient can be improved with nutritional counselling
- An unbalanced diet that lacks fruits, vegetables or proteins and calories can turn perfectly made denture into an unsatisfactory one
- So, a properly guided balanced diet should be included in prosthodontic treatment
- The main objective of nutritional council is to correct nutritional imbalances that interfere with body and oral health.

Five Basic Food Guide Pyramid as Follows

1. Eat diet containing five basic types.
2. Eat at least five servings of fruits and vegetables.
3. Take fish, poultry, lean meat, eggs, or dried peas and beans daily.
4. Eat four servings of calcium rich food daily.
5. Take eight glasses of water.

Question 3

Write a short note on prosthodontic care.

Answer

Nature of Treatment

- Patients in need of prosthodontic care can be divided into three general groups:
  1. Those with natural teeth remaining.
  2. Those wearing dentures who wish or need replacements.
  3. Those who are edentulous.
- The first group of patients may be treated with removable partial denture, or overdentures
- The second and third group of patients may be treated with conventional soft tissue supported complete denture or implant supported complete denture
- Articulator used
- Manufacturer and instrument number
- Control settings: Horizontal condylar guidance (right and left), incisal guide angle, and incisal guide lateral angle (right and left)
- Tooth selection: The shade, mould and material of anterior and posterior teeth should be selected
- Denture base material: Available materials like heat cure or microwave cure or soft base
- Denture base shade: Pink, special pink, veined matching the patient's gingiva
- Anatomic palate including rugae or conventional palate
- Characterization: Choice of stain, drawing proposed plan
- List of items to improve the new dentures
- List of items not to be changed in new dentures.

Question 4

Write a short note on patient appointments.

Answer

- In the first visit, a set of preliminary impressions may be obtained. In addition, surgical procedures are discussed and planned and pre-operative therapy may be given
- This therapy needs the use of any medicine or rest to the mouth to produce ridges which are well healed and the gingiva are in good tonus
- During the second office visit, the final impression is taken and the cast poured using dental stone. Bite rims are made prior to the third visit
- The third visit is concerned with obtaining vertical dimension centric relation and orientation relations which is transferred to an articulator. In addition, eccentric relations are obtained and the condylar guidance is established. The selection of anterior teeth is possible in this stage
- The fourth visit is to trying of dentures to verify records and to satisfy the patient's aesthetic need
- The fifth visit is the insertion of the dentures
- The sixth visit is the first post-operative visit after 24 hours for sore spot adjustment, remounting of casts and final occlusal adjustment
- Then any subsequent visit required for oral examinations and treatments. When the periodic recall for oral examination and the necessary post-insertion appointments are completed the patients are instructed to call for an appointment, if there is any problem
- Every denture patient should be placed on a regular recall programme at a 12 months interval. The necessary occlusal corrections, relining and new denture should be made as required as changes in the mouth occur continuously.

Question 5

Write a short note on prognosis.

Answer

- The determination of the prognosis of every complete denture case is important to both operator and patient. The examination both visual and digital will bring out all the favourable and unfavourable circumstances under which the problem is to solve
- An analysis of the situation will show the operator the extent of favourable and unfavourable conditions and assess his ability to reduce the unfavourable conditions using certain techniques
- The cost of production in this case may increase due to mouth preparations, relining, rebasing, or even remaking the dentures
- The unfavourable oral condition of the patient must be informed before the start of treatment and with the cooperation of the patient the operator can utilize his skill to produce successful dentures
- There are a number of salient features in the mouth to be taken into consideration before determination of prognosis.

CHAPTER 3

Impression and Mouth Preparation

LONG ESSAYS

Question 1

Define complete denture retention. Enumerate the various factors of retention.

Answer

- Retention defined as the resistance in the movement of a denture away from its tissue foundation, especially in a vertical direction
- It is the quality inherent in the prosthesis acting to resist the forces of dislodgement along the path of placement, e.g., the forces of gravity, the adhesiveness of foods, or the forces associated with opening of the jaws. It provides psychological comfort and prevent mental trauma to the patient
- The relation of a complete denture is determined by the fit of the tissue bearing surface so alteration of the dimensions of this surface affects the retention. When the denture is worn, saliva fills the space between the denture and the tissue.

Factors Affecting Complete Denture Retention

- Physical factors: The primary retention of complete denture is obtained from various physical factors. They act just after the insertion of the denture in the mouth
- Biological factors: The secondary retention is obtained by acquired muscular control gradually acquired by the patient after wearing the denture a period of time
- Mechanical factors: Those are aids in retention when applicable.

Physical Factors

The physical forces of adhesion, cohesion, gravity and atmospheric pressure play an important role in denture retention.

Adhesion

- It is defined as the molecular attraction between unlike molecules to bind them together and form a larger mass
- A drop of water introduced on the surface of a solid glass plate will resist movement away from the glass.
- This occurs between the denture base and saliva, and mucosa and saliva. The physical laws of adhesion are as follows:
  - Adhesion is indirectly proportional to the areas in contact, i.e. the more the area covered, the greater the adhesion
  - Adhesion is increased in proportion as the contact is closer
  - Adhesion is increased as the contact is prolonged
  - Adhesion is inversely proportional to the film thickness of saliva.

Cohesion

- It is the physical force of attraction between molecules of the same material
- The viscosity of saliva is important in cohesion. Normal quality and adequate quantity of saliva is cohesive. When the quantity of saliva is excessive and quality is watery, cohesion is decreased
- When the quantity of saliva is decreased and its viscosity is increased, cohesion is decreased due to increase in the film thickness of saliva
- The saliva acts as glue that pastes the denture to the mucosa.

Surface tension

- Interfacial surface tension acts by virtue of a thin film of saliva between two intimately contacted fitting surfaces of denture and oral tissues

Chapter 3 Impression and Mouth Preparation

- It is the resistance to separation in the film of liquid between two well-adapted surfaces of rigid material
- Thinner the fluid film, the greater will be the surface tension
- That is why an accurate fit is necessary.

Gravity

- The force of gravity aids in retention of lower dentures
- Conversely, it acts as a displacing force in upper dentures, but it is not of sufficient magnitude to be considered as an important factor
- In mandibular denture incorporating lead shots in the lingual polished surface of the denture base may increase the weight of the denture
- In maxillary denture, especially large and complicated obturators, gravity acts as dislodging force.

Atmospheric pressure

- It is the physical factor of hydrostatic pressure. It is due to the weight of the atmosphere on the earth's surface
- The physical property of atmospheric pressure is taken as an aid in complete denture retention
- The retention of denture by atmospheric pressure is directly proportional to the area coverage by the denture base
- For atmospheric pressure to be effective, the denture must have a prefect peripheral seal
- The pressure between the denture and basal tissue drops below atmospheric pressure
- The thickness or depth of sulcus varies from mouth to mouth but it should be 1 mm in an average
- A lower denture may be post-dammed at the distal part of the denture on the keratinized tissue of the pear-shaped pad and not on compressible retromolar pad
- The border molding and post-dam will contribute to the retention of denture by atmospheric pressure.

Biological Factors

Neuromuscular control

- Neuromuscular control is the functional force exerted by the muscles in denture retention
- The acquired muscular control developed at the reflex level to retain denture rather displace it as a foreign body
- It becomes effective after the denture has been worn for a period of time
- In younger patients, the required conditioned reflexes will be developed more rapidly than in older patients
- This is one reason why younger people are usually more tolerant of new dentures than are older patients.

Intimate tissue contact

- Intimate tissue contact is a biologic factor that refers to the close adaptation of the denture base to the underlying soft tissues
- The technique of impression will determine the degree of intimate tissue contact obtained with the tissues at rest and during function.

Peripheral seal

- The border seal affected by intimate contact of both the upper and lower denture borders with the surrounding soft tissues
- The seal around the posterior palatal seal area enhances its effectiveness
- The soft tissue area at or beyond the junction of the hard and soft palates on which pressure, within physiologic limits, can be applied by a denture to aid in its retention
- The retention of a complete upper denture is largely dependent upon the establishment of an effective seal against the ingress of air around its border
- The post-dam extends across the pterygomaxillary notches and along the vibrating line
- It should be about 4 mm wide in its widest part.

Shape of the ridge

- The success in denture retention is achieved when the edentulous ridges are firm and regular and covered with firmly attached dense mucoperiosteum. Patients possessing high V-shaped palatal vault present the retention problem
- The processing error may be so severe that post-palatal seal cannot compensate for the resultant lack of intimate tissue contact. In such situation, either a metal base or a cold cure relining will be necessary.

Mechanical Factors

Undercut areas

- The undercuts are frequently found at labial side of maxillary ridge and buccal to one or both tuberosities
- Generally, undercut ridges do not aid in retention of dentures. In case of unilaterally undercut, it is possible to rotate the denture into position
- The presence of undercut helps in retention, if they possess some compressibility to allow the denture to be inserted
- The undercuts exist labial of the maxillary alveolar ridge and buccal to one or both tuberosities prevent vertical displacement of denture.

Denture adhesives

- The adhesive in powder form contains natural gums as tragacanth or acacia or karaya with cellulose
- The powder is sprinkled on the moist fitting surface of the denture and fitted in the mouth where it sticks to the tissues for several hours
- The gum is gradually washed away due to flow of saliva and its effect is lost. So, it is effective in upper denture but not effective in lower denture where salivary flow is more
- Advantages:
  - It is useful during jaw relation records with temporary base and its verification afterwards
  - It can be used to wear old denture when the current denture is being repaired
  - It can be used for short period in immediate denture which becomes loose due to alveolar resorption
  - It can be advantageous to use adhesive by public speakers, e.g. singers, teachers, actors, etc.
- Disadvantages:
  - It is not much effective in lower denture
  - It works as a temporary measure
  - It produces an unpleasant feeling.

Springs

- Coiled stainless steel springs fitted with swivels in the premolar region of both the dentures are used where retention is extremely poor, particularly in hemimaxillectomy or congenital defects in maxilla
- The dentures are attached with each other and have to be inserted in the mouth by holding in intercuspal position.

Suction disks

- These aids in retention by creating partial vacuum. Rubber suction disks are held by a metal stud inserted into the fitting surface of the palate of the maxillary denture
- It often causes ulceration and ultimate perforation of the palate due to bone resorption.

Suction chambers

- A relief chamber is created on the fitting surface of the palate, produce partial vacuum and may help in denture retention
- It should be of no use when tissue grows down into it to obliterate it
- These forces, however, will be negligible when the teeth are separated by a few millimetres.

Question 2

Write about stability and discuss factors effecting stability.

Answer

Stability is defined as the quality of prosthesis to be firm, steady, or constant to resist displacement by functional, horizontal and rotational stresses.

Factors Affecting Stability

- Residual ridge height and contour
- Adaptation of denture base to the underlying tissues
- Residual ridge relationship
- Contour of polished surfaces
- Relationship of the opposing occlusal surfaces
- Tooth position and occlusal plane.

Residual Ridge Height and Contour

- The stability of the complete denture depends upon the anatomic variations of the patient determined by residual ridge height and contour
- A large, square, broad ridge offers a greater resistance to lateral forces than a small, narrow, tapered ridge
- Small rounded irregularities often contribute to better stability than a ridge smoothened by alveoplasty.

Adaptation of Denture Base

- The close adaptation of the denture base to the underlying healthy mucosa is most important for stability
- Adequate extension of the denture base for maximum coverage within ridge physiological limits and positive and intimate contact of the denture base with facial and lingual ridge slopes is essential for denture stability
- The nature of the soft tissue in the palatal inclines is ideal to resist horizontal or rotating forces due to their thickness
- The development of stability is limited by the anatomic variations that determine the residual ridge height
- The lingual slope of the mandible is almost 90 degrees to the occlusal plane
- This successfully resists horizontal forces. Large, square and broad ridges provide a greater resistance to horizontal force than small, round, narrow and tapered ridges
- The surgical removal will decrease stability.

Residual Ridge Relationship

- The horizontal ridge relation is usually rated by Angle's classification

- In class I ridge relation, the stability is better for complete dentures as the maxillary ridge crest is directly above the mandibular ridge
- In class II, the mandibular ridge is narrower and shorter than the maxillary ridge and also often has a large excursive movement
- That causes loss of stability and makes balanced occlusion important.

Contour of Polished Surfaces

- The contour of the external polished surface provides the principal factor for complete denture stability
- The shape of the denture bases should be triangular in cross-section
- The maxillary buccal flange should incline laterally upward
- The mandibular buccal flange should incline laterally and downward and its lingual flange should incline medially and downward
- The general cross-section of the polished surface of a denture through the residual ridge area should be triangular
- This permits forces to direct against these surfaces for best stability.

Relationship of the Opposing Occlusal Surfaces

- The presence of balanced occlusion reduces lateral destabilizing forces and helps in stability of dentures
- The function of speech, swallowing and mastication are considered as the normal range of function
- The premature contacts during various functional and para-functional movements developed lateral forces and affect the stability
- Bilateral occlusal contact in centric relation is essential to limit the dislodging forces.

Tooth Position and Occlusal Plane

- The superoinferior position of the occlusal plane is a factor for stability
- A mandibular occlusal plane that is too high can result in reduced stability
- It is due to two reasons:
  1. First, lateral lifting forces directed against the teeth are magnified as the plane is higher.
  2. Second, the mandibular denture needs to be controlled by the muscles of tongue, lips and cheeks.

Question 3

Define support. What are the methods to obtain support?

Answer

- Support is defined as the resistance to vertical forces of mastication, occlusal forces and other forces applied in a direction towards the denture-bearing area
- Support is the foundation, on which a dental prosthesis rests, or to hold up and serve as a foundation
- This helps in maintaining the occlusal relationships established during tooth setting on the articulator
- A complete denture could perform function ideally as long as the proper support is present to resist tissue ward movement during functional loading.

Methods to Obtain Support

Effective support is realized in a denture as:
- The denture is extended to cover a maximum surface area without impinging on movable or friable tissues
- Selectively loading the tissues most capable of resisting resorption during function
- Tissues most capable of resisting vertical displacement are allowed to make firm contact with the denture base during function
- Compensation is made for the varying tissue resiliency to provide for uniform denture base movement under function and maintain a harmonious occlusal relationship.

Factors Affecting Support

Factors within Tissue

Fit of dentures to the underlying tissues so that occlusal surfaces can correctly oppose one another at the time of initial closure and under functional loading.

Nature of Supporting Tissues

- The soft tissues should be firmly bound to underlying cortical bone and should contain a resilient layer of resilient submucosa
- The bone beneath it should be resistant to pressure induced remodelling.

Health of Tissues

- The maximum support obtained from any denture-supporting area largely depends upon the health of the supporting tissues
- The tissues should be as healthy as possible while supporting prosthesis
- They may have been abused by wearing ill-fitting dentures for many years.

Anatomical Structures of Supporting Tissues

- The success of complete denture depends largely on the relation of dentures to the supporting and limiting structures
- The denture-bearing tissues can be divided into primary and secondary support as well as tissues that require relief to minimize pressure
- The primary stress-bearing areas in mandible include the pear-shaped pad and the buccal shelf area
- The retromolar pad is not a stress-bearing area
- The distal extension of the lower denture is the junction of pear-shaped pad and retromolar pad
- The ridge crest acts at best as secondary stress-bearing area
- The mid-palatine line and incisive foramen are relief areas.

Factors in Denture and its Base

Area of coverage

- The denture is extended to cover a maximum surface area without impinging on movable or friable tissues. These help to distribute forces over a wide area
- The basic snow shoe principal of maximum extension decreases the stress per unit area under the denture base, decreasing tissue displacement and reduces denture base movement.

Area of occlusal table

The force of mastication on supporting tissues is more if the occlusal surfaces are broad than if they are narrow.

Fitting surface of denture base

It should be as smooth as possible or the rough fitting surface of the denture will have sand paper-like rubbing effect on the mucosa causing ulceration.

Impression technique

- A true mucostatic or pressure-less impression is virtually impossible
- The fluid impression material is rigid and causes some pressure
- A composite technique incorporating both pressure-less and selective pressure procedures can provide a desirable impression for a long-lasting prosthesis
- This is done by:
  - Impression materials exhibited least pressure, i.e. zinc oxide eugenol paste
  - Equalization of pressure at crest of the ridge and palatal area by incorporating escape holes or wax spacers.

CHAPTER 4

Primary Impression and Laboratory Procedures

LONG ESSAYS

Question 1

Write in detail about complete denture (CD) impression, types and objectives of CD impression.

Answer

- Complete denture is an appliance which replaces all missing natural teeth and associated structures of the oral cavity
- Impression making is the first and foremost step in CD fabrication
- Impression material is essentially required for making the impression.

Impression

- An impression is a negative likeness or copy in reverse of the surface of an object; an imprint of the teeth and adjacent structures for use in dentistry
- It is made to produce a positive form or cast of the recorded tissues.

Complete Denture Impression

A CD impression is a negative registration of the entire denture-bearing, stabilizing and border seal areas present in the edentulous mouth (GPT).

Types

There are two types of impression:
1. Preliminary impression.
2. Master impression.

Preliminary Impression

- It is defined as an impression made for the purpose of diagnosis, treatment planning, or the fabrication of a tray
- The preliminary impressions of the edentulous mouth are made for producing a diagnostic cast on which special trays will be fabricated

- The preliminary impression should:
  - Record the all denture-supporting area
  - Record the peripheral oral tissues around the denture-bearing area.

Master Impression

- It is the negative likeness made for the purpose of fabricating a prosthesis
- The dentures are fabricated over the master casts.

Necessity of two stages impression

- Due to limitations imposed by the use of standard stock impression trays, it is preferable to record the CD impressions in two stages:
  - The primary impression in first visit and the master or final impressions at a subsequent visit
  - In primary impression, displacement of border tissues is acceptable to obtain certain landmarks
  - The primary impressions are made for producing diagnostic casts and the second or the final impressions are made with more precise border extension in special trays fabricated on these casts.

Advantages of making impression in two stages

- Accurate determination of the peripheral border extensions
- Gaining the control of pressure applied in making final impression
- It helps in easier control of the flow of an impression material
- It helps in dimensional accuracy of the impression material due to uniform thickness inside the tray
- To control the movable soft tissues around the impression with little distortion of these tissues.

Objectives

- There are five primary objectives in an impression making. They are:

1. Retention.
2. Stability.
3. Support.
4. Aesthetic.
5. Preservation of residual ridge.

Retention

- Retention of denture is the quality inherent in the prosthesis which resists the forces of dislodgement along the path of placement
- It is the resistance to the vertical displacing forces that are produced by gravity, adhesive foods, and the forces form the oral musculature
- There are many dislodging forces which cause dislodgement of denture during speech or eating, causing psychologic discomfort and mental trauma
- A retentive denture prevents the embarrassing situation of denture dislodgement
- It also helps in patient's acceptance during delivery of the denture
- Retention of a denture is indirectly proportional to the amount of healthy tissue that can be covered without impingement.

Stability

- Stability is defined as the quality of prosthesis to be firm, steady, or constant, to resist displacement by functional horizontal or rotational stresses
- It is the ability of the denture to withstand horizontal forces
- For this, close adaptation to the undistorted mucosa is the most important
- The lack of stability of denture seems to cause most of the gross soft tissue and bone changes that occur under denture
- Stability of denture is, therefore, very important to the preservation of the ridge
- Stability decreases with the loss of vertical height of the ridges or with the increase in flabby, movable tissues.

Support

- It is defined as the resistance to the vertical forces of mastication, occlusal forces and other forces applied in a direction towards the denture-bearing area
- So, the greater the amount of area covered, the greater will be the support
- The best support for the denture is compact bone covered with fibrous connective tissue
- It is increased by selective placement of pressure on stress-bearing areas and relieving the non-stress-bearing areas of the basal seat that are in harmony with the resiliency of basal seat
- This helps in maintaining the occlusal relationships established during tooth setting on the articulator.

Aesthetics

- Aesthetics begins with the impression
- A well-filled border, particularly in the maxillary impression, will fill out the cheeks and lips and give support to the lip muscles
- In accordance with the amount of residual ridge loss of each patient, the border thickness should be varied.

Preservation of Residual Ridges

- Though some physiological change is expected in edentulous mouths, the preservation of existing ridges is possible
- It is done by maximum area coverage, reducing the force per unit area delivered to the supporting structures and by close adaptation to the tissues minimizing the movement of denture over the basal seat
- The less the horizontal movement, less will be bone resorption under the dentures.

Anatomic Landmarks

- Before fabrication of the CDs, the knowledge of oral anatomy of the supporting and limiting peripheral structures are essential because these are the anatomic landmarks of the denture-bearing area
- Complete dentures have three surfaces
  1. Occlusal surface.
  2. Polished surface.
  3. Basal or fitting surface or impression surface.
- The impression surface is produced from the impression of the denture-bearing area
- The denture base must extend over the denture-bearing tissues as far as possible without interfering the health or function of the tissues.

Question 2

Write in detail about theories of impression techniques.

Answer

Theories of Impression Techniques

- There are various techniques of impression for complete denture construction depending on prosthodontics concept
- They are classified in various ways as follows:

- According to degree of compression
  - Minimum pressure / mucostatic technique
  - Mucocompressive technique
  - Selective pressure technique.
- According to the position of the mouth
  - Open mouth technique
  - Close mouth technique.
- According to the types of impression tray.
  - Spaced tray technique
  - Close-fitting tray technique.

According to Degree of Compression

- The denture-bearing areas are covered by soft tissues that vary in depth and quality in different areas
- There are three basic impression philosophies/theories related to compensation for these differences:
  1. The minimal pressure technique.
  2. The definite pressure technique.
  3. The selected pressure technique.

Minimal Pressure/Mucostatic Impression Technique

- An impression that is registered with a very minimum of pressure is known as a mucostatic impression
- In this technique, an impression is obtained with low viscous material, little or no displacement of the soft tissues overlying the alveolar ridges and palate will occur
- This technique is advocated for two reasons:
  - First, the dentures are under pressure from occlusal load only for a relatively small amount of time, so dentures should fit the relaxed, unloaded tissue surface
  - Secondly, if the tissues are recorded in an undisturbed state with a free-flowing impression material, a thin film of saliva between the mucosa and the fitting surface of the denture increases retention and stability.

Indications

- Evenly thick alveolar mucosa
- Smooth surface alveolar bone
- U-shaped alveolar ridge.

Advantages

- Minute details of resting tissue surfaces are recorded
- An even space of thin film of saliva exists between the mucosa and denture surface contributes to good retention
- Minimum pressure avoids distortion of the soft tissue
- Smaller flanges give comfortable functional wear.

Disadvantages

- The mucostatic principle ignores the principle of dissipating occlusal forces over a large area to maintain the health of the basal seat
- It lacks necessary lip support, as the dentures are not extending into the labial and buccal vestibules
- The musculature is not being utilized fully for retention of the dentures
- The mucosal surface is not static over 24 hours; it is changing so the details of impression will lose during denture insertion
- The mucosa is not a closed vessel, as tissue fluids can escape under the border during chewing with the dentures
- The mucostatic principle does not consider peripheral seal in denture retention.

Techniques

- Primary impressions are made with a low viscosity alginate or plaster to produce mucostatic impression which will include denture-bearing area
- A cast is poured out of these impressions
- A spacer of 3 mm thickness is adapted over the denture-bearing area. Four steps are prepared, two at canine region and two at molar region
- The trays are prepared in shellac baseplate or self-curing acrylic resin
- The trays are checked in the mouth for proper extension and adjusted, if required
- A low viscous impression material is used to record the final impression with minimum pressure. No border moulding is done because adhesion is the only factor considered for retention
- After the material has set, the impression is removed and checked.

Mucocompressive Impression Technique

- It is an impression made under load such that the mucosa is uniformly compressed and evenly condensed
- The denture-bearing areas are not covered evenly with soft tissues but with variable depth and quality
- So, if the denture under no occlusal load touches the soft tissues entirely, on occlusal loading the denture will apply more force to the harder areas covered by thin tissues without submucosa
- This may cause rocking of upper denture in the midline
- This effect, when marked, may result in midline fracture after slight resorption of ridges
- The principal of the pressure technique is to record the soft tissues under a force similar to the occlusion and mastication, so that the softer areas are compressed by the impression

- This is done to compensate the differences in the depth of soft tissue covering from one area to another.

Techniques

The mucocompressive technique can be applied both in open mouth and close mouth techniques.

Open Mouth Impression Technique

- Primary impression is made with a low viscosity alginate to obtain mucostatic impression
- The cast is poured with good surface details
- Special trays are prepared with 3 mm thick spacer of wax over the primary casts
- The trays are loaded with an even thickness of new composition softened
- The surface of the composition is coated with vaseline and impression of the cast is made so that it flows to the sulcus
- The compound is pressed around the tray edge and chilled in cold water
- The excess composition is cut out with a knife
- The surface of the composition is softened by dipping in hot water and seated in the mouth until hardens
- The set impressions are removed from the mouth and chilled in cold water in a bowl
- The impressions are dried, the surface is heated with pinpoint flame for uniform softening, dipped in hot water before insertion in the mouth to record the impression. This produces greater compression than equally soften compound used before
- The retention is tested by asking the patient to dislodge the impression by normal movement of the lips and cheeks
- The refining of the impression is done with a very thin layer of zinc oxide non-eugenol paste (less viscous than eugenol paste).

Close Mouth Impression Technique (Functional Impression Technique)

- This technique utilizes well-fitted occlusal rims prepared on primary cast prepared from a low viscosity alginate
- The jaw relation is recorded first
- The fitting surface of the rims are loaded with impression paste
- The patient closes the mouth and performs functional movements allowing the tissues to be recorded in function
- The completed impression is then transferred to denture base that duplicates the functionally loaded tissues
- It is an impression of tissues purposefully made under a significant load so that the peripheries of the dentures are established during functional loading

- The material of choice is either mouth temperature favourable wax or soft liners.

Indications

- Unevenly thick mucosa
- Flat alveolar ridge
- Even surface of alveolar bone.

Advantages

- Peripheral seal is developed through compression of the soft tissues
- More stable denture during function due to intimate contact during function
- Load distribution is more even
- A more viscous impression material displaces the strong lip and tongue muscles during seating
- The denture made from a compressive impression has better retention as it is doubtful if that the compressed mucosa ever returns to its resting form
- With tissue in resting state an uneven space exists between the mucosa and the denture base, which prevents the development of an intact saliva film essential for good retention.

Disadvantages

- The displaced soft tissues will rebound at rest causing dislodgement of dentures
- The dentures made from such impressions may compress the ridge beyond its physiologic limit, resulting in interfere with the blood supply to the tissues of basal seat and rapid resorption of the residual ridges
- Often the dentures made with closed mouth impression are overextended and need arbitrary trimming. It requires great skill to prevent damage to the residual ridges.

Selective Pressure Technique

- Selective pressure technique is a combination of extension for maximum coverage with intimate contact with the movable tissues and light contact in non-movable tissues
- Selective pressure impression technique is based on the assumption that certain oral tissues can tolerate functional load better than others
- The selection of stress-bearing or supporting and relief area and limiting areas is determined by clinical examination
- Selective pressure impressions are made in custom trays which have less space in the primary denture stress-bearing areas, and greater space (more impression material) in the non-stress-bearing areas

- Stress-bearing areas will be recorded with pressure (over the ridge) whereas the non-stress-bearing areas (middies and incisive papillae) will be recorded with minimum pressure.

Technique

- A preliminary impression is made in a stock edentulous tray to capture the whole denture-bearing areas
- A cast is poured in these impressions. The outline for the spacer is made 2 mm short of tissue reflection point
- A sheet of modelling wax is adapted and trimmed up to this line
- A custom acrylic resin tray is made which is border moulded with stick compound
- A final wash impression is recorded with a free-flowing impression material like zinc oxide eugenol impression paste
- The principle of selective pressure technique is applied here because zinc oxide paste in a spaced tray records the attached mucosa with minimum pressure, while compound pushes the more movable tissues and peripheral sulcus areas with additional pressure to the underlying bone
- The final denture made out of this impression will selectively apply pressure to the peripheral tissues. The ridge crest areas (attached gingival) will receive less pressure.

Areas Requiring Some Pressure

Border seal area

- Areas requiring some pressure are the alveolar mucosa at the border of the denture and the posterior palatal seal area which should be recorded with slight pressure to maintain a valve-like seal for retention
- The pressure may be selectively applied along the border by eliminating the tray relief wax in that area
- It may also be done by using very soft modelling compound applied to the tray border.

Buccal shelf

- The buccal shelf is normally a secondary stress-bearing area for the mandibular denture, whereas the crest of mandibular ridge is the primary stress-bearing area (**Fig. 4.1**)
- But in an excessively resorbed knife edges mandibular ridge covered with soft and easily displaced tissues, the roles of these two areas are reversed, and buccal shelf becomes the stress-bearing area
- The border moulding material can be then extended inward to produce tissue adaptation. The escape holes or slots are employed to provide relief over the ridges.

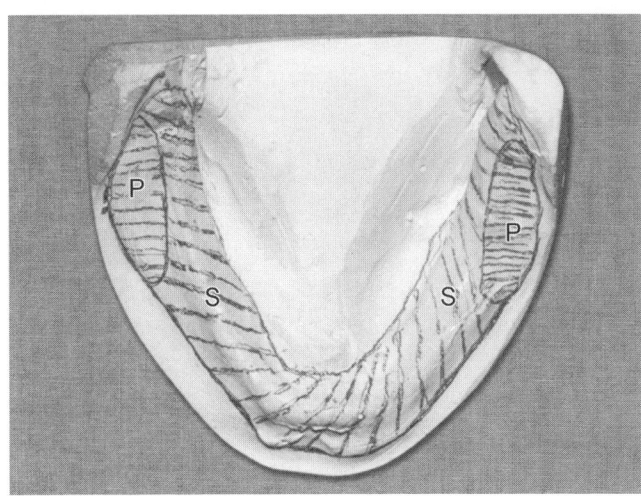

Fig. 4.1: Primary stress-bearing area (P) and Secondary stress-bearing area (S) of mandibular ridge

Retromylohyoid Fossa

The area that needs gentle pressure is the alveolar mucosa of the retromylohyoid fossa which should be in contact of the tray by adding a little soft tracing compound.

Areas Requiring Little Pressure

- Areas requiring little pressure are the residual ridges and palate and the displaceable areas found often in the maxillary anterior ridge which cannot be corrected with surgery should not be displaced during impression
- A tray with relief space and escape holes with least compressible impression material should be used
- The selective pressure technique tries to create a denture base that selectively loads the oral tissues during function of the dentures with maximum stability and retention
- The ridge crest area will be less displaced when the denture is in function (**Fig. 4.2**).

Indications

- Normal healthy ridges
- V-shaped alveolar ridge
- Cancellous and sharp alveolar ridge
- Resorbed ridges.

Advantages

- Tolerance of the basal seat to pressure helps in obtaining maximum support for the denture within the limits of functional adaptation
- Maintenance of the peripheral seal is better
- It takes into consideration the differences in tissue compressibility and produces maximum palatal adaptation of denture base.

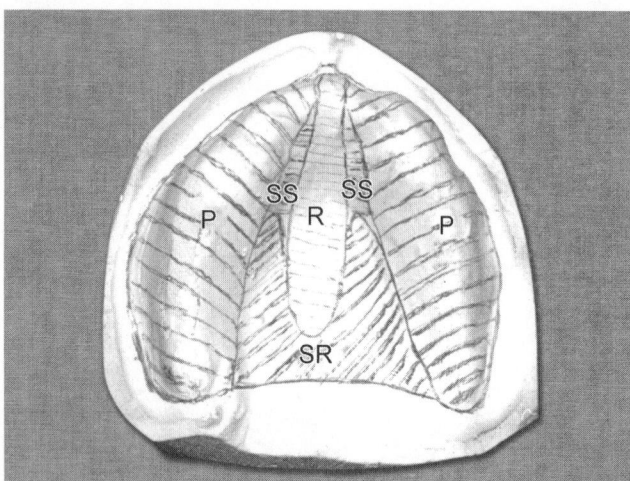

Fig. 4.2: Primary stress-bearing area (P), Secondary stress-bearing areas (SS), Relief areas (R) and Secondary retentive area (SR) of maxillary ridge

Disadvantages

- It is impossible to record some of the areas with different pressure from the others
- A denture base made with functional recording displaces the more resilient tissues
- At rest the denture base may rebound away from the underlying tissues.

According to the Position of the Mouth Impression

- Open mouth impression
- Closed mouth impression.

Open Mouth Impression

- In open mouth technique the operator will support the tray carrying the impression material in the mouth with some degree of mouth opening
- The term open mouth refers to a half-open position and no impression is made with the mouth widely open as this change the sulcus shape
- The facial musculature is stretched and reduces the sulcus width besides making it difficult for insertion of the impression tray
- On half opening the mouth there is no change in sulcus shape
- Open mouth impression is preferred to prevent a displacing force on the denture periphery when opening the mouth.

Advantages

- The operator can see the border moulding procedure
- The border moulding movements can be done more easily
- The denture is retained both in open and close mouth movements.

Disadvantages

- The correct shape of the anterior region of sulcus is difficult to attain as the operator has to hold the tray by handle
- In a few cases, where there is functionally a large difference in sulcus position during contraction of the facial muscles it is difficult to record the functional position accurately.

Closed Mouth Impression

- The impression is recorded with mouth closed in the closely adapted custom tray fitted with occlusion rim. Close mouth technique records the tissues in their functional form. In the first stage of the technique, the jaw relation is recorded
- The rims are trimmed to the correct vertical dimension to support the upper and lower trays during impression procedures.

Advantages

- In a few cases where there is functionally a large difference in sulcus position during contraction of the facial muscles, the closed mouth technique is preferred
- This method helps to border mould the periphery of the impression through the patient's own movements than by the operator and permits to record the exact functionally contracted sulcus through the entire length
- It is argued that close mouth impression causes the tissue compression under the dentures
- This however, is fallacious reasoning as impression material as a viscous fluid does not cause the same amount of force to the underlying mucosa as the denture base does
- In fact, the close mouth impression uses normal closing of the jaws to the centric occlusion.

Disadvantages

- The soft tissues displaced by the impression tend to rebound to their undisplaced position when the forces are removed. This cause unseats the denture
- The denture held in a displaced position limits in the normal blood flow
- The bone resorption due to lack of blood flow
- The resorption causes looseness of denture

- The CDs made with closed-mouth impressions are often overextended and require arbitrary trimming.

Classification of Impression Tray

- Spaced trays
- Close-fitting trays.

Spaced Trays

- These trays are used with elastomeric material or irreversible hydrocolloid impression material needed to accurately record undercut areas frequently buccal to edentulous tuberosities
- The spacing provides sufficient thickness of the material to deform elastically so as to pass over the most bulbous part of tissues and then spring back into a correct negative replica
- Outlined area of the primary cast, thus providing a space between cast and impression tray.

Close-fitting Trays (for use with Zinc Oxide Paste)

- These trays are used to take impressions of non-undercut edentulous arches using a very thin layer (a wash) impression material
- The impression made in trays is adapted directly over the primary casts. The undercut areas are blocked out before making close-fitting tray
- The cast is coated with separating medium and a sheet of self-curing resin is adapted over the cast.

Advantages

- As the trays are less bulky they are more easily inserted into a small oral aperture giving a clear intra-oral view and less discomfort to patient
- As there are less chances of displacement of cheek in sulcus areas, a more accurate impression of the sulcus is obtained
- They are very useful in cases where the mandibular rami are in close approximation to the maxillary tuberosities on both sides. The space is insufficient for a wide conventional tray
- In a case of strong musculature in lips and tongue which contracts reflexly during working in the mouth, placement of the tray is easier when the closely adapted tray is used.

Disadvantages

The limitations of the zinc oxide impression paste are the only disadvantage of the method.

Question 3

Write in detail about procedures of impression making.

Answer

- A method and manner used in making a negative likeness is called as impression making
- The CD impression procedure can be divided into the following steps:

Preliminary Impressions

- Selection of impression tray
- Selection of impression material
- Positioning of the patient
- Positioning of the operator
- Procedure of preliminary impression.

Final Impressions

- Tray adjustment
- Selection of impression material
- Border moulding of trays
- Making of final impressions.

Preliminary Impressions

- A negative likeness made for the purpose of diagnosis, treatment planning or the fabrication of a tray
- The first, the preliminary (or primary) impressions of the edentulous mouth are made in stock trays for diagnosis and for construction of custom tray
- To avoid confusion a standard conventional technique based on selective pressure theory is described, one using impression compound and one using irreversible hydrocolloid (alginate) as the preliminary impression material.

Instruments and materials

- Edentulous impression trays
- Compound knife
- Water bath (composition heater)
- Impression compound
- Bowl for hot water
- Mirror and probe
- Hanau alcohol torch
- Bunsen burner.

Selection of Stock Tray

- The shape, size and form of the alveolar ridges and palate are examined for selection of tray from a range of stock metal trays

- The upper and lower trays should cover the entire denture-bearing area and provide 6 mm space for impression material
- Care should be taken to avoid too large tray that will distort the border tissues and cause patient discomfort.

Upper tray

- Selection of upper tray is done by comparing the measurement between the buccal surfaces of the maxillary tuberosities using callipers
- The tray is inserted into the mouth and the posterior border is raised to contact the hamular notches
- The tray is then slowly raised anteriorly and visualises the width of the tray required to record the functional width of the sulcus when patient half closes his mouth
- The tray should extend 5 mm beyond the external surface of the residual ridge.
- The flanges of the tray must be at least 2–3 mm short of the muscle attachment when the muscle attachments are in a state of rest
- If required, bending of the flanges slightly with pliers will provide adequate space. The tray should be checked for its proper contact with the hard palate without causing rocking.

Lower tray

- Selection of a lower tray is done by comparing the measurement between the lingual surfaces of the retromolar pads
- The lower tray should be held with the handle pointing to the patient's left
- The left heel of the tray is inserted into the mouth with the right cheek retracted and the left heel is rotated and positioned with heels covering the retromolar pads
- The tray is lowered anteriorly to check the adaptation of the tray to the alveolar ridge
- The space of 5 mm should exist between the tray and the ridge
- The flanges of the metal stock tray must be short of the muscle attachments lingually, labially and buccally by 2–3 mm when the muscle attachments are in a state of rest
- The flanges are checked visually for overextension into the labial and buccal sulci
- The lingual sulcus is checked by having the patient to raise the tip of the tongue to the palate
- Only slight finger pressure in the premolar area will be needed to keep tray in position if the tray is not overextended.

Selection of Impression Materials

- The preliminary impression material may be:
  - Impression compound, a thermoplastic material, particularly indicated in the lower jaw with marked resorption where the surrounding tissues encroach the denture space
  - Irreversible hydrocolloid (alginate) where there are large undercuts in the anterior region and around the tuberosities or flabby ridges.

Patient's Position

- The patient should be seated upright with the head in line with the body supported on the head rest in order to prevent the impression material flowing down the throat
- When making the lower impression, the patient's mouth should be at the level of operator's shoulder
- When taking the upper impression, the patient's mouth should be at the level of operator's elbow
- The impression procedure should be explained to the patient to make the patient cooperative.

Operator's Position

- For lower impression, the operator should be in front and on right side
- For the upper impression, the operator should be behind and right of the patient.

Modelling Compound Preliminary Impression

- The preliminary impression with modelling compound allows the complete border moulding procedure in one appointment along with it
- The cast can be poured and custom tray is fabricated for the final impression.

Mandibular Impression

- The mandibular impression should be made first so that patient becomes accustomed with the procedures and materials before the more difficult maxillary impression due to gagging reflex
- The reflex salivation makes the mandibular impression difficult
- The lower impression tray should be inserted by rotating at right angle to its position into the mouth with the cheek retracted by the operator's finger
- The tray is placed in the mouth with the heels covering the retromolar pads. The anterior part of the tray is lowered to see the proper adaptation of it to the alveolar ridge
- The compound is softened in a hot water bath at 55–60°C preferably thermostatically controlled, to maintain the

recommended temperature. The compound is kneaded between the operator's fingers before use, being folded so that any creases produced will go inside the material.

Common Faults in Mandibular Impressions

Underextended in posterior lingual pouch

- Causes:
  - Tray flange is underextended in the region
  - Insufficient compound in the tray
  - Insufficient force in seating the tray
  - Tongue trapped under the tray due to failure of the patient to raise the tongue during the seating of tray.

Underextended in labial, lingual and buccal sulcus

- Causes:
  - Lack of impression compound
  - Insufficient force to seat the tray.

Presence of void in the distobuccal border

- Cause:
  - The cheek trapped beneath the border.

The edge of the tray showing through the impression

- Causes:
  - Tray not centred during seating
  - Use of too large tray or too small size tray.

Maxillary Impression

- The cake compound is heated in a water bath at 55°C and sufficient amount is kneaded into a ball free of folds
- The tray is passed over the flame to dry it so that the compound will stick to it. The ball of compound is placed over the centre of the tray
- The compound is spread over the entire tray and a shallow trough is formed corresponding to the alveolar ridge crest
- The surface of compound is flamed and tempered in the water bath
- The loaded tray is rotated into the half open mouth positioned and centred relative to the maxillary ridge, the upper lip is lifted upwards to expose the whole labial surface of the residual ridge
- The impression tray should be seated gently in place while the patient sucks in the cheeks, pulls down the lip, and moves the mandible from side-to-side and then open wide
- These actions mould the border of the impression so as to record the functional sulcus. The tray is held stationary while the compound cools
- The cheeks are raised and pushed downward to break the seal and the impression is removed by forward pull of the handle of the tray
- The impressions are checked for necessary landmarks. If the impressions are satisfactory, they are dipped in 1 in 20 aqueous solution of chlorhexidine for disinfection and poured with plaster within an hour as the modelling compound flows at room temperature
- Maxillary impression is checked for the following six landmarks:
  1. Residual ridge.
  2. Palate.
  3. Labial and buccal frenum.
  4. Fovea palatinae and vibrating line.
  5. Tuberosities.
  6. Hamular notch.

Common Faults in Maxillary Impressions

A large fold in the midline of posterior third of palate

- Causes:
  - Insufficient compound in the posterior area
  - Insufficient pressure in seating of tray.

Excess compound flowing beyond the posterior border of tray

- Causes:
  - Excessive pressure during seating of tray
  - Excess of compound in the palatal area.

Impression with an underextended periphery

- An underextended periphery can be identified in one of two forms:
1. A sharp periphery in the sulcus
- Causes:
  - Mouth is widely opened and the lips become too tight
  - Failure to pull the upper lip outwards and upwards to allow the compound to flow into the labial sulcus
  - Selected tray is too narrow in the buccal region
  - Anterior portion of the tray is placed too far back into the mouth. The impression should be made again with proper degree of mouth opening, tray positioning, or tray selection
  - Insufficient compound
  - Inadequate pressure.
2. A flat and glazed periphery usually occurs in the tuberosity region
- It is better to rectify the area by adding greenstick compound after drying, flaming, tempering, and reinserting rather than remaking the impression.

Alginate Preliminary Impressions

The material of choice for ridges with undercut is a highly viscous alginate.

Equipments and material:
- Impression trays
- Utility wax
- Tissue clock
- Irreversible hydrocolloid.

Mandibular Impression

- The mandibular impression should be made first so that patient becomes accustomed with the procedures and materials before the more difficult maxillary impression are attempted
- The dental chair is adjusted so that the mandibular arch is parallel to the floor when the mouth is opened
- The border of the tray can be adjusted with utility wax where needed. The labial and lingual posterior borders usually require adjustment
- The alginate is mixed according the manufacturer's instructions and loaded in the tray. Some alginate can be placed in the retromylohyoid spaces labial and buccal vestibule
- The tray is inserted in the mouth and partially seated on the ridge and the patient is instructed to protrude the tongue slightly. The tray is gently vibrated downward
- The lower lip is gently pulled forward to prevent trapping of air in the labial vestibule
- The patient is instructed to close the mouth as far as possible without touching the tray with the upper ridge
- The tray is held to allow the material to set. The impression after setting is removed, washed under tap water and inspected for defects
- The gross excess is removed with a sharp Bard-Parker knife. If the impression is acceptable, cast is poured immediately.

Maxillary Impression

- The patient is seated in the dental chair which is adjusted so that the maxillary arch is parallel to the floor
- The impression is recorded from behind and side of the patient
- The tray borders are modified with wax, if required. The posterior borders along the distobuccal area need often modification
- If the palatal vault is high wax should be added to the palatal vault area of the tray. The mouth should be washed and dried with a gauge piece just before the impression is recorded
- The impression material is mixed according to the manufacturer's instructions and loaded into the tray. A small amount of material is placed in the palate and the buccal and labial vestibule
- Tray is inserted into the mouth and seated posterior first by centring on ridge until the impression material flows into the sulcus
- The lips and cheeks are pulled outward to prevent trapping of air. The patient is directed to close the mouth as far as possible without touching the mandibular ridge.
- The impression is removed after setting, rinsed with tap water and excess is cut with a sharp Bard-Parker knife. If acceptable, it is poured immediately.

Patient Instructions

- The patient must be instructed to keep the existing dentures out of the mouth for at least 48–72 hours prior to the final impression
- If it is not possible due to social or business obligations, tissue conditioning material should be placed in the existing dentures and repeated several times till optimum health of the tissue is restored before the final impression.

Final Impressions

- The impression that represents the completion of the registration of the surface or object
- The final impressions are commonly recorded in special trays using a two-stage technique
- This is done first making a record of the functional sulcus, using greenstick compound traced on the tray periphery
- The final overall impressions are recorded in the modified tray with zinc oxide eugenol paste
- Elastic or elastomeric material can be used in case of large undercuts and in a very dry mouth.

Custom/Special Tray

- A special tray is defined as a custom-made device prepared for a particular patient which is used to carry, confine and control an impression material while making an impression
- The design of these trays varies with the impression technique. They should be rigid, evenly spaced from the tissues, and capable of adjustment to proper extension.

Instruments and Materials

- Handpiece and acrylic trimmer
- Mirror and spatula

Chapter 4 Primary Impression and Laboratory Procedures

- Greenstick compound
- Alcohol torch
- Hot water bowl
- Bard-Parker knife
- Scissors
- Bunsen burner.

Impression Materials

The following impression materials are now used for CD final impressions:

Border moulding materials

- Low fusing greenstick compound
- Polyether.

Final/Wash impression materials

- Zinc oxide eugenol pastes (tray: acrylic, spacer 0.5 mm):
  - These are the most commonly used final impression material now. It is rigid material and cannot be used in presence of bony undercuts. It is useful in highly resorbed ridges in closed fitted tray as wash impression.
- Silicone elastomers (tray: acrylic, spacer 1.5 mm):
  - These materials and alginate materials are used in spaced custom trays in presence of undercuts. A low-viscous alginate or silicone elastomers may be used for this purpose. The high-viscous materials are used for preliminary impression.
- Impression plaster (tray: acrylic, spacer 2 mm):
  - It was one time used frequently as a final impression material but it is not used now due to messy handling characteristic.

Border Moulding

Border moulding is defined as the shaping of an impression material by the manipulation or action of the tissues adjacent to the borders of the impression.

Importance of Border Moulding

- Border moulding records the three-dimensional form of the peripheral sulcus by functional means. The border or periphery of the denture provides ample opportunity for the ingress of air
- Correct adaptation of the denture border to the gingival sulcus and the inside of cheeks and lips ensures border seal
- The soft tissues of the lips and cheeks move inwards due to atmospheric pressure and maintain contact with the dentures
- This prevents ingress of air through the border to break the seal.

Methods of Border Moulding

- One step border moulding
- Sectional border moulding.

One step border moulding

- The whole border is recorded simultaneously in one step
- It has some advantages:
  - Number of insertion of tray is reduced to one
  - Prevents the effect of error from one area to the other.
- Polyether is the material of choice for this method.

Sectional border moulding

- This method utilizes the border moulding of custom tray section by section using stick compound
- The stick compound also known as low fusing compound, is the most common material used for border moulding. It is available in several colours like green, gray and white
- Accurate border moulding depends upon the fit of the tray. It should be 2 mm short of the reflections
- A pointed flame should be used preferable from an alcohol torch to soften the compound so that it is softened properly to adhere to the tray and has sufficient flow during moulding against the tissues
- It should be tempered in warm water bath before inserting in the mouth to prevent burn
- The compound should be dried when reheated to ensure uniform heating of the material. Border moulding is completed in two stages:
  1. First a slight overextension is allowed.
  2. Then the excess is removed by trimming from the inside of the tray and excess from outside.
- The final moulding should represent an accurate impression of the peripheral tissues
- A knife trimming around the frenum and retromolar pads is required after the refinement is completed as compound will be distorting these very displaceable tissues.

Mandibular Custom Tray Border Moulding

- The buccal extension of the lower tray is checked in patient's mouth to ensure that it is 2 mm short of the functional sulcus
- If overextended, the tray should be reduced until it has the correct extension
- It should extend across the retromolar pad until it lies just anterior to the ascending ramus of the mandible
- It should not extend beyond external oblique ridges

- The lingual extension of the tray is checked by asking the patient to protrude the tongue, to wipe across the vermilion border of the upper lip without noticeable displacement of the tray
- If the tray lifts, this indicates overextension. It should be reduced until only slight finger pressure is needed to hold the tray in position.

Border moulding

- Greenstick compound is then traced along a section of the dry lower impression tray, tempered in water bath for 3–5 seconds and the tray is inserted into the mouth
- The impression of the functional buccal sulcus is made by asking the patient to suck in the cheeks.

Distobuccal area and retromolar pad

- The patient is asked to open and close the mouth when a downward pressure is exerted by the operator over the posterior aspect of the tray causes the masseter muscle to contract
- This forces the buccinator muscle to push the softened modelling compound medially and creating the masseteric notch on the distobuccal border of the mandibular impression.

Anterior lingual flange (premolar to premolar)

This area is moulded by asking the patient to move the tongue from one corner to other corner of the mouth to use the mylohyoid muscle and genioglossus muscle to determine the lingual border extension and anterior lingual border extension, respectively.

Distolingual flange (premolar to retromylohyoid fossa)

- This area is moulded by moving the tongue from one corner of the mouth to the opposite corner of the mouth which activates the palatoglossus muscle
- The tray should be kept in position with two fingers placed on finger rests. The thumb is used to support the mandible during these procedures
- Completed border moulded tray is checked for retention.

Maxillary Custom Tray Border Moulding

- The final impression trays are examined in the mouth to verify that trays should be 2 mm short of the functional sulcus
- If the tray is overextended, it should be reduced until it has correct extension
- The posterior border of the upper tray should extend up to the vibrating line, the fixed and movable parts of the palate
- The posterior border of the tray is then trimmed to the line
- Labial and buccal flanges (greenstick compound is warmed above a flame until it is soft)
- It is then traced quickly on the dried tray along the labial and buccal flange periphery upto tuberosity to a height of 3 mm
- The material is adapted with the fingers to the tray border
- The compound is re-softened with alcohol torch, gently to prevent burning
- It is tempered in the water bath for 3–5 seconds, and the tray is seated in the patient's mouth and the patient is asked to suck in the cheeks, pull down the lip, and move the jaw from side-to-side so as to mould the distobuccal flange by the action of the coronoid process.

Final Impression

- Several different materials are used to refine the tissue-fitting areas of which zinc oxide eugenol paste is seldom used due to its advantages:
  - A thin mix of zinc oxide eugenol paste is smeared on the greenstick compound
  - The impression tray is then placed in the mouth, seated with positive pressure and the functional movement used to mould the compound is repeated, so that any minor errors can be corrected
  - Areas of heavy contact will be visible by piercing of the paste by the underlying compound.
- The underlying compound should be cut back gently in these areas before the final impression is made
- Some dentists prefer to place holes over the medial palatal raphe and over the ridges especially over the displaceable soft tissues in the maxillary impression tray and along the crest of the ridge in case of mandibular tray with a no. 8 round bur to provide escape ways for the final impression material
- The reason for it is not to displace the denture-bearing tissues during recording.
- The entire impression tray is loaded with a fresh mix of zinc oxide eugenol paste
- It is seated firmly in the mouth, anteriorly first and then posterior, and the patient opens his mouth wide
- The mucous secretion in the posterior palatal seal area should be wiped dry with gauge just before the insertion of the loaded tray.
- The paste is allowed to set:
  - The impression is removed by lifting the lip and cheek to break the seal and checked for defects.
- Small defects may be:
  - A thin layer of impression paste in the post-dam area indicates a proper sitting; a thick layer of paste in that area indicates failure to seat the tray fully.

Chapter 4 Primary Impression and Laboratory Procedures

- An adequate post-dam seal will have to be produced by trimming the master cast at the latter stage
- An impression of the edentulous ridge must be compared with the structures of the mouth. Unless this is done, the whole procedure will be useless and fruitless
- Impression making may give rise to gagging in susceptible patient both for upper and lower jaws.

Question 4
Write in brief about maxillary denture stress-bearing areas?

Answer

Denture-bearing Areas

- The denture-bearing area covered by denture base consists of two areas:
  1. Stress-bearing or supporting area which is a relatively static area and present minimal problems to record.
  2. Peripheral or limiting area although they are inseparable, they will be discussed separately for convenience.

Maxillary Denture-bearing Area

Average denture-bearing area of edentulous maxilla is 24 cm^2.

Maxillary Supporting Structures

- Residual ridge
- Hard palate
- Rugae area
- Incisive papilla
- Median palatine raphe or suture
- Zygomatic process/crest
- Maxillary tuberosities
- Torus palatinus.

Maxillary Peripheral or Limiting Structures

- Labial frenum
- Labial vestibule
- Buccal frenum
- Buccal vestibule
- Pterygomaxillary (hamular) notch
- Post-palatal seal area
- Fovea palatine.

Anatomy of Maxillary Supporting Structures

Residual Ridge

- The crest of the residual ridge is considered as the primary support area for the maxillary denture as it is covered with a layer of masticatory mucosa and the underlying bone is compact cortical bone
- The palate is usually regarded as the primary stress-bearing (support) area, as it is resistant to resorption.

Hard Palate

- The anterior one-third of hard palate, the rugae area, the crest and slope of the residual ridges including the attached gingiva is composed of masticatory mucosa
- It is composed of highly keratinised stratified squamous epithelium and a thick dense layer of connective tissue and the lamina propria supported by firm submucosa. In the middle one-third of the hard palate.

Median Palatal Raphe or Suture

- It is the area extending from the incisive papilla to the distal end of the hard palate. It forms an irregular groove anteroposteriorly in or near middle of the palate
- The submucosa covering this area is very thin. The mucosa is tightly attached to the periosteum giving no cushioning effect.

Rugae Areas

- These are raised areas of dense connective tissue radiating from the midline in the anterior one-third of the palate
- The rugae appear as small grooves radiating from a central groove like branches of a tree.

Incisive Papilla

- It is a pad of fibrous connective tissue overlying the opening of the nasopalatine canal for corresponding nerves and vessels
- It is located between the two central incisors on palatal side in edentulous mouth
- In edentulous mouth, it may lie on or labial to the crest of the ridge as a small round depression.

Zygomatic Process/Crest

- It is a process of maxilla inferior and lateral to the first molar
- This crest like the buccal shelf area of mandible is a stress-bearing area in maxilla
- Though the bone is good, yet the mucosa covering is very thin and failure to provide relief may cause ulceration in the area.

Maxillary Tuberosity

It is the bulbous extension of the residual ridge in the second and third molar region ends in hamular notch.

Torus Palatinus

It is a hard bony mass that occurs in the midline of the palate in about 20% of patients.

Maxillary Limiting Structures

Labial Frenum

- The maxillary labial frenum may be single or multiple, narrow or broad, fold of mucous membrane extending from lips to crest of the residual ridge at the median line
- It contains no muscle fibres, and therefore, can be surgically removed, if attached very near to the crest of the alveolar ridge.

Labial Vestibule

It is located between the labial and buccal frenum and contains no muscle fibres. It extends on both sides from the labial frenum to the buccal frenum.

Buccal Frenum

It may be single or multiple, contains no muscle fibres usually, but occasionally includes fibres of the caninus muscle, buccinator and orbicularis oris muscles.

Buccal Vestibule

It is the space between the ridge and the cheek distal to the buccal frenum to the hamular notch.

Pterygomaxillary (Hamular) Notch

- It is the depression distal to the alveolar ridge and mesial to the pterygoid hamulus indicating the lateral posterior border of the maxillary denture
- The pterygomandibular raphe remains in close proximity as it arises from the hamular process.

Post-palatal Seal Area

- The posterior palatal seal area is defined in the glossary of Prosthodontic terms as the soft tissues along the junction of the hard and soft palates on which pressure within the physiologic limits of the tissues can be applied by a denture to aid in the retention of the denture
- It is not straight but follows the contour of the palatine bones
- In the mouth we observe vibrating line across the posterior part of the palate marking the division between the movable and immovable tissues of the soft palate.

Fovea Palatini

- The coalescence of the minor salivary gland ducts generally located slightly posterior to the junction of hard and soft palate near the midline
- Their position is variable and therefore, cannot be used to delineate the posterior border of the denture.

Question 5

Write in brief about mandibular denture-bearing area.

Answer

- Mandibular dentures like maxillary should be extended as far as possible within the limits of health and function of the tissues and structures that support and surround them
- The support for the mandibular denture comes from the body of the mandible. Average denture-bearing area for edentulous mandible is 14 cm^2.

Mandibular Supporting Structures

- Residual ridge
- Buccal shelf area
- Mylohyoid ridge
- Mental foramen
- Genial tubercles
- Torus mandibularis.

Mandibular Limiting Structures

- Labial frenum
- Labial vestibules
- Buccal frenum
- Buccal vestibules
- Masseter muscle
- Retromolar pad
- Lingual frenum
- Alveolingual sulcus
- Retromylohyoid space.

Mandibular Supporting Structures

Residual Ridge

- The mandibular ridge crest is covered by a keratinised mucosa and firmly attached submucosa to the underlying periosteum providing good support to the denture
- But the underlying bone is cancellous and not favourable as primary stress-bearing area for lower denture
- It acts as secondary stress-bearing area.

Chapter 4 Primary Impression and Laboratory Procedures

Buccal Shelf Area

- It extends anteriorly from mandibular buccal frenum, posteriorly to the anterior border of the masseter muscle
- It is bounded medially by the crest of the residual ridge and laterally by the external oblique ridge.

Mylohyoid Ridge

- It is a rough bony crest extending from the third molar to second bicuspid region
- The mylohyoid muscle is attached to the mylohyoid ridge. In the anterior region the mylohyoid ridge with attached mylohyoid muscle lies close to the inferior border of the mandible
- Posteriorly, it is superior in position and the lingual flange of the denture may extend below the mylohyoid ridge if it drops vertically or slopes at 45 degrees toward the tongue.

Mental Foramen

- The foramen in a resorbed ridge will locate close to the crest in the premolar region
- Through this passes the mental nerves and vessels, which may be compressed to cause numbness of the lower lip.

Genial Tubercles

- The depth of the anterior lingual is influenced by the muscles attached to these
- The resorption causes the genial tubercles to move upward which causes soreness in tissues in this area.

Torus Mandibularis

- It is the bony prominence usually found bilaterally in the premolar region lingually in dented mandible
- In edentulous mandible, where resorption has taken place it is on the crest of the ridge
- As it is often covered by thin mucosa, it needs surgical removal because it is difficult to provide relief.

Anatomy of Mandibular Limiting Structures

Mandibular Labial Frenum

- It is a fold of mucous membrane between the alveolus and labial mucous membrane
- It may be single or multiple and usually not as pronounce as the maxillary labial frenum
- It may contain a band of fibrous connective tissue attached to the orbicularis muscle and may be very active during speech and mastication
- It forms labial notch when careful relief is given.

Mandibular Labial Vestibules

- It is extended from the labial frenum to the buccal frenum in the premolar areas
- It is limited in extension because the fibres of the orbicularis oris, incubus inferioris, and mentalis lie close to the crest of the ridge.

Buccal Frenum

- It is a fold or folds of mucous membrane extending from the lip to buccal mucosa of the residual ridge in the premolar region
- It overlies the levator anguli oris, the buccinators and orbicularis oris muscles so must be functionally moulded. The notch formed should allow relief for the frenum, will prevent dislodgement during facial expression.

Buccal Vestibule

- It runs downwards and outwards from corner of the retromolar pad to the buccal frenum following the attachment of the buccinator muscle which extends from the modiolus anteriorly to the pterygomandibular raphe posteriorly
- The buccinator muscle forms a pouch in the cheek and the denture can be extended laterally to produce a large posterior buccal flange
- The polished buccal surface faces outwards and upwards so that the contracting buccinator forces the cheek inwards to keep the denture in place
- The buccinator affects both the lateral and the distal extension of the denture with the help of the pterygomandibular ligament.

Masseter Muscle

The periphery at the distobuccal corner of the buccal vestibule, the masseter muscle overlies the buccinator muscle and influences the denture border forming the masseteric notch.

Retromolar Pad

- Distal to the crest of the edentulous ridge there is an elevated soft pad of mucosa, the retromolar pad. It is oval or round in outline lying on the retromolar fossa
- The submucosa contains loose glandular and areolar tissue, pterygomandibular raphe, buccinator, superior constrictor, and temporal tendon fibres
- Failure to extend the denture up to the pad may increase resorption of alveolar ridge.

Pear-shaped Pad

- In front of the retromolar pad and often attached with it is a firm fibrous pear-shaped pad
- It arises from the collapse of the distal papilla into the socket on extraction of the last molar tooth.

Mandibular Lingual Frenum

- It is wide midline fold of mucous membrane as the anterior attachment of the tongue to the alveolar mucosa and the floor of the mouth
- It lies over the genioglossus muscle. It is well above the genial tubercles, the attachment of genioglossus muscles in case of normal ridge, but at the level of the genial tubercles in case of extreme resorption
- It should be recorded in function as it is often close to the crest of the ridge during function though much lower at rest.

Lingual Vestibule/Alveolingual Sulcus

- The space between the tongue and the alveolar ridge is called alveolingual sulcus
- It extends from lingual frenum to the retromylohyoid curtain. It is divided into anterior and posterior parts:
- The anterior part extends from the lingual frenum to the premylohyoid fossa
- The structures in that area are the sublingual fold and the sublingual papilla (opening of Wharton's ducts) and sublingual glands rest on the mylohyoid muscle
- The posterior part extends from the premylohyoid fossa to the postmylohyoid fossa
- The mylohyoid muscle determines the lingual flange of the denture. The lingual flange may extend 4–5 mm below the mylohyoid ridge, if it drops vertically or slopes towards the tongue at 45 degrees
- It should not be extended below the mylohyoid ridge forming an undercut.

Retromylohyoid Space

- It lies at the end of the alveolingual sulcus. It extends from end of the mylohyoid ridge to the retromylohyoid curtain
- It is bounded lingually by anterior tonsillar pillar, distally by the retromylohyoid curtain and superior constrictor muscle, and on the buccal side by the mylohyoid muscle, the ramus, and the retromolar pad
- The denture border should be extended posteriorly to contact the retromolar curtain when the tip of the tongue is touching the anterior maxillary residual ridge.

CHAPTER 5
Secondary Impression and Laboratory Procedures

LONG ESSAYS

Question 1

Define preliminary cast. Write about mounding method.

Answer

A cast formed from a preliminary impression for use in diagnosis or fabrication of an impression tray is called a preliminary cast.

Uses

- Analysis of possibility of various forms of treatment
- Analysis of the relationship between maxilla and mandible when casts are mounted on articulator
- Analysis of static and dynamic relationship of the occlusal surfaces of opposing teeth
- Communication between the dental surgeon and patient or laboratory technician
- Construction of special trays
- Making records of various anatomical structures
- Survey of oral structures.

Laboratory Preparation

Pouring the Cast

The preliminary impression may be poured in one of three ways as follows:
1. Mounding method
- It is a two stage pour technique which is acceptable for preliminary edentulous impression.
2. Boxing method
- It is the enclosure of an impression to produce the desired size and form of the base of the cast and to preserve desired details
- Strips of soft boxing wax are wrapped around the impression to form a mould for the gypsum
- Generally, wax is extended 1 cm beyond the tissue side of the impression to form a base for the cast
- The mixed gypsum is vibrated into the impression to enhance the flow of the material into the impression and avoid the entrapment of air bubbles. It is usually recommended for final or master impression.
3. Model former method
- Pouring a cast using a container called model former to form the base for the impression.

A double pour mounding method is acceptable for preliminary edentulous impressions and boxing method is required for final impressions.

Mounding Method

Steps

- The impression is washed under cold running water to remove traces of blood or mucosa from its surface by shaking and dried with compressed air or a piece of gauze
- The impression is placed on the plaster bench in such a way that the posterior end does not contact the bench
- This will prevent distortion of the impression and placing the tray parallel to the bench makes it easy for pouring
- The cast may be poured in plaster of Paris or a mixture 50:50 plaster of Paris and dental stone or only dental stone. Usually 150 gm of gypsum is adequate for single cast
- Water is poured and measured in a calibrated glass according to the plaster or dental stone mix used and placed in a plaster bowl
- The plaster or dental stone is weighed and sifted slowly into the water (dental plaster of 100 gm is required to shift in 50 ml of water)
- The gentle taps on the side of the bowl helps to prevent air inclusions
- The mixing is done with hand held spatula or a mechanical spatulator with a vibrator. The procedure is known as spatulation

- The impression tray is held in one hand with its handle touching the vibrator and small increments of plaster may be introduced with a spatula into the impression from the posterior region
- The vibrations continued until the impression has been filled to its periphery and it is placed with the tray parallel to the bench again
- The remaining plaster or stone is added to a height of 5 mm above the highest part of impression
- Rough protrusions of gypsum are added to the surface to provide locking undercuts for the second stage of pour
- After the initial set, the impression is soaked in a bowl of clear slurry water for 4–5 minutes to thoroughly wet the first pour gypsum
- A second mix of gypsum mixed with same water powder ratio and placed in a 12 mm thick mound on a glass slab and formed into the shape of the impression
- The filled impression is inverted and seated into the mass
- The excess of plaster is drawn up over the outer periphery of the impression with sufficient bulk to allow for trimming later
- Excess plaster is removed from the tongue space and allows the cast to harden
- Care should be taken to avoid locking the impression tray into the stone or plaster.

Separation of Impression

Compound Impression

- When the cast material has reached its initial set, excess is cleaned from the tray
- After the final set of plaster (minimum 30 minutes) excess compound is removed from the outer surface of the tray by a plaster knife
- The cast is held firmly with the fingers supporting the tray, and the thumb on the base of the cast
- The metal tray is removed by tapping it sharply at the base of the handle with a wooden mallet or by handle of knife
- If it not separated easily the cast is immersed in hot water of 65°C for 5 minutes and the tray may be removed easily by lifting up the buccal area all rounds and then the palatal or lingual area
- It should not be placed in too hot water to prevent sticking of melted compound to the cast
- The compound overheated and adhering to the cast may be removed by pressing a ball of softened compound over the area and then removing it.

Alginate Impression

- Alginate impression should be poured within 12 minutes after removal from the month.
- Alginate impression if taken in perforated tray, material extended through the holes is first cut away before attempt to separate the cast from impression material
- The alginate is then lifted from the cast on the buccal and labial sides with fingers
- The cast should be separated from impression after 45–60 minutes of pouring and is allowed for final set.

Trimming Casts

- It is the procedure of shaping the cast
- It is normally carried out on a model trimmer in the following ways:
  - The wet cast is placed on its base on the platform of the model trimmer with posterior surface moved gently through the opening against the rotating carborundum or diamond wheel
  - The wheel is lubricated with water which disposes off the removed cast material. It should be trimmed about 5 mm from the hamular notch and retromolar pad
  - The cast is then placed upright on its posterior surface and the base is trimmed so that the edentulous ridge lies approximately in the same plane as it would in the mouth. The base of the cast should be at least 10 mm thick for adequate strength
  - The outer surface is trimmed 3 mm from maximum depth of the sulcus by placing the base on platform. The sharp corners produced are removed by knife to form a 45 degree chamfer about 1.5 mm wide
  - The excess plaster on the lingual space of a lower cast is removed with a flat blade sculptor to leave a 2 mm deep lingual sulcus.

Disinfection

To prevent cross infection impressions should be thoroughly rinsed in water and then socked in 0.5% sodium hypochlorite solution diluted 1:10 for 10 minutes before pouring the cast.

Question 2

Define and classify impression trays. Write about functions and requirements.

Answer

Impression tray is a device that is used to carry, confine and control impression material while making an impression.

Chapter 5 Secondary Impression and Laboratory Procedures

Parts of Impression Tray

The stock tray consists of a body and handle. The body consists of a floor and flanges. The maxillary tray has a vault.

Functions of Impression Tray

- To support an impression material in planned contact with oral tissues
- To allow placement of additional stress in selected regions of the residual ridge while recording other regions in a displaced state
- To support the set impression material when removed from the mouth so that a cast can be poured.

Requirements of Impression Trays

- The tray should be rigid but not abnormally thick
- They should be clean and smooth
- To support the impression material when removed from the mouth so that a cast can be poured
- They should allow the correct thickness of impression material to be used
- The shape of the handle should not displace the lip during impression making
- They must hold the impression material against the whole areas to be recorded
- They should support the lips and cheeks in their pre-extracted position so that the recording of the sulcus is in its original shape and size
- They should be capable of modification by trimming and binding
- They should retain their original shape during construction and pouring of cast
- It should be easy to construct and require minimum time and cast.

Types of Trays

- According to the patients status:
  - Dentulous (box tray)
  - Edentulous (anatomical).
- According to design:
  - Perforated
  - Non-perforated.
- According to material of construction:
  - Metallic
  - Non-metallic.
- According to method of fabrication:
  - Stock trays
  - Custom/special trays.

Advantages of Impression Tray

- Accurate peripheral extension is assured
- The border of the tray can be so adjusted that the movement of soft tissues around the impression remains undistorted
- The space provided inside the tray may be varied according to the nature of the impression material
- A uniform space may be created for impression material for dimensional accuracy
- There is less discomfort to the patient while making impression due to proper size of tray and reduced mass of impression material
- There is economy in impression material.

Fabrication of Special Tray (Laboratory Procedures)

- An individual impression tray provides a support for obtaining a wash impression which accurately records tissue details and peripheral extension
- These trays can be made best from tray material or from cold-cure acrylic resin
- These can be made either by adapting a sheet of dough over the cast or by preparing a wax pattern on the cast, investing, boiling out, and packing the mould with cold-cure acrylic resin
- The outline of the tray should be marked on the primary casts by the dentist
  - The line is placed 2–3 mm short of the vestibular sulcus and all frenum
  - If the tray is shorter more than 3 mm it will be very difficult to control and manipulate the compound during border moulding
  - In the maxillary cast the outline should connect the hamular notches passing through just 2 mm posterior to the fovea palatinae
  - If fovea is not visible the line is drawn straight from one hamular notch to the other. In the mandibular cast it should cover the retromolar pads.

Forming the Tray

- A uniform spacer of one thickness of modelling wax is provided over the outlined areas. The use of wax as spacer enables stops to be incorporated into the inner surface of the tray
- These stops contact the mucosa before the rest of the tray.
  - These enable the proper placement of tray in the same position every time when placed on the ridge
  - These stops also help to maintain uniform 2–3 mm thick impression material

- The stops are made by cutting holes in wax 2–3 mm wide extending from a point slightly palatal to the ridge across to the gingival sulcus
- They are located over the molar and canine area on both sides.
- An acrylic resin handle should be added in the midline of the crest of both upper and lower trays before the tray material has set. It should be joined by moistening with a small amount of monomer
  - Two narrow fingers, rests (1 cm × 1 cm × 4 cm) are attached to the lower tray in the region of first molars.

Separation of Tray and Cast

- After the tray acrylic resin sets completely, the cast and tray is immersed in warm water to soften the spacer wax
- The tray is removed from the cast by gently pulling by the handle.

Trimming the Tray

- The borders of the tray are trimmed to round all corners and edges. They should have smooth border but not polished as the greenstick compound used for border moulding will adhere to a course surface
- The special tray can be prepared with shellac base, visible light cure material or vacuum formed thermoplastic sheets
- Shellac trays need reinforcement to reduce distortion and improve strength
- In the maxillary a wire is adapted across the palatal seal area
- In the mandibular tray the wire is adapted along the lingual flange
- The handles are made with self-cure acrylic resin.

Question 3

Write in detail about boxing and pouring of master casts.

Answer

Boxing Impression

- It is the process of enclosure of an impression to produce the desired size and to form the base of the cast and to preserve desired details
- It is usually utilized for pouring the master cast of edentulous ridges.

Wax Boxing

- This boxing can be used for zinc oxide paste final impressions and also for rubber base as well as plaster impressions of edentulous ridges
- A strip of beading wax or soft modelling wax may be used for beading. The wax is rolled into 5 mm diameter rod, long enough to encircle the impression tray
- It is wrapped around the tray 5 mm short of the depth of the sulcus and sealed to it by the use of a hot wax knife
- A sheet of modelling wax of 12 mm wide is adapted and sealed outside the beading wax to box the impression
- The lingual aspect of a mandibular impression is filled with a sheet of modelling wax cut into size and sealed to the wax roll
- Zinc oxide eugenol paste and rubber base impressions need no separating media and they are cast immediately.
- In case of plaster impression the liquid soap should be applied with a soft camel hair brush to form lather which is then washed off
- This is repeated until sheen is visible on the surface of the impression. Soap forms an insoluble calcium deposit by reaction with the plaster which should be washed off.

Pouring of Cast

- The cast is poured in dental stone mixed to a water power ratio of 30 cm^2/100 gm
- Small increments of stone is vibrated into the impression until the stone reaches the top of the box. The cast is allowed to harden for one hour
- The cast on removal from the impression is trimmed in the manner similar to the primary cast.

Pumice-plaster Boxing

- This method can be utilized with most of impression materials especially for hydrocolloids where wax will not adhere to the impression surface
- A mix (1:1) of plaster and pumice is formed into a patty approximately 12 mm thick and the impression is seated into this mix with the tissue side up and horizontal to the table
- The mix is then taken up to the level of 3 mm inferior to the buccal borders
- For the mandibular impression, the lingual side is flattened to form a platform 3 mm inferior to the lingual border. The mix when set is trimmed to form a 3 mm land area around the labial, buccal and lingual borders
- A thin layer of plasticine (modelling clay) is applied on the whole land areas of the base around the impression
- The impression is then boxed with boxing wax attached to the vertical wall of the plaster-pumice base with hot wax knife and sticky wax

- Dental stone is mixed using appropriate water powder ratio and vibrated into the boxed impression till it is filled up
- After one hour, the cast is separated by immersing in hot water to soften zinc oxide impression material
- The master cast is trimmed similar to the primary cast.

Indexing the Cast

- Indexing cast prior to mounting in articulator permit removal of the cast and accurate replacement in the articulator
- It is helpful in remounting for removing processing errors of a denture and for verifying jaw relation records
- Grooves, notches, or metal or plastic remounting plates may be placed in the cast for indexing.

Groove indexing method

- The bases of the casts are indexed groove with a lathe mounted wheel
- It will produce a smooth V-cut without producing undercut so that they may be remounted accurately in the articulator after processing to allow for the correction of minor processing errors
- The bases of the casts should be lightly painted with petroleum jelly or soap solution before mounting them in an articulator.

Notch indexing method

- The notches are cut in the base of the cast at three or more points to provide positive index
- The main disadvantage is that in case of reduction of cast to fit in a flask it will be lost.

Split remounting indexing method

- It is done by mounting one part of Hanau remounting plate in the base of final cast during pouring and the other part in the mounting stone on the articulator
- It is more precise than other methods and permits rapid removal and replacement of the cast on the articulator.

Requirements of Record Base

- When selecting a material for a record base one should consider the following:
  - Strength and rigidity
  - Dimensional stability
  - Ease of fabrication
  - Cost
  - Colour.

Strength and Rigidity

- A record base should be rigid so that it is not affected by pressures while the jaw relation registration is made and as a result a faulty recording transferred to the articulator
- So, rigidity of the record base is essential for an accurate record to be registered and transferred.

Dimensional Stability

- During the whole course of treatment the record base will be subjected to heat during the laboratory procedures
- So, the material selected should be one that will remain stable when subjected to difference of temperatures
- Since variable time period is involved in making the dentures, a base material is required that will not distort with time.

Ease of Fabrication

The relative ease of fabrication will reflect the cost of material, ease of manipulation and the final result.

Cost

A material should be selected for a good performance at a reasonable expense.

Colour

The colour of the base should be of the same pink colour as the denture base material as it acts as a background when the teeth are seen during the try-in stage.

Types of Bases

It is agreed that jaw relations are difficult to record accurately with poorly fitting bases made from material that is subject to distortion and dimensional change. Bases may be temporary or permanent.

Temporary Bases

- These are made of shellac or cold cure acrylic resin
- Hard base plate wax is occasionally used but is unsatisfactory as got distorted when kept in the mouth for more than a few minutes
- Vacuum formed vinyl or polystyrene are also used.

Permanent Bases

- These are made of heat cure acrylic resin and chromium cobalt alloy made on the master cast
- This usually causes destruction of the master cast during deflasking

- The teeth are attached to them either with cold cure or heat cure acrylic material
- Many prosthodontists believe that it is only by the use of permanent bases that accurate intra-oral records can be made and transfer to the articulator
- Permanent bases ultimately become part of the complete denture.

Materials

Shellac

- The most commonly used base material is available as flat sheets shaped as upper and lower arches
- The forms are heated in the open flame to soft pliable state after which they can be adapted to the cast with either the fingers or an instrument or a combination of both.

Wax

Hard wax (base plate) adapted on cast dusted with talcum powder and reinforced with ten gauge wire.

Acrylic Resin Base

Autopolymerising acrylic resin base: It is prepared by any of the following three methods:

1. Heat cure acrylic resin base: A wax pattern of requisite thickness is prepared on the cast (3 mm).
2. Compressed air or vacuum-formed bases: It can be used to form bases very quickly but it is very expensive and a machine is required for that.
3. Light cure composite bases: It can be used within short period but material is very expensive.

Laboratory Procedures

- Instruments
- Wax spatula
- Base plate wax
- Separating media
- Cold cure acrylic resin monomer and polymer
- Carbide acrylic trimmer
- Rubber bowl/pressure pot
- Lathe, felt wheel and pumice
- Plaster spatula
- Hot plate.

Fabrication of Occlusion Rims

- A little moltened sticky wax is placed over the crest of the ridge of the base
- A half sheet of base plate wax is passed over the flame until soft and pliable throughout and rolled into a rod and its cross-section formed into a 12 mm square by pressing the wax between finger and thumb of both hands simultaneously
- The rim is sealed to the base using a hot spatula. The excess of length posterior is cut off. The labial surface is contoured to blend with the periphery of the base
- The occlusion rims are trimmed to the dimensions as described below:

Maxillary Rim

- Anteriorly, the occlusion rim should be 20 mm from the periphery of the base lateral to the labial frenum and posteriorly, at the molar area 16–18 mm high and 10 mm anterior to the hamular notch
- The buccal surface is contoured at the posterior part distal to the canine slightly, towards the palate to create space between the buccal surfaces of the posterior teeth and the cheeks
- The width of the rim anteriorly should be 6 mm:
  - The width of incisal edge seldom exceeds 3 mm
  - The width of the posterior rim should be 8–10 mm to ensure contact with the lower rim
  - The labial surface of the rim should be 10 mm anterior to the posterior end of the incisive papilla.

Mandibular Rim

- The lower rim should be even with the centre of the retromolar pad and parallel with the mean plane of the residual ridge
- The height of the mandibular occlusal rim in anterior region should be approximately 16 mm from the sulcus through the rim.

Chapter 6: Maxillomandibular Relations

LONG ESSAYS

Question 1
Write in brief about vertical dimension and discuss its mechanical methods.

Answer

Vertical Dimension at Occlusal

- It is defined as the length of the face, when the teeth (occlusal rims, central bearing points or any outer stop) are in contact and the mandible is in centric relation or the teeth on in centric relation
- It can be recorded by using following methods:
  - Mechanical methods
  - Physiological methods.

Mechanical Methods

- Ridge relation
  - Distance from incisive papilla to the mandibular incisors.
- Parallelism of ridges
  - Pre-extraction records
    - Profile photographs
    - Profile silhouettes
    - Radiography
    - Articulated cast
    - Facial measurements.
- Measurements from the former dentures.

Ridge relations

- It is defined as the positional relationship of the mandibular ridge to the maxillary ridge
- It can be measured by:
  - Distance from the incisive papilla to mandibular incisors.
  - They are stable landmarks which even after the resorption of alveolar ridge do not change a lot
- The distance between papilla to the maxillary incisor edge is 6 mm
- The vertical overlap is mostly 2 mm between upper and lower incisors
- Therefore the distance between the incisive papilla and lower incisors will be around 4 mm.

Ridge parallelism

- At occlusion the mandible is parallel to the maxilla
- This factor can used to figure out the vertical dimension at occlusion
- The mandible should be parallel to the maxilla with 5° opening of the jaw in the temporomandibular joint
- This in turn gives a right amount of jaw separation
- In case where the teeth of both upper and lower are extracted at the same time the ridges will be parallel to each other as the length of crown of opposite anterior and posterior teeth will be equal
- Patients with periodontal diseases are not considered for this method as they lost teeth at different periods of time.

Pre-extraction records

Extraction records are of following types:
- Radiographs
- Profile photographs
- Articulated cast
- Profile silhouettes
- Facial measurements.

Radiographs

- The jaw recreation is determined by specific radiographs like cephalometric profile or condylar fossa radiographs
- Due to inaccurate technique there use is limited.

Profile photographs

- These photographs are taken before extraction. There should be maximum occlusion present as it is easy to maintain position during photographs
- Photographs should be made to the size of the real facial measurement
- So that anatomical landmarks should be measured and compound with the photographs to avoid any possible errors.

Articulated cast

- An inter-occlusal record is made from patient's mouths. Which is used to articulate the mandibular cast with the maxillary cast
- This is done by mounting the cast in articulator and than transferring to face-bow
- They are used as pre-extraction records.

Profile silhouettes

- Using patient's photographs a outline is drawn using a cardbound and wire
- They are used as template
- This show's vertical dimension at rest as they were taken before extraction
- It should be make sure that the chin is always 2 mm above the level of the lower border of the silhouette.

Facial measurement

- This is done just before extraction as two points are marked on upper and lower part of the face
- At occlusion the vertical dimension is measured. The distance is measured before extraction from the chin to the base of the nose.

Physiological Methods

- Power point
- Using wax occlusal rims
- Physiological rest position
- Phonetics
- Aesthetics
- Swallowing threshold
- Tactile sense or neuromuscular perceptions
- Patient's perception of comfort.

Power point

- Record plate is attached to a metal plate. In addition to this a bimeter is attached to the maxillary record base
- Bimeter contains a dial which has the significance to show the amount of pressure acting on it
- Procedure:
  - Patient is asked to bite on record base at different degrees of jaw separation after being inserted in the mouth
  - The biting forces are than transferred to the bimeter from the bearing point
  - The reading is noted till the highest point and this is called as power point.

Using wax occlusal rims

- Cast is articulated in a tentative centric relation and vertical dimension is measured with the occlusal rims
- For graphic tracing a tracing device is attached to the occlusal rim
  - Procedure:
    - The points between the nose and chin are recorded while the vertical dimension is at rest
    - The facial expression is an alternative to be used as a guide for getting this value
    - The occlusal rim is than placed in the mouth before that apply petroleum jelly. So it does not disturb any soft tissue
    - When there is no retention adhesive powder is used
    - Place the modelling wax over the mandibular occlusal rim which is softened in hot water at 130°F
    - The apex should be towards the maxillary rim
    - Vertical dimension at occlusion is attained after patient closed his mouth slowly and the point where he is comfortable gives the dimension
    - The wax is let to cooled and removed from the mouth and articulated.

Physiological rest position

- Niswonger's method
  - This is not a very accurate method as it is based on the patients cooperation and alteration of movement
  - There can be a lot of errors at the time of procedure because of alterations in jaw position
  - Procedure:
    - Patient is mode to sit upright with no support to head and looking straight
    - Upper and lower occlusal rims that were modified and inserted into the mouth
    - Lips are parted away and space between the occlusal rim is created
    - This space is caused as free-way space
    - Vertical dimension (VD) at rest = VD at occlusion + free way space.

- Silverman's closest speaking space
  - This space is attained when sounds like ch, s, j are made by the patient
  - In these words when pronounced the upper and lower teeth reach their closet relation without contact
  - This minimal space between upper and lower teeth is called Silverman's closest speaking space.
- Pound and Murrel technique
  - In this method the anterior teeth are arranged on the occlusal rim which is then modified according in patients mouth
  - The patients are made to speak letters like F or V to determine the position of anterior teeth.

Aesthetics

- It plays an important role in determining the correct vertical dimension
- This can be achieved by selecting teeth of the same size as the natural teeth and by analysing the amount of residual ridge resorption
- Skin
  - High vertical dimension can cause stretching of the skin of the cheeks along with increased nasolabial angle.
- Lips
  - The thickness of the labial flange affects the contour and fullness of the lip. The occlusal rims should be contoured in order to provide adequate lip support.

Swallowing threshold

- At the beginning of swallowing, the teeth of the upper and lower jaws almost come in contact, which in turn can be used as a guide to determine vertical dimension at occlusion
- For recording the vertical dimension, the upper and lower record bases are inserted in the patient's mouth
- Salivation is stimulated and the patient is asked to swallow
- Then, the height of the conical wax rim is decreased due to the pressure developed while closing the mandible during swallowing.

Tactile sense or neuromuscular perception

- In this method, patient's tactile sense or sense for comfort aids in determining the vertical dimension at occlusion
- Procedure
  - The occlusal rims with the central bearing screw and plate are inserted into the mouth of the patient
  - The central bearing screw is slowly tightened which will bring both the occlusal rims towards each other
  - After a certain limit, the patient will start feeling discomfort in his jaws due to over-tightening
  - This point at which discomfort starts, it is recorded
  - The same procedure is repeated with the central bearing plate in the mandibular rim and the central bearing screw in the maxillary rim
  - The central-bearing point is reduced until the patient specifies a comfortable jaw relationship.

Patient's perception of comfort

- It is a very easy and simple method of determining the vertical relation
- The record bases with excessively tall occlusal rims are inserted in to the mouth of the patient
- The excess base plate wax is removed step wise till the patient perceives the occlusal height as comfortable.

Question 2

Write about horizontal jaw relation and write in detail about centric relation.

Answer

Horizontal Jaw Relation

This is a relationship of the mandible to the maxilla in the horizontal plane.

Centric Relation

It is defined as the most posterior relation of the lower to the upper jaw from which the lateral movement can be made at given vertical dimension.

Significance

- The position like learnable, repeatable and recordable remains same throughout
- The movement of mandible to any eccentric position and than back can be attained
- The movement like swallowing and chewing can be done at this position
  - Condylar guidance can be adjusted to give balanced occlusion
  - Retruding mandible
  - The patient should be without any systemic disorder to get the position.
- Mandible should be in to most posterior position procedure:
  - The upper jaw of the patient is protruded forward while occluding on the posterior teeth
  - Ask the patient to touch the posterior border of the upper record base by using tongue.

Recording Centric Jaw Relation

Physiological Methods

Tactile or Intra-occlusal check record method procedure:
- Patient is asked to retrude the mandible by taking the approximate jaw relation the cast is mounted
- Intra-occlusal registration is done after the teeth arrangement is done.

Pressure Less Method

- At the centric relation position the patient is asked to close mouth till he is comfortable after the occlusal rims are customised
- This position is than sealed.

Nick and Notch Method

- For recording in centric jaw relation this is the most common method
- Try-in is done without occlusal check
- It is done by removing 3 mm of wax from either side of the mandibular occlusal rim
- A V-shaped notch can be seen across the width
- The nick and the notch are lubricated and inserted in mouth and patient is asked to close the mouth at maximum retruded position
  - After it is removed 4.5 mm of aluwax is placed on the trough
  - It is than softened by dipping in the water and inserted in the mouth again
  - Patient is asked to close his mouth the aluwax flows into the nick and notches
  - The excess aluwax is taken out
  - Place both occlusal rims against each other
  - The occlusal rims are placed on the articulated casts
  - The centric relation is than verified by tracing device than can be intra or extra oral.

Pressure Method

- After vertical dimension is done the occlusal rim is inserted into the patient's mouth
- There is excess height given to the lower occlusal rim which is fabricated and softened and again inserted into patient's mouth
- The mandible is guided when patient closes his mouth. Both the rims are taken out after gaining the vertical dimension, which is than articulated.

Functional Methods

Needle house method

- The fabrication of the occlusal rims are made of impression compound
- In the premolar and molar area of maxillary occlusal rim metal beads are fixed (four in number)
- This is than inserted into patients mouth
- After inserting, the patient is asked to close mouth and lateral movement, protrusive and retrusive movements are done in all the positions
- A diamond shaped marking can be seen otherwise a line is seen in other cases.

Graphic Method

The use of tracing and records are mostly used in this method:
- Types
  - Arrow point tracing
  - Pantograph.
- Arrow point tracing:
  - This is a one dimensional graphic tracing
  - They are recorded in the horizontal plane
  - The procedure involves the mandibular movement which draws pattern on the recording plate
  - They are called as central point.

Pantographic tracing

- It is defined as graphic record of mandibular movement in three planes as registered by the styli on the recording tables of a pantograph tracing of mandibular movement recorded on the plates in the horizontal and sagittal planes
  - This is a three dimensional method and mostly very accurate.

Chapter 6 Maxillomandibular Relations

SHORT ESSAY

Question 1

What are the types of mandible movements?

Answer

Types of Mandibular Movements

Based on the Dimension Involved in the Movement

- Rotation around the transverse or hinge axis
- Rotation around the anteroposterior or sagittal axis
- Rotation around the vertical axis
- Translation in time.

Based on the Type of Movement

- Hinge movement
- Protrusive movement
- Retrusive movement
- Lateral movement.

Lateral Rotation or Laterotorsion

Right and left lateral movement

Lateral Translation or Bennett Movement

- Immediate side shift
- Recurrent side shift
- Progressive side shift.

Based on the Extent of Movement

- Border movements
- Extreme movements in the horizontal plane
- Extreme movements in the sagittal plane
- Extreme movements in the coronal plane
  - Envelope of motion
    - Intra-border movements.
  - Functional movements
    - Chewing cycle
    - Swallowing
    - Yawning
    - Speech.
  - Para-functional movements
    - Clenching
    - Bruxism
    - Other habitual movements.

SHORT NOTES

Question 1

Define bennett movement.

Answer

- It is defined as the bodily lateral movement or lateral shift of the mandible resulting from the movements of the condyles along the lateral incline along the mandibular fossae in lateral jaw movements
- There is a movement about 1–4 mm of the mandible towards the working side. This shift is called as Bennett movement.

It can be classified as:

- Immediate side shift
  - There is a lateral translation that happens before the forward movement of the non-working condyle.
- Recurrent side shift
  - There is lateral translation during first 2–3 mm in forward movement of the non-working condyle.
- Progressive side shift.
  - The lateral translation which continuous even after 2–3 mm of forward movement of the non-working condyle.

Question 2

Discuss vertical relation at increased and decreased dimensions.

Answer

- Increased vertical dimension:
  - There is increased trauma that occurs in the denture-bearing area
  - There is difficulty in speech and swallowing
  - There is stretching of facial muscle
  - Lower facial height is increased
  - Check biting can be seen.
- Decreased vertical dimension:
  - There is less trauma to the denture bearing area

- ○ Lower facial height is decreased
- ○ There is difficulty is swallowing
  - ➤ Due to corners folded angular cheilitis can be seen
  - ➤ TMJ pain, neuralgia and headache can be felt.

Question 3

What is U-shaped frame?

Answer

- It is a metallic bar which is U-shaped
- It is the main frame of the face-bow
- The different components are attached to this U-shaped frame
- This is a large assemble which extend from the region of the TMJ to atleast 2–3 inches anterior to the face
- This is wide enough to avoid any contact with the sides of the face
- This is used in recording the plane of the cranium.

Question 4

Explain hinge method.

Answer

- The rotational movement of the joint is known as hinge movement
- It happens around a horizontal axis till patient opens his mouth to about 20–25 mm
- The hinge movement according to studies have been at from 10° to 13° of the TMJ
- This movement can be established while crushing food items or swallowing
- The muscles that produce hinge movements are lateral pterygoid and suprahyoid.

Question 5

Explain jaw relation record and terminal jaw relation record.

Answer

- Jaw relation record is defined as registration of any positional relationship of the mandible in reference to the maxilla
- These records may be any of the many vertical, horizontal, orientation relation
- Terminal jaw relation record is defined as the relationship of the mandible to the maxilla made at the vertical dimension of occlusion and at the centric relation.

Question 6

Mention different factors while making eccentric jaw relations.

Answer

- During eccentric jaw movement condyles do not travel in straight lines
- Eccentric movement are reproduced by semi-adjustable articulators. In these articulators condyles travel on a flat path
- Condylar path cannot be altered
- Using a pantographic tracing the condylar and incisal guidance are fabricated individually with acrylic in fully adjustable articulators.

Chapter 7: Laboratory Procedures Prior to Try-In

LONG ESSAY

Question 1
Write in brief about articulators. Add their types and uses.

Answer

Articulator is a mechanical device which represents the temporomandibular joint (TMJ) and jaw members to which maxillary and mandibular casts may be attached to simulate jaw movements (**Fig. 7.1**).

Parts of Articulators

- Upper member
- Lower member
- Condylar guidance
- Incisal pin
- Incisal guide
- Extension stud
- Mounting plate.

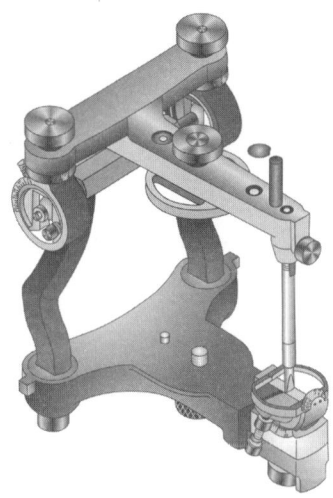

Fig. 7.1: The Hanau H2 articulator

Purpose of an Articulator

- To place the upper and lower casts in the same positional relationship as that of the normal dentition and to reproduce the centre-relation position
- To simulate mandibular movements
- The basics are acquired from the patient and transferred to the articulator:
  - Facebow, to relate the maxilla to the hinge axis
  - Maxillomandibular record to relate the mandibular cast to the maxillary cast
  - Eccentric registration to set the condylar controls of the articulator.

Uses of an Articulator

- It is used in absence of the patient to facilitate fabrication of restorations outside the patient's mouth
- For diagnosis of occlusal conditions both in natural and artificial dentition
- To perform treatment planning and patient presentation
- To fabricate the occlusal surfaces of dental appliances
- To correct and modify finished restorations.

Requirements of an Articulator

- The articulator should accept centric and eccentric relations
- It should hold the casts in the correct vertical relationships
- It should be able to perform open and close hinge movement
- It should be rigid in construction
- It should have an incisal guide pin and table
- It must have independent adjustable condylar paths and be able to accept protrusive record to set it
- A normal person should be capable of handling it
- It should not be expensive.

Classification of Articulators

- Articulators have been classified in the following ways:
  - Based on the theories of occlusion
  - Based on the type if inter-occlusal record used
  - Based on the ability to stimulate jaw movement
  - Based on adjust ability of the articulator.

Based on the Theories of Occlusion

- It was designed by WGA Bonwill
- Bonwill's theory states that the teeth move in relation to each other as it is guided by the condylar controls and incisal point
- This is called as theory of equilateral triangle
- In this there was a 10 cm distance between the condyles and incisal point.

Conical theory of occlusion

- It was designed by R.E Hall
- This theory states that the lower teeth move over the surface of the upper teeth which generates a angle of 45 degrees with the central axis of the cone tipped to the occlusal plane
- This also states that the teeth having 45 degree cusp and necessary when the dentures are built on this articulator.

Spherical theory articulators

- This was designed by G.S Monsoon
- It is based on the spherical theory of occlusion in which the lower teeth that lower teeth move over the surface of upper teeth as over a surface of sphere with a diameter of 20 cms
- The centre of the sphere which is in the glabella and the surface of the sphere passing through the glenoid fossa along with the articulating eminence.

Based on the Type if Inter-occlusal Record used

Inter-occlusal record adjustment

- These are the records that are made
- Zinc oxide eugenol paste
- Cold cure acrylic resin base plate wax
- They are adjusted by inter-occlusal records.

Graphic record adjustment

- They are used to reproduce the border movements of the mandible and also the records of the extreme positions of the movements of mandible
- Records are transferred by pantograph.

Based on the Ability to Stimulate Jaw Movement

Class I

- Barndoor articulator, Hinge articulator
- Simple holding instruments capable of accepting a single static registration with possible vertical motion.

Class II

- Instrument that Permits horizontal as well as vertical motion but do not orient the motion to the temporo-mandibular joint (TMJ) via facebow transfer as:
  - Eccentric motion permitted is based on average or arbitrary values, e.g., Grittman articulator, Gysi adaptable articulator, Gysi simplex articulator
  - Eccentric motion permitted is based on theories of arbitrary motion, e.g. Manson articulator
  - Eccentric motion permitted is determined by the patient using engraving methods, e.g. House articulator.

Class III

- Instruments that simulate condylar pathways by using mechanical equivalent for all or part of motion and allow facebow transfer
  - Instruments that accept static lateral protrusive registration and use equivalents for the rest of motion, e.g. Hanau H2, Dentatus
  - Instruments that accept static lateral protrusive registrations and use equivalents for the rest of motion, e.g. Truebyte articulator, Stanberry articulator, Ney's articulator, Hanau 130–21. Teledyne articulator, Panadent articulator.

Class IV

- Instruments that accept three-dimensional dynamic registrations with facebow, e.g. TMJ instrument of Kenneth Swanson
- The cams representing condylar paths are formed by registrations engraved by the patient
- The condylar paths can be angled and customized, e.g. Denar articulator, Staurt articulator.

Based on Adjustability of the Articulator

Non adjustable

They are divided into two types:
- Simple hinge type
  - They records only the occlusal position and do not accept lateral or protrusive registration. It has a hinge

- to enable the casts to be separated and returned to the correct relation
  - The movement of the hinge does not contributes to the opening and closing movements of the jaws
  - The freedom from interference and occlusal balance is not achieved by this articulator
  - At the time try-in or finishing stage the occlusal adjustment should be made.
- Average value type
  - They allow horizontal and vertical motion but cannot be altered to accommodate individual patient variations
  - Average values for condyle angle and tooth-condyle relations are used in this method
  - The teeth are arranged against the template which is supplied with these articulators.

Adjustable articulators

- They can be adjusted to accept records from the patient.
- They contain an adjustable sagittal condylar guide which can be attached to either the lower or upper part of the instrument
- The adjustable articulators are of different types.

Semiadjustable articulators

- Dentatus, Hanau, Whip-Mix articulators
- They work on the fact that the posterior control mechanisms are set by means of inter-occlusal records.

Highly adjustable articulators

- Denar, Stuart articulators
- They work on the principle that the posterior condylar control mechanisms are set in three plane of motion and accept kinematic facebow transfer
- The simulation of the movements of the mandible is achieved with greatest accuracy. They are of two types:
- Arcon articulators
  - They are the articulators having the condylar path elements attached to the upper jaw member and condylar element in lower member
  - For example, Hanau arcon H2.
- Nonarcon articulators
  - These articulators have the condylar paths attached to the lower jaw member, and the condylar elements attached to the upper member
  - For example, Hanau H2, Dentatus.

Articulation

- It is contact relationship between the occlusal surfaces of teeth during function
- It is the dynamic sliding contact of cusps of upper and lower teeth that takes place during closed gliding movements of the mandible
- Articulation is a continuous change from one occlusal position to the other. The term occlusion and articulation are often interchanged.

Centric Relation

- It is a maxillomandibular relationship in which the condyles articulate with the thinnest avascular portion of their respective disks with the complex in the antero-superior position against the slopes the articular eminence
- The position is independent of tooth contact. This position is clinically desirable when the mandible is directed superiorly and anteriorly. It is restricted to a purely rotary movement about the transverse horizontal axis.

Balanced Articulation

- The glossary of Prosthodontic terms defined balanced occlusion as the bilateral, simultaneous, anterior and posterior occlusal contact of teeth in centric and eccentric positions
- The more appropriate definition of balanced occlusion would be the occlusal contacts of maxillary mandibular teeth initially in maximum intercuspation and their continuous contacts during movement from this initial position along specific working, balancing and protrusive guidance pathways developed on the occlusal surfaces of the teeth.

Laws of Articulation of Balanced Occlusion

- The laws of articulation are purely physical laws which must be observed in the formation of the masticatory surfaces of natural and artificial dentures, whenever it is the aim to establish or produce that function which we accept as balanced articulation
- ADA journal in 1926. Of these nine factors the most important in practice are the following five factors which is known as Hanau's Quints:
  - The inclination of the condylar guidance
  - The prominence of the compensating curve
  - The inclination of the plane of orientation
  - The inclination of the incisal guidance
  - The height of the cups.

Condylar guidance

- It is an anatomical concept transferred to the mechanical device on a articulator intended to produce guidance in

articulator movement similar to the paths of condyles in the temporomandibular joints
- It is not the geometrical replica of anatomical inclination, but the equivalent for it and due to relief of the tissues
  - The registration of horizontal condylar guidance is obtained from the patient by means of protrusive record and transferred to a semi-adjustable articulator such as Hanau, Whip-mix or Dentatus articulator
  - It is made with recording material placed between the teeth at try-in stage after the vertical and horizontal relationships are confirmed
  - A minimum six millimeter of protrusion will produce a record for setting the articulator
  - The horizontal condylar setting of 0–20° is low, 20–30° medium and above 30° is high
  - For lower or medium 0°, 20° or 30° or combination and for high setting 20° or 30° or combination are chosen.

Arrangement of Anatomic (Cusp) Teeth to Balanced Articulation

- Anteroposterior and mediolateral are arranged for the bilateral balance compensating curves
- The cusps are tilted mesially or buccally to for the arrangement
- Selective grinding is done for the final adaptability
- The two methods to obtain stability are protrusive and lateral balance.

Protrusive Balance

- Protrusive balance is not achieved at the expense of having unstable tooth positions, or unaesthetic appearance
- Only in cases where the anterior teeth can be set with an incisal angle of 20 degrees or less (with little overbite) protrusive balance can be obtained with advantage.

Lateral Balance

- The lateral balance obtained between the lower buccal and upper lingual cusps with a slight lateral tilt because correctly set posterior teeth have very little buccal overbite
- Neutralization of the inclines is achieved by use of flat ('0' degree) teeth and abandoning all attempts to secure balance by setting teeth in a flat plane

- Centralization of forces is achieved by reducing the size and number of artificial teeth
- This concept in practice is used on four parameters:
  - Position: Teeth are positioned in as per as centrally with respect to medial and lateral forces, i.e. in the neutral zone as described by fish
  - Proportion: The teeth size is required to be reduced up to 40% to achieve centralization of forces
  - Pitch: The inclination or tilt of teeth and the occlusal plane is pitch. It has to be eliminated
  - Form: The cuspless 0 degree teeth or rational posterior teeth (low cusp) are used to avoid cusps or projections that may cause interference with eccentric movements.

Lingualized Articulation

- It is defined as the form of denture occlusion articulates the maxillary lingual cusps with the mandibular occlusal surfaces in centric working and nonworking mandibular positions (Fig. 7.2)
- In a balanced arrangement maxillary tooth with sharp and pointed lingual cusps are used against shallow cusped occlusal table
- In nonbalanced arrangement monoplane mandibular teeth are used
- It is stated that the maxillary buccal cusps of posterior teeth should be reduced so that only lingual cusps would be in contact.

Advantages

- Flexibility
- Artificial teeth with cusp forms that lock against their antagonist during articulation are unacceptable for a patient with compromised muscle control
- The lingualized articulation is a better choice because it permits development of maximum intercuspation at centric jaw relation position yet provides some freedom of movement forward from this recorded position
- Edentulous patients rarely present classic class I jaw relationship
- When using anatomic teeth some freedom of movement must be provided by occlusal reshaping procedures during. It is possible in lingualized articulation
- Patients with resorbed ridge or flabby ridge usually restored with monoplane occlusion and zero incisal guide angle presented with unaesthetic appearance
- The lingual cusp of posterior teeth penetrates the bolus in a holding and grinding fashion similar to the action of a mortar and pestle.

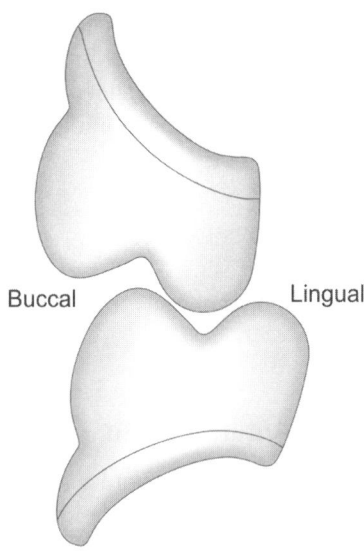

Fig. 7.2: Lingualized articulation

Selection of Upper Anterior Teeth

- There are four main considerations when selecting anterior teeth:
  1. Size.
  2. Shape.
  3. Colour (shade).
  4. Material.

Selection of Size

- The size and shape of the anterior teeth especially the maxillary central incisors are extremely important to the overall visual effect of the teeth
- Teeth are judged to be too large or small, too narrow or wide, or of ethically disproportionate in shape when compared with the overall proportion of the other facial structures leading to aesthetic disharmony
- To select the appropriate size of maxillary anterior teeth there are two dimensions to consider:
  1. Length.
  2. Width.

Length

- The length of the maxillary bite rim is first established by phonetics pronouncing the "F" and "V" sounds
- The second method of tooth length selection is based on the proportional size between the face and tooth
- There is a harmony in the proportion of the maxillary anterior teeth and the face. The length of the maxillary central incisor is 1/16 of the length of the face from the hairline to the tip of the chin.

Width

- Several anatomic guides are there to select correct width of maxillary anterior teeth. These are extreme variable guidelines. It is therefore, suggested that several of these can be compared before coming to conclusion
  - Intercommissural distance: The corners of mouth can be marked on the correctly contoured maxillary occlusal rim. The combined width of the six upper anterior teeth represent the measurement between these marks
  - The width of six maxillary anterior teeth equals to the bizygomatic width divided by 3.3. The facebow can be used to measure the bizygomatic width
  - The width of the maxillary central incisor is usually 1/16 of the bizygomatic width (Sears, 1941). The lateral incisors are 2 mm narrower and the canine 1 mm wider than the central incisors. The chart supplied by the manufacturer should be consulted to find the mould that possess the same width.

Selection of Shape

Faces are classified into four types as square, tapering, and ovoid facial forms to determine the most pleasing size and shape of a maxillary central incisor (**Fig. 7.3**).

Dentogenic Concept

Age

- The amount of anterior teeth visible in rest or in function often related to age. With increase in age, the amount of the maxillary central incisors showing with lip just parted will decrease
- Natural teeth wear with ages in most patient and the wear can be simulated by grinding the incisal edges of the denture teeth. With age there is exposure of roots and interdental papillary become blunt.

Sex

The shape of anterior tooth differs in sex. The masculine characteristics are flat labial surfaces, square in shape, incisal edges are flat whereas the female characteristics are more curved in shape.

Personality

The personality ranges from delicate to medium pleasing to vigorous. A delicate personality is very small in percentage of population.

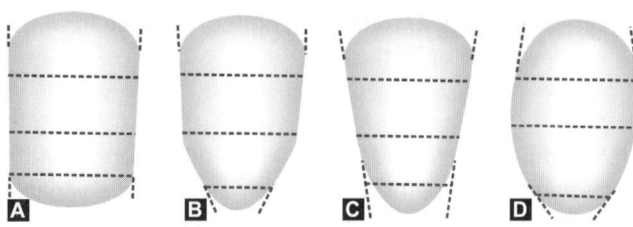

Fig. 7.3: Face form: (A) Square, (B) Square tapering, (C) Tapering and (D) Ovoid

Number System of Artificial Teeth

Three Digit Number System

- 1st Number gives classification of mould:
  - Square
  - Square tapering
  - Square ovoid
  - Tapering
  - Ovoid
  - Square tapering ovoid.
- 2nd Number length + curvature of profile
  - Long straight
  - Medium straight
  - Short straight
  - Long curve
  - Medium curve
  - Short curve.
- 3rd Letter (inter-canine width)
  - B – Less than 44 mm (six anterior teeth on a curve)
  - C – 44–46 mm
  - D – 46–48 mm
  - E – 48–50 mm
  - F – 50–52 mm
  - G – 52–54 mm
  - H – 54–56 mm
  - J – Above 56 mm.

The natural teeth are polychromatic and consists of three distinct shades:

- Cervical
- Incisal
- Transitional middle third. The shade possesses three qualities:
  - Hue: It is the specific color of the object, e.g. a tooth classed as red, yellow and grey
  - Value: The relative brightness or darkness of the color. There is a transition of the shade from the central incisor to canines
  - Chroma: The amount of concentration of color. In most of the shade guide, yellow is the prominent hue, chroma is the amount of yellow in each tooth. The canines have more chroma than the central incisor.

Materials

A choice must be made between:
- Conventional acrylic resin
- Interpenetrating polymer network (IPN) acrylic resin
- Composite resin
- Porcelain.

Arrangement of Anterior Teeth

- There are four factors that govern the basic positions in arrangement of anterior teeth:
  1. Horizontal position.
  2. Vertical position.
  3. Inclination.
  4. Aesthetic arrangement and customisation.

Horizontal Position

The horizontal positions of anterior teeth in edentulous arch usually follow the form and shape of the arch. Arch forms are classified as:
- Square
- Tapering
- Ovoid.

Adjustments for functional requirements are made depending upon the ridge relation are as follows:

- In class I relation the lower incisal edges should be no further anterior than mucobuccal fold
- In class II relation the upper anterior have to be set slightly lingually
- In class III relation the upper anterior have to be set on the upper ridge and inclined forward while lower anterior should be moved to ridge crest.

Vertical Position

The correct vertical positioning of teeth should provide:
- Denture stability
- Lip support
- Aesthetic
- The length of the maxillary central incisors is established by aesthetic and phonetics.

The vertical positioning of lower anterior depends on:
- Phonetic and aesthetic requirements

Chapter 7 Laboratory Procedures Prior to Try-In

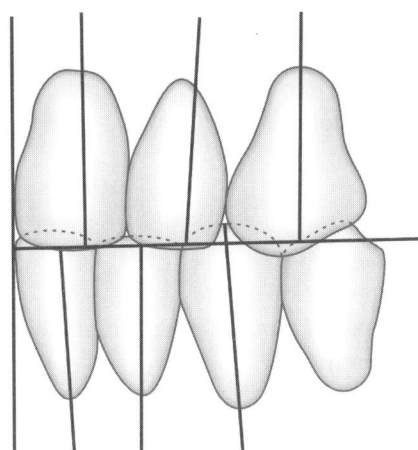

Fig. 7.4: Sketch showing the normal relationship between the upper and lower anterior teeth in class I jaw relationship when viewed form the front

- Ridge relations
- Occlusal scheme
- Inter-ridge distance.

Inclinations

- Central incisors
  - Its long axis is parallel to the vertical axis when viewed from the front, and sloping slightly labially when viewed from the side. The incisal edge is in contact with the horizontal plane.
- Lateral incisors
  - The long axis is sloping towards the midline of the mouth when viewed from the front, and is inclined labially to a greater degree than the central when viewed from the side. The incisor edges are about 2 mm above the horizontal plane.

Aesthetic Arrangement and Customisation of Anterior Teeth

- Normal arrangement
  - The central incisors of normal size and normal arrangement.
- Soft arrangement
  - The central incisors with prominent mesial sides and set back distal sides.
- Bold arrangement
  - The central incisors are positioned straight across or slightly ahead of the adjacent teeth.
- Modification of a central can be done by:
  - Squaring the incisal edges and corners
  - Rounding the incisal edges.

SHORT ESSAYS

Question 1

How to determine jaw relationship?

Answer

- The relationship of the teeth of lower denture to those of the upper will be decided by the relationship of the jaws
- Angle's classification is usually used to designate the three basic jaw relationships as follows:

Class I (Normal)

- The maxillary ridge crest is directly above the mandibular ridge. This is the most favourable relation for complete dentures (Fig. 7.4)
- About 70% of edentulous cases belong to this class.
- In this case anterior teeth are set with an overjet and overbite of 1–2 mm
- In this case usually the posterior teeth can be set in normal position with 1 mm overjet buccally.

Class II (Retrognathic)

- The mandibular ridge is narrower and shorter than the maxillary ridge. The maxillary posterior ridge crest is buccal to the mandibular ridge crest that makes the setting of posterior teeth difficult
- About 25% of edentulous cases belong to this class. In this case anterior teeth are set with an over-jet and overbite of 2–4 mm
- In this the posterior teeth are set with more overjet than normal (> 1 mm).

Class III (Prongathic)

- The mandibular ridge is larger and wider than maxillary ridge. It projects beyond the maxillary ridge. This patient shows no excursive movement but only open and close hinge jaw movement
- This makes balance occlusion unnecessary. About 5% of edentulous cases belong to this class

- In this case anterior teeth are set with overbite 0 mm and overjet 1 mm
- In this case posterior teeth are set with cross-bite, i.e. negative overjet.

Question 2

Discuss number system of artificial teeth.

Answer

Three Digit Number System

- 1st Number gives classification of mould:
  - Square
  - Square tapering
  - Square ovoid
  - Tapering
  - Ovoid
  - Square tapering ovoid.
- 2nd Number length + curvature of profile:
  - Long straight
  - Medium straight
  - Short straight
  - Long curve
  - Medium curve
  - Short curve.
- 3rd Letter (inter-canine width)
  - B – Less than 44 mm (six anterior teeth on a curve)
  - C – 44–46 mm
  - D – 46–48 mm
  - E – 48–50 mm
  - F – 50–52 mm
  - G – 52–54 mm
  - H – 54–56 mm
  - J – Above 56 mm.

Chapter 8: Laboratory Procedures for Insertion

LONG ESSAYS

Question 1

Write about causes of occlusal discrepancies.

Answer

Causes of Occlusal Discrepancies

- Incorrect registration of jaw relations
- Errors occurring during mounting of casts on articulator
- Errors in the setting of the denture teeth
- Tooth movement occurred during flasking packing and polymerization
- Incomplete flask closure.

Methods of Correcting Occlusal Discrepancies

- Two methods are generally used in correcting occlusal discrepancies. In both the methods occlusal surfaces of teeth are altered by selective grinding
    - Method I
        - Laboratory remounting and correction of occlusion due to processing errors by selective grinding before recovering the dentures from their casts.
    - Method II
        - Clinical remounting dentures with check-bite records (a new jaw relation records) and adjustment of the occlusion is necessary at the time of delivery of complete dentures to eliminate errors, which may not be found at the try-in of the trial denture.
- The laboratory remounting procedure will not correct for clinical errors in recording maxillomandibular relation records
- So, corrections of occlusal discrepancies are done preferably by patient check record remounting and selective grinding at the time of delivery.

Laboratory Remounting Method

- This is done by using split cast mounting plates or by notching casts to create keys in the mounting plaster
- The split cast has got several advantages:
    - Processing errors introduced by movement of teeth are easily detected
    - Deflecting contacts can be removed easily by grinding
    - Original vertical dimension can be restored
    - The centric occlusal relation position of cusps to the opposing teeth can be re-established.

Procedure

- Any chips of investment or acrylic flash that prevent accurate sitting of the casts should be removed first from the base of the casts
- The upper and lower dentures on their original casts are remounted on the articulator. They are attached to the original plaster mountings with sticky wax added to the sides
- The remounting shows the changes that occurred in the teeth during processing and makes it helps to restore the original vertical dimension of occlusion that exist in wax-up dentures. It may be found that the incisal pin fails to contact the incisal table to about 0.5–1 mm
- It is corrected by placing a fine articulating paper in between the teeth and the articulator is closed in centric position several times
- The marks are ground by the process of selective grinding until the original vertical dimension is restored as evident by the contact of the incisal guide pin to the incisal guide table
- When the occlusion is perfected on the articulator, the amount of work in the mouth is reduced substantially.

Clinical Remounting Method

- The clinical remounting method is to remount the dentures on an articulator by means of inter-occlusal records made in the patient's mouth
- This is most accurate method. It has the following advantages:

- It allows the dentist to observe the procedures better
- It eliminates patient participation
- It provides a stable mounting casts and bases those are not shifted on resilient tissues
- The saliva will not remove the markings of articulating paper
- The correction made in absence of the patient is advantageous
- It may be done in recall appointments from 24 hours adjustment to one year appointment
- Of course delay of occlusal adjustment until the denture settle in patients mouth may cause excessive tissue injury, instability and unsatisfactory retention.

Procedure

- This method maintains the articulator settings for various records used in setting and the face bow index of the maxillary waxed cast before processing
- After processing the dentures are recovered from investment and carefully finished and polished. All the undercuts are blocked with modelling clay. The fitting surface is lubricated with petroleum jelly and mounting casts are poured
- The maxillary cast is attached with plaster to the articulator with face bow index produced on the remounting jig. With both the dentures a wax check-bite centric relation record is obtained from the patient are joined securely with sticky wax
- The upper arm of the articulator is opened up and maxillary denture is seated on the upper mounted cast on the articulator
- The plaster is placed on the lower mounting disk and the articulator is inverted and closed as plaster sets.

Selective Grinding

- The intentional alteration of the occlusal surfaces of teeth to change their form
- Grinding of the occlusal surfaces of the artificial teeth at selected points is carried out to ensure that the centric occlusion of the teeth coincides with the centric relation and also to have balanced eccentric contact in all position
- The elimination of the deflective contacts of the teeth with provision of balanced occlusion is one of the most important stages in the fabrication of dentures carried out as a clinical remounting after the dentures have been tried in the patient
- It is a corrective process that should be carried out after a thorough knowledge of balanced occlusion
- This procedure is to correct minor errors in clinical and/or laboratory procedures
- It is not effective in elimination of gross error where a wrong centric relation has been obtained.
- Selective grinding helps in preservation of tooth form and occlusion. The process is carried out in two stages:
  1. Correction of centric occlusion at a correct centric relation.
  2. Development of eccentric balancing contacts.

Correction of Occlusal Errors in Anatomical Teeth on Articulator

Instruments

- Red and blue thin articulating paper
- Green stones or diamonds
- Laboratory handpiece
- Rubber points
- Gauze moistened with alcohol.

Rules for selective grinding

- A centric cusp tip should never be grind unless prematurely in all excursions of the mandible. The opposing fossa should always be grind
- The Bull rule should be used for working occlusion by grinding the buccal cusp inclines of the upper and lingual cusp inclines of the lower
- In balancing occlusion, cusp inclines should be grind and not the cusp tips
- In protrusive interferences in anterior teeth grinding of lower labial and upper lingual teeth is recommended. In posterior teeth the upper buccal cusp slopes and lower lingual cusp slopes should be grind.

Centric occlusion

- Articulating paper of minimum thickness is placed between the posterior teeth bilaterally and the teeth are tapped together. The articulator should be locked with centric lock so as to make centric closure only
- The markings are observed for premature contacts that are to be relieved depends both in centric and eccentric relationships as follows:
  - If tip of cusp is high in centric contact only, the opposing fossa should be deepened
  - If tip of cusp is high both in centric and lateral excursions, it is reduced
- The marking and reduction is repeated until even, bilateral, cusp/fossa markings occur. The marking of premature contacts should be identified as dark spot with a light centre

Chapter 8 Laboratory Procedures for Insertion

- The anterior contact, if any, should be removed as required. There should be no contact of anterior tooth in centric relation
- The incisal guide pin is set against the incisal table and locked in this position.

Working and balancing occlusion contacts

- The articulating paper is placed bilaterally between the teeth. The articulator is moved in right and left lateral excursions placing articulating paper between the teeth bilaterally
- Blue colour articulating paper is placed between the teeth and tapped sharply together in centric relation. The marks should not be removed during selective grinding for eccentric balance
- The premature areas are identified and removed by grinding according to the following rules:
  - On working side: It is essential that the proper alignment of the opposing cusps and their opposing embrasures are re-established
  - It is done by reducing the lingual inclines of the upper buccal cusps and the buccal inclines of the lower lingual cusps (Bull rule)
  - On the balancing side: The buccal inclines of the upper palatal cusps are reduced and the lingual inclines of the lower buccal cusps are saved
  - The process of marking and grinding is repeated until there is even bilateral contact for both right and left lateral movements.
- The anterior contact occurs, the lingual surface of the maxillary anterior teeth and labioincisal surface of mandibular anterior are reduced.

Protrusive balance

Protrusive balance is least important in denture occlusion. It is desirable but not so important to sacrifice aesthetics.

- The red articulating paper is placed between the teeth bilaterally and the articulator is moved anteriorly in edge-to-edge position
- The blue articulating paper is placed between the teeth in centric relation contacts
- The premature contacts are identified and removed by grinding according to the following rules:
  - If teeth contact anteriorly only and not posteriorly, the lingual surface of the upper incisal edges of anterior teeth and the labial surface of the incisal edges of lower anterior teeth are reduced
  - If the teeth contact posteriorly but not anteriorly, the distal inclines of upper buccal cusps and mesial inclines of the lower buccal cusps are reduced.

Evaluation of Occlusal Adjustment

- After the occlusal adjustment is over it should be checked observing the following points:
  - Maximum tooth contacts bilaterally in centric and eccentric positions
  - No contact of anterior tooth in centric closure
  - Incisal pin remains in contact with incisal table during its movements
  - Light contact between posterior teeth during protrusive movement
  - Tooth contact when incisal pin moves 2 mm on incisal table
  - The occlusion is fully balanced during the movements of the articulator.

Correction of Occlusal Errors in Non-anatomical Teeth

After the centric relation mounting of the lower cast has been proved to be correct, the occlusal grinding should be done in the laboratory. This is done as follows:

- The flat occlusal table of the mandibular denture is grounded by gently rubbing the occlusal surfaces and incisal edges over flat sandpaper block. This is done as the mandibular teeth are arranged to a flat plane and the maxillary anterior teeth may be set slightly below the occlusal plane for aesthetic reasons
- The dentures are placed on the articulator and a 10 cm square articulating paper is placed between the teeth, and tapped together gently several times
- The premature contacts of the denture bases between the tuberosities and retromolar pads are removed by grinding
- The premature contacts of the maxillary teeth are removed with a large diameter wheel instead of a small diameter bur as it will removes the contacts between two flat occlusal surfaces of teeth
- All the anterior contacts are removed by grinding the lingual surfaces of the maxillary teeth
- The gross lateral interferences are removed without sacrificing the aesthetics although no horizontal condylar inclinations are usually when using cuspless teeth and monoplane occlusion.

Providing Smooth Articulation

- All the ground tooth surfaces should be smoothened with a brush wheel applying wet pumice

- This will remove any uneven contact along the paths between the centric and eccentric position. In case of porcelain teeth silicon carbide paste No. 150 is applied on the lower posterior teeth and lateral and protrusive movements are performed to produce smoothness.
- Milling
  - It is a process of removing the irregularities of grinding with a slight abrasive paste.
- Polishing
  - The surfaces of teeth is then polished using rubber wheels, with pumice.

Question 2

What are the effects of complete dentures on oral tissues?

Answer

- The wearing of complete denture may have some adverse effects on the oral environment particularly to the denture-bearing tissues
- These effects can be divided into two types of sequelae:
  1. Direct
  2. Indirect.

Direct Sequelae

- Residual ridge reduction
- Mucosal reactions
- Denture stomatitis: The pathological reactions of the denture-bearing palatal mucosa
- Angular cheilitis
- Soft tissue hyperplasia
- Flabby ridges: It is mobile and extremely resilient alveolar ridge due to replacement of bone by fibrous tissue
  - It is often seen in long-term denture wearers due to residual ridge resorption
  - It has been observed in 24% of edentulous maxilla and 5% of edentulous mandible and most frequently in anterior region
  - It is seen most commonly in the anterior part of the maxilla, when anterior teeth remain in the mandible causing excessive loading.
  - Surgical removal is the common mode of treatment.
- Denture irritation hyperplasia
- Traumatic ulcers: The small painful ulcers or sore spots commonly develop within 1–2 days after placement of dentures due to overextended borders or deflective occlusal contacts
  - A sequelae of wearing ill-fitting dentures causing tissue hyperplasia in denture border due to chronic injury by unstable dentures, thin or overextended borders.
- Oral cancer: It may develop in wearing ill-fitting dentures in alcoholic or tobacco use with uneducated and low socioeconomic groups of people
- Burning mouth syndrome: It is a burning sensation in one or several oral structures in contact with the denture with a feeling of dry mouth
  - It may be due to instability in denture, Vitamin deficiencies, and iron deficiency anaemia, xerostomia induced by radiation or drugs or psychologic factors.
- Gagging: It is triggered by tactile stimulation of the soft plate, the posterior part of tongue, tonsils and psychologic factors
- Altered taste perception.

Indirect Sequelae

- Atrophy of masticatory muscles: Atrophy of masseter and the medial pterygoid muscle occur in complete denture wearers particularly women with lessoning of bite forces progressively
  - The reduced biting force and chewing efficiency is sequel of wearing complete dentures, resulting in impaired masticatory function
  - The placement of new denture will not cause improvement in masticatory efficiency. The old denture wearer gradually changes their food habit to softer food.
- Nutritional deficiencies: In healthy adults there is no evidence that the nutritional intake is impaired in denture wearers of complete dentures so replacement of ill-fitting dentures with well-fitted new dentures will not improve the nutritional status
  - However, nutritional deficiencies occur in patient with poor general health, poor absorption, intestinal, metabolic, and catabolic disturbances, anorexia and salivary gland hypofunction, or altered taste perception.
- Temporomandibular disorders: Complete denture patients and patient with other types of dentition can be affected by temporomandibular disorders in a similar way
  - But as the severe signs and symptoms are rare there is relatively less number of complete denture wearer with temporomandibular disorders
  - Treatment with new complete dentures relieves the patient of signs and symptoms of the diseases.
- Masticatory ability: A study shows that the great majority (70–85%) of edentulous patients was satisfied with the masticatory ability of their complete dentures
  - Older patients have been more satisfied with poorly fitting dentures and will not seek new denture

Chapter 8 Laboratory Procedures for Insertion

- Measurements of masticatory force and ability to comminute a test food are drastically reduced in complete denture wearers in comparison to the people with natural teeth, as well as with implant supported dentures
- Only 8% of totally edentulous patient would prepare to accept dental implants, if available
- The main reason for declining implant prosthesis was that they were satisfied with their present dentures.
- In edentulous cases, the placement of implants and the insertion of an implant-supported prosthesis reduce bone loss.

SHORT ESSAYS

Question 1

Describe residual ridge reduction (RRR).

Answer

Definition

Residual ridge reduction is a chronic, progressive, irreversible and cumulative disease.

Aetiology

- Anatomic factors:
  - Size and shape of ridge
  - Type of bone
  - Type of mucoperiosteum
  - Ridge relation.
- Metabolic factors:
  - Age: The older the patient more the resorption of bone
  - Sex: The female at menopause are more prone to osteoporosis which increases bone resorption
  - Hormonal balance: Higher amount of parathyroid hormone causes more bone resorption
  - Vitamins: Deficiency of vitamin D can cause bone resorption, deficiency of vitamin A and C affects bone growth.
- Mechanical factors:
  - Functional factors: Cancellous bone can withstand compressive forces better than any other type of bone.
  - Prosthetic factors: Form of teeth, arrangement of teeth, inter-occlusal distance.

Treatment

- Many prosthodontics and surgical treatments are performed in case of several residual ridge resorptions, but without much success
- The best treatment is preventive, i.e. avoiding total extraction, preservation teeth and treatment with overdentures which cause much less bone resorption

Question 2

Write about denture stomatitis.

Answer

- Denture stomatitis is caused by a yeast or fungus called candida
- It is not an infection that we get or pass on to others, because we all have some candida in our mouths
- Thrush can appear in other parts of the body, but when it affects the mouth it may be called 'denture stomatitis'
- It can be seen as a red area under the denture. There may also be red sore areas at the corner of the lips.

Aetiology

- Candida infection results in microbial plaque on the fitting surface of the denture
- Traumatic factors, e.g. mechanical, thermal and chemical irritations
- Allergic reactions to denture base material
- Immunological disorders.

Treatment

- Good oral hygiene: It is important to keep your mouth as clean as possible and rinse your mouth and dentures after meals. Smoking encourages the growth of further yeast infections
- Keeping your dentures as clean as possible: Keep your dentures out of your mouth as much as possible, and definitely overnight
- Some yeast infections will clear up completely, if you don't wear your dentures at night for two weeks
- Clean your dentures by brushing, soaking and then brushing again. Dentists recommend using a soft toothbrush so you do not damage the material of your dentures. You can also soak your dentures in any solution used to sterilise babies' bottles

- If your denture has metal parts, do not use anything that contains bleach, but use chlorhexidine, instead. Do not use chlorhexidine every day as it will stain your denture. Use it once a week
- Medication: If good oral hygiene and careful cleaning have not helped, you will be given some treatment
- There are many treatments available, most of them involving sucking tablets or lozenges slowly in your mouth. You may need to continue the treatment for one month.

Question 3

Explain flabby ridge.

Answer

- A flabby ridge is one which becomes displaceable due to fibrous tissue deposition. Most frequently seen in the upper anterior region
- Usually occurs when natural teeth oppose an edentulous ridge
- A flabby ridge causes instability of the denture. There are a number of different methods to overcome this problem, 3 of which will be discussed.

Treatment

Surgery

- This involves removal of the fibrous tissue to leave a firm ridge. However removing the shock absorbing flabby ridge may lead to trauma of the underlying bone, and an increased bulk of denture material
- The other technique involves constructing a denture over the flabby ridge
- The impression may be either mucostatic or mucodisplacive where a mucostatic impression technique, good retention obtained when the teeth are out of occlusion and when the denture is put under load, instability may occur
- With mucodisplacive impression techniques, the denture will only fit well when the denture is under load, it may be unstable at rest because the flabby ridge tends to recoil back into its original position displacing the denture.

Window Technique

- A primary impression is taken in alginate loaded in a stock tray. The impression is then poured and a special tray is constructed on the model.
- The special tray is close fitting and has a hole or window over the area corresponding to the flabby ridge. An impression is taken in impression paste (mucodisplacive). Once this has set it is left in place and impression plaster (mucostatic) is painted over the flabby ridge and allowed to set and removed as one impression. The impression is removed as one, cast and the denture constructed on the resulting model.

Selective Displacive Technique

- This techniques aims to displace but not distort the flabby ridge, as if in function. A primary impression is taken in a mucostatic impression material, (e.g. impression plaster or alginate) and cast in stone
- A spaced special tray for an impression compound impression is then constructed on this model. The tray is loaded with compound and an impression taken of the model of the patient's mouth
- This reduces the risk of displacing the flabby ridge. The tray is then warmed and placed in the patient's mouth. It is adapted and border moulded to the tissues and should be quite retentive
- The impression is removed and warmed all over apart from the flabby ridge area. The impression is retaken, the flabby ridge is compressed but not distorted as the other portions of the impression compound sink into the tissues
- The impression is removed inspected and re-tried in the mouth to check that it is stable. If any instability occurs then the impression should be reheated and re-taken
- A wash impression may be taken in impression paste to obtain maximum and retention and stability.

Question 4

What is the burning mouth syndrome (BMS)?

Answer

The burning sensations of structures of mouth in contact with the dentures. It occurs most frequently in tongue. It is more frequent in middle-aged men and women.

Aetiology

Local Factors

- Mechanical irritation
- Tongue habits
- Allergy: True allergies to acrylic are rare. Allergy can be confirmed by a patch test on denture-bearing tissues or skin. If positive result is obtained the denture can be remade using another resin such as polystyrene, nylon, or polycarbonate, or cast chrome-cobalt. Free monomer present in incompletely cured denture may be the cause

- Pressure on nerve. A burning sensation in anterior part of palate may be due to excessive pressure from the denture on incisive papilla. Proper relief will cause immediate relief
- *Candida albicans* and bacterial infections
- Unstable dentures
- Smoking, tobacco chewing, mouth breathing, chronic alcoholism
- Intake of excessively seasoned foods
- Use of denture adhesives, cleansers, etc
- The patients with reduced tongue space, incorrect level of occlusal plane and increased vertical dimension of denture are more susceptible to BMS.

Systemic Factors

- Vitamin deficiency anaemia
- Menopause
- Xerostomia
- Systemic diseases
- Drugs
- Psychological and/or psychosocial disturbances like depression, anxiety
- Metabolic and circulatory disturbances, pernicious and iron deficiency anaemia, gastrointestinal disorders, and hormonal imbalance.

Treatment

- Optimization of deficient dentures
- If there is no denture deficiencies the psychological evaluation is essential in collaboration with psychologist
- An implant supported denture fabrication may be carried out along with psychotherapy.

SHORT NOTES

Question 1
Write about gagging.

Answer

It is a normal reflex to prevent foreign bodies from entering the trachea.

Aetiology

- The tactile stimulation of the soft palate, posterior part of tongue and tonsil
- The sight, taste, noise, as well as psychological factors or combination of all these factors
- Persistent complaints of gagging may be due to overextended borders particularly at the posterior part
- The unstable occlusions or increased vertical dimension of occlusion may trigger gagging reflex.

Treatment

- Correction of overextended dentures by proper trimming
- Correction of occlusal vertical dimension and occlusal prematurities
- Psychological: The patient who is wearers of old dentures, gagging may be due to some systemic diseases of the gastrointestinal tract, tonsil and alcoholism.

Question 2
What is angular cheilitis?

Answer

Angular cheilitis is a common inflammatory condition affecting the corners of the mouth or oral commissures. Depending on underlying causes, it may last a few days or persist indefinitely. It is also called angular stomatitis and cheilosis.

Aetiology

- Dribble of saliva causing eczematous cheilitis, a form of contact irritant dermatitis (perlèche)
- Overhang of upper lip resulting in deep furrows (marionette lines)
- Dry chapped lips
- Proliferation of bacteria (impetigo), yeasts (thrush) or virus (cold sores).

Clinical Features

Angular cheilitis may result in the following symptoms and signs at the corners of the mouth:
- Painful cracks / fissures
- Blisters / erosions / ooze / crusting
- Redness
- Bleeding.

Treatment

In many cases, no treatment is needed and angular cheilitis resolves by itself. Depending on the specific cause, the following treatments may be useful:
- Lip balm or thick emollient ointment, applied frequently
- Topical antiseptics
- Topical or oral antistaphylococcal antibiotic
- Topical antifungal cream
- Oral antifungal medication
- Topical steroid ointment
- Nutritional supplements
- Filler injections or implants to build up the oral commissures.

Question 3

Write about control of sequelae of wearing complete dentures.

Answer

- The consequences of complete denture wearing are reduction of the residual ridges, and oral pathological changes.
- This results in discomfort, insufficient mastication and poor aesthetic problems
- The patient may be unable to wear the denture completely and will be levelled as prosthodontically maladaptive.
- These sequelae cannot be prevented but can be delayed as follows:
  - The treatment with complete denture by total removal of teeth should be avoided except in poor periodontal health. Instead partial denture should be planned. Some teeth or at least roots should be preserved to act as an abutment for the over denture
  - The complete denture patients should be placed on routine yearly recall and check-up plan so as to maintain the fit and occlusion
  - The complete denture patients should be aware of benefit of implant-supported dentures
  - The patient should be advice not to wear the dentures during the night
  - The patient should be properly advised to clean and maintain the denture regularly and if necessary patient may be seen every three monthly intervals.

Chapter 9: Relining and Rebasing

LONG ESSAYS

Question 1

Write in brief about repair, types of fracture and techniques for repairing dentures.

Answer

It is the procedure by which the fractured parts of a denture are assembled and joined together using denture-base material of same type.

Causes of Fracture

- Intraoral causes: Resorption of alveolar bone, causing denture rocking and fracture
- Faulty construction: These may be due to incorrect setting of teeth, inadequate polymerisation time, denture base too thin or large labial frenum relief
- Accident of drop, during cleaning.

Treatment

- Repair
- Relining.

Materials

- Broken acrylic resin complete denture can be repaired using heat curing or cold curing materials. The use of heat cured resin with flasking often results in dimensional change of the base material at the curing temperature
- Nowadays self-curing resin is used to make fast, easy and very satisfactory repair. A broken tooth can be replaced with selfcure resin without flasking. A light cure resin may be used.

Types of Fractures

- Simple: Single or several tooth facture or dislodgement
- Complex: Fracture of denture based in two or more pieces.

Techniques

Replacing broken teeth/tooth

- A reduction is made in the denture base material on lingual/palatal surface of the denture base where the tooth/teeth are broken or missing
- Tooth/teeth of correct mould and shade are placed or ground in position and held with sticky wax at the incisal edge. The denture may be articulated against opposing cast and teeth set up to ensure that no occlusal interferences occur
- Separating medium is applied to the labial surface and adjacent teeth, and an index is made of plaster or silicone putty
- The area of repair is moistened with cold-cure monomer with the help of a small glass dropper two or three times to make the area tacky
- The polymer is spread over the area from a small plastic bottle. This is followed by alternate applications of monomer and polymer until the area is slightly over-filed
- Always slight excess of monomer should be present there to assure complete polymerisation. A wet sheet of cellophane is placed on the acrylic and pressure is applied with the index finger for few minutes
- The denture is bench cured for about 20 minutes and polishing and finishing is done in the usual way.

Repair of midline fractured dentures

- Repair is not advisable, if the fractured fragments cannot be accurately approximated
- The technique for maxillary or mandibular denture is similar. The fracture parts are assembled together with sticky wax in correct position and the fragments are held together with one or more wooden match sticks to the occlusal surfaces of the teeth

- The denture is tried in the mouth if possible for accuracy of reassembly. Any undercuts on fitting surface is blocked out with moist cotton wool and a plaster cast is poured into the denture and allowed to set
- The pieces of denture are removed. The pieces are prepared by removing 3 mm of acrylic from the fracture line
- A long rounded bevel (4–5 mm) is used to produce a bond of acceptable strength
- Tin foil substitute is applied on cast to the area beneath the fracture. When dried, the pieces are placed on the casts. The edges of the bevel are wetted with monomer
- Monomer and polymer powder is placed in the areas of bevel incrementally
- The plaster matrix is placed in position and held there for 10 minutes. It is allowed to stand for another 10 minutes for bench curing
- In case if pressure curing unit is used to quicken curing and preventing porosity, the repair job is placed in the pressure unit and covered with water at 100° F. Compressed air is introduced in curing unit at 30 lbs/sq for 10 minutes
- After curing, the excess material is trimmed and polishing of denture is done.

Light-cure repair

- First two fractured parts of the denture are rejoined with cyanoacrylate and stabilized with sticky wax and wooden sticks
- Then stone cast is poured to maintain the orientation of two parts
- Gap of 2–3 mm is created and edges were bevelled to 45°
- Then space for fibres is made and the fracture, site is prepared with monomer/bonding agent
- A thin layer of flowable composite resin was applied. It is not polymerised as it creates an adhesive surface that allows for the fiber-reinforced composites (FRC) to be tacked down
- Multiple strips of FRC are cut, tacked across the fracture site and light cured
- FRC repair is then covered with cold cure resin to mask the color of FRC. It is slightly overfilled to compensate the polymerisation shrinkage
- Then prosthesis was placed is warm water and allowed to polymerise in a pressure pot at 20 psi. After 15 minutes, the prosthesis is removed, pumiced and polished
- Advantages:
  - Long lasting service due to enhance of strength of repaired denture
  - Frequency of fracture of maxillary complete denture opening a natural dentition is reduced
  - It is a simple straightforward procedure and can be easily done in dental office
  - Esthetic is not compromised
  - There is no increase in weight and bulk.

Question 2

Define relining and rebasing. Write in detail about clinical and laboratory procedures.

Answer

Relining

Relining is the process of resurfacing by adding base material in a quantity to fill the space between the tissue and the denture base created by the resorption of the supporting ridges.

Indications

- Immediate dentures at three or six months after construction
- When residual alveolar ridges have resorbed and the adaptation of the denture bases to the ridges is poor
- When the patient cannot afford the cost of having new denture construction
- When the construction of new dentures with series of appointments can cause physical or mental stress in geriatric or chronically ill patients
- When the occlusal vertical dimension is satisfactory
- When centric occlusion coincide with centric relation
- Patient's appearance is acceptable to the patient and the dentist
- The oral tissue is in optimum health
- The posterior limit of the maxillary denture is correct
- The denture base extensions are adequate
- Speech is satisfactory with the existing tooth arrangements
- There should be no severe bony undercuts or flabby tissues.

Contraindications

The denture should not be relined:

- When an excessive resorption has taken place
- When abused soft tissue is present
- When patient complain of temporomandibular joint problem—until treatment of problem is accomplished
- If the denture have poor aesthetics or unsatisfactory jaw relationships
- If the denture creates speech problem
- When severe bony undercut present
- Absence of freeway space.

Chapter 9 Relining and Rebasing

Clinical and Laboratory Procedures

- The clinical procedures for both the relining and rebasing is same, only the laboratory procedures are different
- Impressions may be made either by the functional (close mouth) or by the static technique, depending upon the need of the patient and the decision of the dentist
- Before impression is made, the mucosa should be free from irritation and it should be in healthy state
- The denture should be left out the mouth for a minimum 2–3 days.

Functional Impressions

- Tissue treatment material may be used for making a functional impression
- This type of impression is indicated in dentures which require no modification of the vertical dimension of occlusion
- The denture is prepared by removing all undercut areas so that the denture may be removed from the cast without damaging the latter
- The denture border, in specific location such as frena, need to be relived, it is not necessary to cut away a portion of the entire border because the impression material should record the original relation of the border with the muscular borders
- The vertical dimension may be altered by more or less than this relation
- The dentures are first relined with tissue treatment material (using a percentage of 1:1 powder liquid ratio) and placed in the mouth, and the patient is allowed to close lightly with teeth in centric occlusion
- Border molding is accomplished by functional movements
- The denture is removed from the mouth after 5 minutes for evaluation of the impression
- It should have a smooth rounded border and surface free from imperfections, and accurate reproduction of the patient oral tissue
- After removing the excess material from the facial surface of the denture, the patient is allowed to wear for 24 hours
- The patient should return for evaluation of the denture. If the dentures have develop adequate stability and retention and tissues do not show any sign of irritation, the dentures are relined with the same ratio of powder liquid (1:1)
- The upper and lower are loaded with the material at the same time inserted in the mouth and closed without much pressure on the teeth, and make open and close for 2 minutes
- The dentures are kept in the mouth for 45 minutes. If they are removed earlier, the material is not properly set and sticks to the tissues and gets distorted
- The maxillary denture is removed by asking the patient to blow with his mouth closed to preserve the peripheral border
- The excess material which has flowed on the denture base 4 mm beyond the peripheral border is removed
- The occlusion is recorded with a plaster buccal key for remounting
- The dentures are removed from the mouth and stone cast is poured by carefully covering the borders
- The buccal keys are secured to the dentures for remounting on an articulator
- The keys are removed, the dentures are cleaned and occlusion examined
- The dentures are invested usually without removing the dentures from the casts
- To avoid distortion of the old denture base during processing, all the acrylic resin should be removed from the maxillary denture and rebasing is done, whereas relining is done in a mandibular denture.

Static Impressions

- Separate impressions are made without utilizing the existing centric occlusion
- The dentures should be left out of the mouth for at least 24 hours before impressions are made. All the undercuts are eliminated
- The denture borders are checked. Any overextension must be removed by grinding away the denture periphery in that area until they are at least 1 mm short of tissue reflection point
- Any area of the denture base that impinged on soft tissue should be relieved before the entire fitting surface is reduced from 0.5 to 1.0 mm, depending upon the impression material used
- Four composition stops are placed in the alveolar groove area of the denture, one each in each canine and one each in the molar areas
- The dentures are placed in the patient's mouth and addition or subtractions from the stops are made until the desired vertical dimension is obtained
- The dentures are border moulded with green stick composition as a new denture impression. If close mouth method is used, patient closes the mouth each time border molding is done

- After the border moulding is completed, the dentures should be retentive. All borders except, the posterior palatal seal area on the maxillary denture and buccal shelves on the mandibular denture should be reduced 1.0 mm
- A wash impression is made with zinc oxide paste or light body rubber base
- The denture will now be retentive and stable. The vertical dimension and centric relation and appearance are rechecked. If correct the denture is boxed and cast is poured
- The denture may be relined either with autopolymerising acrylic resin or heat cure resin in laboratory. This is performed using any of the two methods:
  1. Hooper duplicator method.
  2. Jectron jig method.
- The maxillary and/or mandibular casts are not separated and mounted in the top of jig or duplicator
- A layer of plaster is placed in the lower member of the jig, and the upper member with the denture to it attached is closed into the soft plaster
- So that the teeth penetrate the plaster surface to a depth of 3 mm approximately. The set plaster formed a key into which the teeth can be set repeatedly
- The denture is now removed from the cast by dipping in hot water to soften the impression material. Now it should be decided whether to reline or rebase the denture
- The post dam groove is cut in the maxillary cast. Self-curing resin is mixed up as per manufacturer's direction and poured in the space created by removal of the impression material
- The gig or duplicator is closed to its original position
- The denture is finished and polished as usual. The intraoral checking of occlusal contacts and relationship should be performed during delivery.

Chairside Relining

- Research continues to develop some material that can be added to the denture base and allowed to set in the mouth
- Two types of material available temporary soft liner and permanent soft liner
- The former is used to treat abuse tissue developed from wearing faulty denture without leaving the denture out of the mouth.

Procedure

- The tissue fitting surface (except the posterior palatal seal area) and the denture borders are reduced about 2 mm
- Two anterior steps may be placed in canine region without relieving two (3 × 3 mm) areas
- The material is mixed (powder and liquid) according to the manufacturer's directions
- The material is evenly spread on the fitting surface of the dentures including the borders
- The dentures are placed in patient's mouth and the patient is advised to tap his teeth lightly together without putting excessive pressure
- Border moulding is done functionally
- The denture is removed from the mouth and checked for voids, if found and new material is to place over them and dentures returned to the mouth to correct these areas
- The pressure spots are relieved with round bur or carbide burs
- The centric relation must coincides centric occlusion at correct vertical dimension
- The patient is dismissed for 72 hours and asked not to brush the fitting surface and avoid hard food
- Additional treatment may be needed after 72 hours and the material is replaced by new material till tissues become normal.

Rebasing

Rebasing is the process of refitting a denture by replacing all the old denture base material with new material, without changing the occlusal relations of the teeth.

Objectives

- The purpose of such process is to close contact between the supporting tissue and the denture base created by the resorption of tissues
- If the change in the oral tissue is not great, relining rather than rebasing is required.

Indications

- In case of excessive resorption of ridge
- When a denture has been repaired many times
- When a denture has been fractured into many pieces.

Procedure

- When the denture is intact an impression is taken in the denture. When the denture is fractured, an impression is obtained from mouth in a stock tray
- A cast is poured into the impression and the polished surface is cleaned

Chapter 9 Relining and Rebasing

- The denture and the cast are flasked in the shallow section of a flask
- When the plaster has set, the denture is removed from the flask and cleaned of impression material along with the cast
- Denture base material is removed with a grinding wheel mounted on lathe until only teeth remain on a 5 mm of wide acrylic giving a horseshoe appearance. The denture base from interpoximal areas are removed with a No. 3 flat fissure bur
- A post dam is cut on the maxillary cast. The teeth one firmly seated into the flask and acrylic resin dough is packed.
- The curing, deflasking, finishing and polishing done before delivery.

Chapter 10: Special Complete Dentures

LONG ESSAYS

Question 1

Write in brief about overdentures and its types.

Answer

- Overdenture may be defined as a removable partial or complete denture that covers and rests on one or more remaining natural teeth or roots and/or dental implant
- Tooth supported complete overdentures are actually referred as overdentures or hybrid dentures
- Overdentures were initially prescribed for patients with congenital or acquired defects where the need for maximum support is required.

Indications

- The overdentures are indicated for patient with badly mutilated teeth
- They are indicated in patient with congenital or acquired intraoral defects
- They are indicated for patient with abnormal jaw relation and abnormal jaw size.

Contraindications

- In high caries index and poor oral hygiene
- In abutments with poor periodontal conditions
- Bony undercuts adjacent to the supporting teeth
- In case of endodontic treatment produces poor prognosis
- Failure to establish a sufficient zone of attached gingiva
- Aged and uncooperative patients.

Advantages

- Conservation of natural teeth and concomitant reduction of or slowing of residual ridge resorption
- Stability and support of overdenture is better than a conventional denture. In a patient with natural teeth the occlusal forces are sustained by the periodontal membrane. After the loss of teeth, the area of mucosa left for support is almost ¼th of the area of periodontal membrane
- Sensory feedback of the periodontal receptors is maintained and masticatory efficiency is better
- The procedures of overdenture are simple as conventional complete dentures
- The repair, alterations or relining of overdenture can be easily performed as the conventional complete dentures
- The overdentures generally have better retention than conventional complete dentures
- The overdentures due to their same positioning of teeth as the natural teeth produces more aesthetic results
- The maxillary overdentures without palate is possible, if both anterior and posterior teeth are saved. The time and cost of treatment is less than alternative fixed partial dentures
- The overdentures may be converted to transitional or treatment denture when patient lose the teeth or roots. It is possible to produce a large vertical overlap of anterior teeth without displacing the denture during function
- Excellent patient acceptance, needs minimum adjustments, can be converted to complete denture
- The procedure is reversible, ease to clean than fixed partial denture, helps maintaining stability of existing oral structures
- It is particularly useful in patients with congenital defects, e.g. cleft palate, difficult class III occlusion and cleidocranial dysostosis.

Disadvantages

- Maintenance of good oral hygiene is difficult and caries susceptibility and plaque accumulation is increased
- The additional time and cost due to additional preparation of copping

- Lack of the inter-occlusal distance leads to difficulty in tooth arrangement and weak dentures
- Maintenance of the abutments and dentures are time consuming
- Aesthetics may have to be compromised
- It may be difficult to insert the denture flanges due to bony undercuts.

Types of Overdentures

- Overdentures are of three basic types:
  1. Immediate overdenture.
  2. Transitional overdenture.
  3. Remote overdenture.

Immediate overdenture

- It is the overdenture constructed for insertion immediately after the removal of hopeless natural teeth
- The clinical and laboratory procedures are similar to the immediate denture, except the selection, retention and preparation of the abutment teeth
- Most patient first receive an immediate overdenture.

Transitional overdenture

It is an overdentures obtained by modifying an existing removal partial denture. It is worn for an interim period and is replaced, if required later.

Remote overdenture

- A remote overdenture is constructed some time later, usually a year or more after the removal of the last hopeless teeth
- It may be used for replacing an immediate or transitional overdenture following satisfactory use.

Techniques

- Simple tooth modification and reduction: It is used in partially endodontic cases or in severe attrition cases. The remaining teeth are reshaped to eliminate undercuts and reduced in height, if required, to create inter-ridge space for the overdenture
- Tooth reduction and cast coping: This is done because of sensitivity or prevention of caries. This is usually done with teeth with adequate bony support and good periodontal prognosis
- Endodontic therapy with amalgam filling
- Endodontic therapy with cast coping
- Endodontic therapy with cast coping using some attachment, e.g. stud attachments.

Treatment Procedure

Immediate Overdenture

- The hopeless posterior teeth are removed
- During the healing period, prerequisite endodontic and periodontal treatment is completed
- Final impressions are made
- Recording of jaw relations and casts mounted on articulator
- Selection of acrylic anterior and posterior teeth is done
- Try-in with posterior teeth setting
- The anterior teeth are arranged using an adjacent stone tooth as guide
- The over-reduced abutment preparation is done on stone cast
- The acrylic abutment tooth is modified and set over the prepared stone abutment
- The denture is waxed, flasked, packed with high impact resin and cured in a conventional manner
- The denture is finished and polished and stored in water until insertion
- Abutment teeth in the mouth are reduced in a similar manner as done on the cast, but little smaller in size to allow placement of the overdenture without interference using the reference cast as a guide
- The clear acrylic stent is placed intraorally to judge the tissue impingement
- The abutment prepared teeth are treated with fluoride gel such as acidulated phosphate fluoride (APF) for 2 minutes, which is followed by application of 4% stannous fluoride gel
- The anterior hopeless teeth are removed and the overdenture is inserted. The peripheral extension and occlusion is checked
- The post-insertion instructions are provided and the patient is advised to report for 24 hours post-surgical appointment
- The 24 hours evaluation and necessary adjustments are made. The overdenture is adapted to abutments with tooth color autopolymerizing resin
- Follow-up care with application of fluoride on abutments
- Evaluation of oral hygiene, need for relining after six to eight weeks
- Yearly evaluation of oral hygiene and progress.

Tooth Supported Complete Denture

- Preparation of abutments for copings
- The impression is made and dies are poured
- The waxing, investing, casting and polishing of copings

- Checking the fit of copings on teeth and cementation with glass ionomer cement
- The existing overdenture is relined with autopolymerising resin to adapt the lubricated coping restored abutments.

Question 2

Write in brief about single complete dentures.

Answer

- The making of a maxillary or mandibular denture as distinguished from a set of complete denture
- Since in single denture only one arch is involved, it appears to be easy and require half as much work and time in comparison to a complete denture
- It is not so easy to fabricate and it requires much skill and experience to produce a successful prosthesis.

Indications

- Opposing the natural dentition only
- Opposing a combination of fixed and partial denture and natural teeth
- Opposing a removable partial denture and natural teeth
- Opposing an existing complete denture.

Contraindications

- A mandibular single complete denture opposing maxillary natural teeth is usually contraindicated as less basal seat area to support the mandibular denture than a maxillary denture
- The mucosa is thin and delicate, and a rapid loss of supporting bone. So, it may be necessary to extract healthy upper teeth looking after the long-term health of the mouth
- The overdenture may be a better option to the problem of a mandibular denture opposing natural teeth
- But mandibular denture opposing natural teeth may be considered in the following situations:
  - In class III jaw relationship mandibular complete denture against opposing upper natural teeth as the mandibular supporting tissues is able to resist the forces from upper natural teeth
  - The patient with cleft palate the upper teeth are preserved as the prognosis of an upper complete denture is not good. A lower complete denture may be made against it.

Problems of Single Complete Denture

- The firmness and rigidity of the natural teeth are due to their anchorage in the bone
- The force recorded on a single molar tooth is 198 lb where as a complete denture exerts a load of 26 lb. Therefore, the denture will be loose when natural teeth occlude against it
- The occlusal inclination and form of the remaining natural teeth will guide the occlusal form of the denture
- The unfavourable occlusal form results in shunting of denture.

Precautionary Measures

- Full use of every factor of retention and stability for success
- The forces applied on the denture must be reduced as far as possible by preparation or restoration of the remaining natural teeth so as to provide an acceptable occluding surface. The occlusal plane should exhibit no more than a gentle curve anteroposteriorly and mediolaterally
- The location of the occlusal plane in relation to the opposing supporting structures is below the middle of the interarch space, undesirable leverages may occur to either maxillary or mandibular complete dentures
- Teeth placed facial to the crest of the residual ridge induce torqueing and dislodging forces on denture during function.

Occlusal Modification

- In conventional complete dentures, upper and lower teeth are be arranged to obtain occlusion and articulation. In case of a single complete denture the occlusal pattern of the natural teeth is already present
- The natural teeth are modified by grinding or restoration to produce a more suitable occluding surface and grossly malpositioned teeth are extracted or orthdontically repositioned.

Methods

Swenson's method

- The maxillary and mandibular casts are prepared. The recording of tentative jaw relation is done without making any adjustments to the natural dentition
- These casts are mounted on an articulator and artificial teeth are set. The interferences in the natural occlusion is adjusted on the cast with a knife or bur and marked with pencil
- The occlusal adjustments of natural teeth are carried out in the mouth, using the marked study cast and the trial dentures as guide

Chapter 10 Special Complete Dentures

- A new impression of the natural teeth is made, cast prepared and a definitive jaw relation record is made. The new cast is mounted on the articulator, and the artificial teeth are reset and adjusted for trial
- The technique is accurate but time consuming as several impressions and casts are to be made.

Yurkstas method

- The mandibular study cast is evaluated with the help of U-shaped metal template with slight convex lower surface
- The template is placed on the occlusal surface of mandibular teeth. The cusps high or low are observed. They are marked using articulating paper
- The high cusps are judiciously equilibrated by removing a little of stone with knife on the study cast. This procedure is repeated by remarking and trimming until equalization is obtained
- In most patient the natural teeth modifications requires enameloplasty only
- The grinding should not be restricted to the tips of cusps but should extend on the buccal surface to prevent increase in occlusal table size.

Bruce's method

The method of tooth modification is done using same template, but marking is done with the help of pressure indicating paste instead of articulating paper.

Methods used to Obtain Balanced Occlusion

- Functional chew-in techniques (Stansbury, 1928)
- Articulator-equilibration techniques.

Functional Chew-in Technique (Stansbury, 1928)

- A compound maxillary rim is prepared against the mandibular natural teeth. It is trimmed buccally and lingually for freedom in lateral excursions
- Soft carding wax is added on the compound rim and the patient is asked to perform lateral and protrusive chewing movements
- The wax is abraded or reshaped to represent the functional paths of movement where as the compound preserve the vertical dimension
- The paths are known as functionally generated path and occlusion developed by this method is known as functionally generated occlusion
- The occlusion obtain is free from lateral and protrusive interferences. Stone is poured into the occlusal surfaces of the wax paths and without separation
- The mandibular cast mounted on the articulator is replaced by functionally generated cast. All interfering spots are ground until the incisal guide pin touches the incisal table and prevents further closure.

Articulator-equilibration Technique

- This is the most common method indicated when the denture base lack stability or the patient is unable to perform eccentric movements to form a chew-in record
- The maxillary and mandibular casts are mounted on articulator with a tentative jaw relation without making any adjustments to the natural dentition
- The relationship between the upper and lower posterior teeth are studied and following adjustments are done:
  - If the posterior denture teeth are to be placed too far lingually when articulated with the lower lingual cusps, they are reset to oppose the lower buccal cusps
  - If the posterior denture teeth are to be placed too far lingually when articulated with the lower buccal cusps, they are reset to oppose the lower buccal cusps.
- In this technique, only the functional cusps are allowed to contact the central fossa. The inclines of the nonfunctional cusps are reduced
- If the lower buccal cusps are selected as the functional cusps, the lingual cusps are reduced. If the lower lingual cusps are selected as the functional cusps, the buccal cusps are reduced
- At the wax try-in, eccentric records are made and the condylar inclinations are set on the articulator with the upper posterior teeth arranged in balanced occlusion. The denture is processed
- At the time of delivery, a new centric record is made and balancing of occlusion is achieved on articulator.

Occlusal Materials for the Single Complete Denture

- The single denture is usually opposed to different types of teeth in the opposing arch, so selection of occlusion forms for single denture should be done judiciously
- The occlusal surface will be such so that it should not wear too fast or it should not cause wearing of the natural dentition
- The following teeth may be considered with their relative advantages and disadvantages:
  - Vacuum fired porcelain
  - Acrylic resin
  - Gold occlusal
  - Acrylic resin with amalgam stop
  - Interpenetrating polymer network (IPN).
- The use of maxillary porcelain teeth, will lead to rapid wear of the opposing natural teeth. Silver amalgam

inserts or stops on occlusal surface wears out rapidly against the natural teeth
- Gold occlusals are very effective against natural teeth to maintain vertical dimension without undergoing wear but very expensive and time consuming preparations are necessary. The use of acrylic resin or IPN teeth is the best alternative.

Clinical Procedures for Single Complete Denture Opposing Natural Teeth

- An impression of the natural mandibular teeth is made in alginate hydrocolloid and cast is poured in stone
- A preliminary impression of the maxillary arch is made with modelling compound. The special tray is fabricated on the preliminary cast
- The final impression is made with zinc oxide paste. The master cast is poured in artificial stone
- A stabilized base plate with wax occlusal rim is constructed
- The occlusal rim is shaped to provide aesthetic lip support, the preliminary vertical dimension of occlusion is established. The tentative centric relation is determined
- The facebow record is made and the maxillary cast is mounted on the articulator which is programmed with protrusive record
- The anterior artificial teeth are arranged to provide aesthetic. The posterior teeth are arranged in centric occlusion
- The posterior teeth are rearranged to produce balanced occlusion. The occlusal surface of the mandibular cast is modified for balancing. The modified surfaces are marked with pencil to serve as a guide to accomplish the same in the patient mouth
- After modifications of the natural teeth, a new impression of the mandibular ridge is obtained in alginate hydrocolloid and a stone cast is poured
- A new centric relation record is made, and the mandibular cast is remounted on the articulator
- The anterior teeth are reset to provide proper aesthetic. The posterior teeth are reset in balanced occlusion
- The waxing and processing is done in usual manner and the facebow transfer is preserved
- The denture is processed, a new centric relation record is made by cheek-bite and the lower cast is remounted on the articulator and occlusal correction is done
- The denture is delivered with proper instructions
- The post-insertion check-up and adjustment are made as for conventional complete denture.

SECTION 2

REMOVABLE PARTIAL DENTURES

CHAPTER 11

Introduction to Removable Partial Dentures

LONG ESSAYS

Question 1

Discuss the steps required in the fabrication of a removable partial denture.

Answer

The fabrication of a removable partial denture comprises of various stages, which are as follows:
- Diagnosis
- Pre-prosthetic procedures
- Primary impression and cast preparation
- Designing the prosthesis
- Prosthetic mouth preparation
- Secondary or final impression and cast preparation
- Fabrication of the framework
- Try-in of the framework
- Fabrication of the trial prosthesis
- Try-in of the trial denture
- Processing the trial denture
- Insertion of denture.

Diagnosis

- According to GPT, diagnosis is defined as the determination of the nature of the disease
- It includes numerous procedures which determine the requirements and present oral condition of the patient
- It is basically classified as:
  - Personality
  - Clinical
  - Laboratory evaluation.
- This evaluation in turn aids in treatment planning, e.g. the type of denture that is best suited to the patient
- For better planning and implementation of treatment, diagnostic casts are made which help in the determination of inter-arch space and occlusal contacts.

Pre-prosthetic Procedures

- Pre-prosthetic procedures includes all the non-prosthetic procedures that are performed before the beginning of prosthetic treatment
- These process are undergone to remove interferences like any pathosis, undercuts, etc.
- These procedures adds to the success of the prosthetic treatment
- Other procedures can be extraction, periodontal treatment, orthodontic realignment of abutment teeth, conservative and/or endodontic treatment of damaged teeth.

Primary Impression and Cast Preparation

- Primary impressions, after six weeks of any pre-prosthetic surgical procedures is made by using alginate or irreversible hydrocolloid impression material
- Alginate, an economical, elastic and easy to manipulate material is used to prepare primary cast which is further used to design the prosthesis.

Designing the Prosthesis

- Designing the prosthesis plays a crucial role in the fabrication of a removable partial denture
- It involves selection of the type of components and the type of material for each component and determination of the location of various components and the path of insertion
- It is done with the help of an instrument known as surveyor.

Prosthetic Mouth Preparation

- Prosthetic preparation of the mouth involves construction of the rest seats and guide planes

- Rest seat, a depression on the occlusal surface of the teeth is prepared to receive a rest in order to shift the occlusal load of the partial denture to the abutment teeth
- However, guide planes are the parallel surfaces along which the different parts of the partial denture slide across during its insertion and removal
- In addition, they offer tensofrictional resistance or indirect retention to the proximal plate of the partial denture.

Secondary or Final Impression and Cast Preparation

- The secondary impression, alike primary impression is made from alginate after prosthetic mouth preparation
- The impression is taken after applying a small quantity of alginate over the occlusal surfaces so that the rest seat and guide plane preparations get recorded accurately
- Furthermore, special impression techniques are used to record distal extension cases
- The impression is thus, poured with dental stone for producing master cast with high strength and better surface reproduction
- This master cast then in turn, is surveyed and is used to fabricate the prosthesis.

Fabrication of the Framework

- The metallic framework is fabricated by casting the wax pattern on a refractory cast, which is a replication of master cast
- The choice of material of framework is established during treatment planning
- The framework, after casting should be finished and polished before try-in.

Try-in of the Framework

- The polished framework should be tried-in before the fabrication of the trial denture to eliminate any occlusal interferences
- The process is also performed to check the fit of the frame work in the patient's mouth.

Fabrication of the Trial Prosthesis

- The framework attached to an acrylic temporary denture base is used for the trial prosthesis whereas the master cast is used to fabrica-te the trial denture
- Occlusal rims are fabricated over the temporary denture base to record the jaw relationships
- In cases such as full mouth rehabilitation, removable partial denture's opposing fixed partial denture's, a kinematic face-bow and a fully adjustable articulator should be used
- Subsequent to the recording of jaw relation, the master casts are articulated in an articulator
- Furthermore, teeth selection and arrangement is done on the occlusal rims followed by the waxing up of the trial denture.

Try-in of the Trial Denture

- This stage is required to assess the aesthetic and functional aspects of the denture in patient's mouth
- Any error can be modified in this phase depending on the requirements of the patient.

Processing the Trial Denture

The denture should be waxed up followed by flasking dewaxing, packing, curing, finishing and polishing procedures.

Insertion of Denture

- The denture is inserted and is determined for premature occlusal contacts and minor errors
- Post-insertion instructions are given to the patient and is followed-up for evaluation of the success of the denture.

Question 2

What are the objectives and requirements of classification of partially edentulous arches? Describe Kennedy's classification along with Applegate's modifications and rules.

Answer

Objectives of a Classification

A classification must satisfy the following requirements:
- Should be universally accepted
- Should allow visualization of the type of partially edentulous arch, being reviewed
- Should discriminate between tooth-supported and tooth-tissue supported partial dentures
- Should act as a guide to the type of design, being considered.

Requirements of a Classification

Classification of partially edentulous arches should be done for following reasons:
- To intercept the complications occurring frequently for that particular design

Chapter 11 Introduction to Removable Partial Dentures

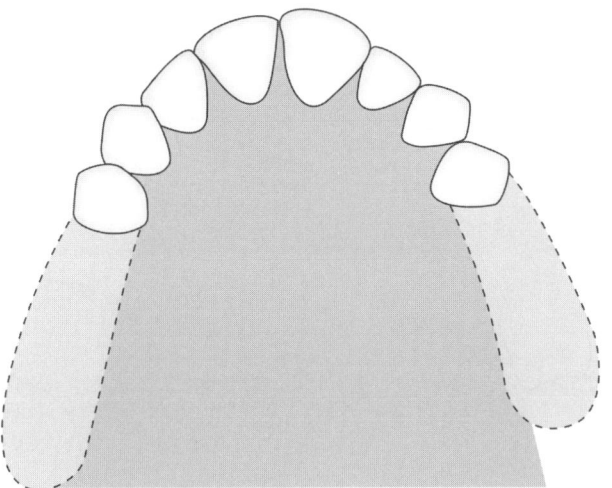

Fig. 11.1: Class I Kennedy's Classification

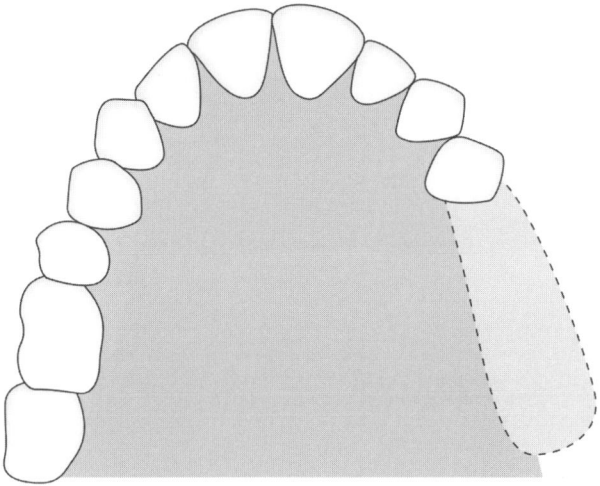

Fig. 11.2: Class II Kennedy's Classification

- To communicate about the case with a professional dentist
- To design the denture according to the occlusal load.

Kennedy's Classification of Partially Edentulous Arches

In 1923, Dr. Edward Kennedy of New York proposed this most commonly used classification. The classification is positional or anatomical and imparts knowledge about certain teeth and their relationships. However, it provides little information about the teeth present and their positional relationships.

- Class I: Bilateral edentulous areas located posterior to the remaining natural teeth. For example, there are two edentulous spaces located in the posterior region without any teeth posterior to it **(Fig. 11.1)**
- Class II: Unilateral edentulous area located posterior to the remaining natural teeth. For example, there is a single edentulous space located in the posterior region without any teeth posterior to it **(Fig. 11.2)**
- Class III: Unilateral edentulous area with natural teeth anterior and posterior to it. For example, there is a single edentulous area which does not cross the midline of the arch, with teeth present on both sides (anterior and posterior) of it **(Fig. 11.3)**
- Class IV: Single, bilateral edentulous area located anterior to the remaining natural teeth. For example, there is a single edentulous area, which crosses the midline of the arch, with remaining teeth present only posterior to it **(Fig. 11.4)**

Applegate's Modification

On the basis of the condition of the abutment, Applegate in 1960 modified the above classification by adding two more groups:

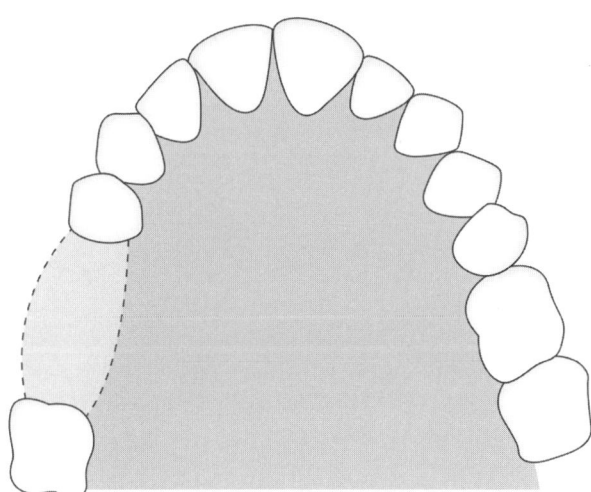

Fig. 11.3: Class III Kennedy's Classification

- Class V: Edentulous area bounded anteriorly and posteriorly by natural teeth but in which the anterior abutment like lateral incisor is not suitable for support. It is primarily a class III situation without the support of the anterior abutment. Therefore, it is not considered and treated similarly like a conventional class III edentulous space **(Fig. 11.5)**
- Class VI: Edentulous area in which the teeth adjacent to the space are capable of total support of the required prosthesis. This denture does not need any tissue support. Most of the removable partial dentures are tooth tissue-supported. Hence, this condition is categorised as a separate group **(Fig. 11.6)**.

Essential Quick Review: Prosthodontics

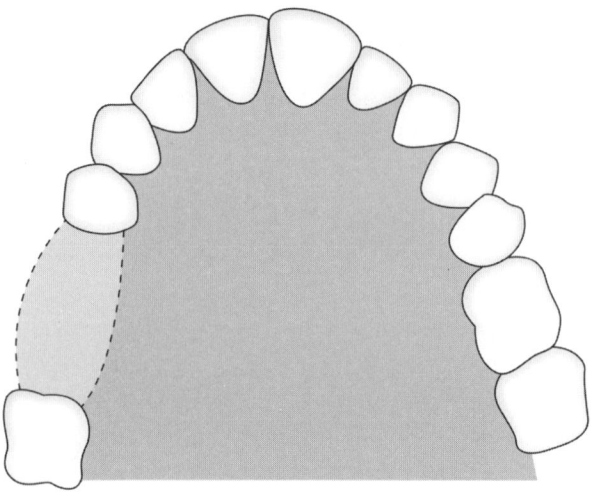

Fig. 11.4: Class IV Kennedy's Classification

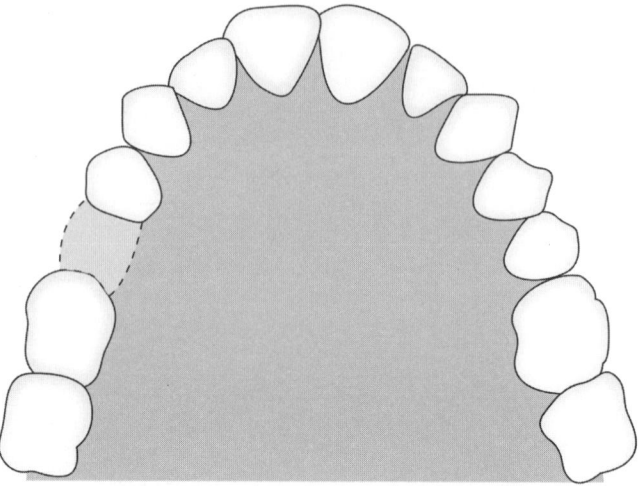

Fig. 11.6: Class VI Kennedy's Classification

- Rule 6: Edentulous areas other than those determining the classification are referred to as modifications and are designated by their number
- Rule 7: The extent of the modification is not considered. Only the number of additional edentulous areas is considered
- Rule 8: There can be no modification areas in Class IV arches.

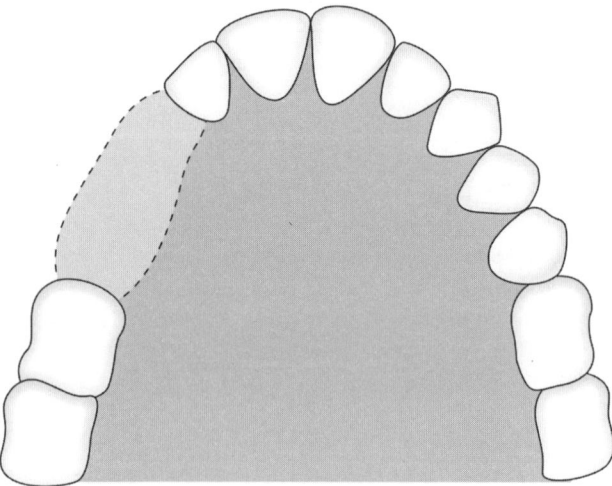

Fig. 11.5: Class V Kennedy's Classification

Applegate's Rules

Given by Applegate, the following eight rules should be taken into consideration while classifying partially edentulous arches based on Kennedy's classification.
- Rule 1: Classification should follow rather than precede any extractions of teeth that might alter the original classification
- Rule 2: If a third molar is missing and not to be replaced, then it is not considered in the classification
- Rule 3: If a third molar is present and is to be used as an abutment, then it is considered in the classification
- Rule 4: If a second molar is missing and is not to be replaced, then it is not considered in the classification
- Rule 5: The classification is always determined by the most posterior edentulous area or areas

Question 3

What are the indications of removable partial dentures?

Answer

Length of Edentulous Ridges

- For long span edentulous arches, removable partial dentures are preferred treatment of choice
- They are considered as they aid in distributing forces around the ridge evenly unlike fixed partial dentures, which exerts excessive force on the abutment teeth.

Age

- Removable partial dentures are indicated in patients under the age of 17 years as the teeth have large dental pulps and insufficient clinical crown height
- Moreover, owing to reduced life expectancy and recurrently deteriorating health of the old patient, these economical dentures are desired.

Abutment Tooth

- Removable partial dentures are used in cases when there is no available tooth posterior to the edentulous space to act as an abutment

- Removable partial dentures are indicated in patients when the periodontal support of the remaining teeth is poor as they do not require support from the abutment teeth.

Cross-arch Stabilisation

- Removable partial dentures are used in patients when the forces, distributed by the denture base, acting on one side of the arch has to be stabilised on the opposite side
- These denture provide stabilisation against lateral and anterior-posterior forces unlike fixed partial dentures which only offer antero-posterior and limited lateral or buccco-lingual stabilisation.

Excessive Bone Loss

Teeth in removable partial dentures can be easily placed, even in case of excessive residual ridge resorption or bone loss in comparison to fixed partial denture, where it is difficult to place teeth in an ideal bucco-lingual position.

Aesthetics

- Teeth in removable dentures have a life-like appearance in comparison to pontics with dull and flat appearance
- Therefore, these have better aesthetics in contrast to fixed prosthesis due to natural appearance given by the denture base to the tooth arising from the gingiva
- In addition, the denture base also re-establishes the normal facial contours by providing good lip and cheek support
- Moreover in these dentures, artificial tooth can be placed according to the operator's preference to impart adequate phonetic and aesthetics unlike fixed dentures.

Immediate Teeth Replacement after Extraction

- Immediate teeth replacement after extraction can be achieved only in removable prosthesis as in cases of fixed partial denture, ridge resorption occurs after extraction which further leads to unaesthetic appearance
- Moreover, the process of relining can be performed, if the resorption occurs in these dentures.

Emotional Problems

- Removable partial dentures do not impose physical and emotional problems to the patients as the appointment is shorter and less demanding
- In addition, the treatment is economical and less tedious in comparison to fixed prosthesis.

Patient Desires

At times, patients prefer removable prosthesis instead of fixed prosthesis owing to the reasons namely; prevention of healthy teeth from operative procedures and economical treatment.

SHORT NOTES

Question 1

Mention disadvantages of Kennedy's classification of partially edentulous spaces.

Answer

Disadvantages of Kennedy's Classification of Partially Edentulous Spaces

- Kennedy's classification does not give any idea about length, span or number of teeth missing and also provides less knowledge about the location of the missing teeth
- Kennedy Class II does not give any idea about the side of missing teeth and where the edentulous areas are located
- Moreover, it does not offer enough information about supporting structures such as the condition of the abutment teeth, which is a fundamental factor in achieving support for a prosthesis
- The classification also offers no difference between modification spaces which occurs in the anterior to those of posterior segment. This plays an important role while designing and constructing the prosthesis
- The classification cannot be applied in single standing tooth
- This classification is incomplete without Applegate's modifications.

Question 2

Mention the objectives and requirements of acceptable classification system in partially edentulous arches.

Answer

Objectives of a Classification

A classification must satisfy the following requirements:
- Should be universally accepted
- Should allow visualization of the type of partially edentulous arch, being reviewed

- Should discriminate between tooth-supported and tooth-tissue supported partial dentures
- Should act as a guide to the type of design, being considered.

Requirements of a Classification

Classification of partially edentulous arches should be done for following reasons:
- To intercept the complications occurring frequently for that particular design
- To communicate about the case with a professional dentist
- To design the denture according to the occlusal load.

Question 3

Write Kennedy's classification of partially edentulous arches.

Answer

Kennedy's Classification

Kennedy's classification has four main groups with modifications of each of the first three of these:
- Class I: Bilateral free-end edentulous spaces posterior to the natural teeth
- Class II: Unilateral free-end edentulous space posterior to the natural teeth
- Class III: A bounded unilateral edentulous space having natural teeth at each end
- Class IV: A bounded edentulous space anterior to the natural teeth.

Modifications of Kennedy's Classification

All classes, except Class IV, have modifications. Each modification is an additional edentulous area.

Examples of Modifications
- An additional edentulous area in Class I would be called as Class I modification 1
- If two additional edentulous areas are present, then it could be called as Class I modification 2
- A unilateral saddle with one additional edentulous area is Class II modification 1
- A unilateral bounded edentulous area with three additional edentulous areas is Class III modification 3
- Class IV has no modifications.

Question 4

What are the various parts of a removable partial denture?

Answer

The various parts of a removable partial denture are:
- Major connector
- Minor connector
- Rest
- Direct retainer
- Indirect retainer
- Denture base
- Artificial tooth replacement.

Question 5

What are the contraindications of removable partial dentures?

Answer

The various contraindications of removable partial dentures are as follows:
- Patients with macroglossia having tendency to push the denture away
- Cannot be used successfully in mentally retarded patients
- Should be avoided in patients with poor oral hygiene.

Chapter 12: Diagnosis, Treatment Planning and Mouth Preparation

LONG ESSAYS

Question 1

Explain the role of clinical diagnosis and treatment planning in removable partial denture.

Answer

Clinical Diagnostic Procedures

- They play a crucial role for the planning of appropriate treatment in patients requiring partial dentures
- Clinical examination of the remaining teeth as the primary supporting structure is essential for the successful fabrication of the removable partial denture.

Periodontal Condition of the Teeth

- Periodontal condition of the existing tooth such as inflammation of the gingiva, bleeding on probing, periodontal breakdown and mobility of the teeth etc. should be examined
- Various indices like oral hygiene index for determining oral hygiene, gingival index for evaluating gingival inflammation and bleeding, Russel's index for assessing periodontal breakdown and mobility are used
- Other instruments such as forcemeters and periodontometers can aid in measuring mobility of teeth
- In addition to these, radiographical examination of amount of horizontal or vertical bone loss and furcation involvement can assess the prognosis of supporting tooth
- In addition, the structure of the basal bone in the denture bearing area should also be analysed
- Therefore based on the diagnosis, a clinician can plan for periodontal therapy or extraction in the pre-prosthetic phase of treatment.

Occlusion Relationship of the Teeth

- Correct occlusal relationship of the existing teeth hold importance as tilted and/or malaligned teeth are unfit to support the prosthesis
- Therefore, these teeth should be either extracted or orthodontically realigned to prevent the interference in the prosthesis
- Moreover, occlusion should be analysed to diagnose trauma from occlusion, which is typified by premature contacts (high points), mobility of teeth and buttressing bone formation, wear facets, etc.

Conservative and Endodontic Status of the Teeth

- Teeth involving carious lesions such as pit and fissures, deep caries, gross tooth decay, etc. should be evaluated and treated accordingly during pre-prosthetic phase
- Radiographical examination can aid in determining the extent of lesion and presence of retained root stumps
- Endodontic therapy is instituted if the caries has pulpal involvement
- Retained root stumps should be either extracted or a post core preparation can be done in order to accept occlusal load from the partial denture
- In addition, the teeth should also be determined for cracks, chipped corners and fractures.

Treatment Planning

After formulating the correct diagnosis, appropriate treatment planning is done based on the needs of the patient.

- Phase I:
  - Collection and determination of diagnostic data such as diagnostic impressions

- Management of emergency conditions including relief of pain and infection
- Evaluation of the type of prosthesis to be fabricated
- Motivation of the patient.
☐ Phase II:
- Pre-prosthetic mouth preparation
- Primary impression making
- Motivation of the patient.
☐ Phase III:
- Designing the removable partial denture.
☐ Phase IV:
- Prosthetic mouth preparation
- Final impression making
- Motivation of the patient.
☐ Phase V:
- Fabrication of the removable partial denture.
☐ Phase VI:
- Insertion
- Instructions to the patient for post-insertion management
- Periodic reviewing of the patient.

Question 2

Write in brief about the various types of pre-prosthetic mouth preparation procedures involved in removable partial denture.

Answer

☐ Mouth preparation comprises of procedures performed to change the existing oral condition of the patient so that it can assist in the appropriate placement and functioning of the removable prosthesis
☐ This is categorised into:
- Pre-prosthetic mouth preparation
- Prosthetic mouth preparation.
☐ Pre-prosthetic mouth preparation forms the second phase of the treatment and is performed to facilitate the prosthetic treatment
☐ This includes procedures of preparing the oral cavity by eliminating any interference such as frenectomy, excision of tori, etc.
☐ The various procedures involved in pre-prosthetic mouth preparation are as follows:
- Oral surgical procedures
- Relief of pain and infection
- Conditioning of irritated and inflamed tissues
- Periodontal treatment
- Treatment of incorrect occlusal plane
- Endodontic therapy
- Support for periodontally weakened teeth
- Treatment of malaligned teeth.

Oral Surgical Procedures

☐ Oral surgical procedures include extraction of teeth with poor prognosis, residual root stumps, impacted and severely malposed teeth
☐ The soft tissues should be examined for pathologies and can be diagnosed with help of radiographs
☐ Ridges should be palpated for bony spicules and knife-edged ridges
☐ Along with these, muscle and frenal attachments should also be examined for any abnormality
☐ These procedures of removing cysts, tumours, exostoses, tori, hyperplasia, etc. should be done minimum 6 weeks before impression making for adequate healing
☐ Various dentofacial deformities like cleft lip, etc. should also be corrected prior to the fabrication of removable denture
☐ Ridge augmentation and vestibular extension procedures are performed, if required.

Relief of Pain and Infection

☐ The treatment of pain and infection should be done immediately in the initial phase of the treatment to prevent their progression
☐ The numerous conditions that should be treated are listed below:
- Potential conditions leading to emergency such as acute pain, abscess etc.
- Carious teeth with symptoms of pain and discomfort
- Excavation and an intermediate restorative material should be used for restoring asymptomatic teeth with deep carious lesions
- Infectious gingival diseases like acute necrotizing ulcerative gingivitis, acute herpetic gingivostomatitis, gingival abscess, etc. should also be managed
- Additionally, removal of calculus and plaque accumulations should be done to facilitate oral hygiene conditions

Conditioning of Irritated and Inflamed Tissues

☐ Various factors such as ill-fitting dentures, nutritional deficiencies, diabetes, blood dyscrasias, etc. can cause irritation and inflammation of soft tissues
☐ They should be treated prior to the making of primary impression due to changes occurring in tissue contour after healing
☐ The different symptoms for which the patient should be treated can be:
- If the inflammation and irritation of the soft tissues persist in the denture bearing areas

- Burning sensation in the residual ridge, tongue, cheeks and lips
- If the normal anatomical structures like incisive papillae, rugae and the retromolar pads get distorted.

Periodontal Treatment

- The therapy is typically carried out in conjugation with oral surgical procedures and aims at restoring health of the peridontium of existing teeth for proper functioning of the prosthesis
- The various procedures should be performed before primary impression making, which are as follows:
  - Oral prophylaxis procedures involving the removal of aetiological factors like calculus are performed for improving gingival health
  - Other processes like root planning and curettage, and eradication of local irritant factors such as overhanging restorations, food impactions should be done as a part of periodontal therapy
  - Flap surgery can be used to eliminate of periodontal pockets and gingival inflammation
  - Procedures such as bone resection or reconstruction can be done to restore normal alveolar architecture whereas other procedures like coronoplasty can aid in the correction of functional occlusion
  - Patient should be thoroughly instructed for the maintenance of oral hygiene.

Treatment of Incorrect Occlusal Plane

- One of the major problem encountered while fabrication of removable partial dentures is its uneven plane of occlusion
- This occurs due to supra-eruption of the teeth opposite to the edentulous space
- Moreover, mesial migration and tipping of the teeth adjacent to the edentulous spaces is the common occurrence
- The following methods by which occlusal plane can be corrected are:
  - Supra-eruption of tuberosity is seen in association with maxillary molars in few cases. Surgical intervention can be done to achieve proper plane of occlusion.
  - Enameloplasty, a procedure of re-contouring a portion of the enamel to obtain a desired morphology is used to reduce the correct the occlusal plane. However, in case with excessive supra-eruption, extraction or over denture is used.

Endodontic Therapy

- Endodontic therapy is essential to retain abutment tooth that are important to the design of a removable partial denture
- For example, retaining a 2nd or 3rd molar can aid in imparting support to the denture and can thus, a distal extension condition can be avoided
- Moreover, these teeth can be used to prevent vertical displacement of the denture base
- However, in case of supra-erupted tooth and insufficient inter-arch space, a crown can be prepared over post-endodontic tooth.

Support for Periodontally Weakened Teeth

- Teeth with reduced alveolar bone support in a partially edentulous condition warrant the need for the procedures namely; removable splinting, fixed splinting and over denture abutments
- These treatment provide adequate support for abutment teeth.

Treatment of Malaligned Teeth

- Malaligned teeth should be treated before the initiation of fabrication of removable partial denture
- They play a vital role in designing the prosthesis by causing poor oral hygiene
- Malalignment of teeth also offers hindrance in accessing proximal surface of crowded teeth
- They also impose complications in establishing guide planes and the path of insertion of denture
- Therefore, orthodontic realignment is the preferred treatment approach.

SHORT ESSAY

Question 1

Describe splinting in detail.

Answer

Splinting

- According to GPT, splinting of abutments is defined as the joining of two or more teeth into a rigid unit by means of fixed restorations
- Whereas a splint is a prosthesis, which maintains a hard and/or soft tissue in a predetermined position
- Splinting in a partially edentulous condition is a process to protect, immobilise or support teeth which have reduced alveolar bone support
- The process aids in the retention of the teeth and maintenance of the continuity of the arch, so as to avoid extraction of the periodontally weakened teeth
- Moreover, this can prevent inclusion of additional modification spaces into the design of the removable partial denture
- Splints can be made of rigid such as wood, metal, plaster or flexible like fabrics, or adhesive tape materials
- Splinting is further divided into two types:
  1. Removable splinting.
  2. Fixed Removable splinting.

Removable Splinting

- Its success is largely dependent on the patient's cooperation
- The process results in either reduced mobility or prevention of increase in mobility of the periodontally weakened teeth.

Fixed Splinting

- The prognosis is better as compared to removable splinting as it does not require patient's cooperation
- Indicated for supporting teeth that do not offer sufficient amount of support for the removable partial denture
- However, a tooth with strong periodontal support should not be included in splinting as it may cause weakening of the tooth
- Moreover, teeth with more than 50 % loss of alveolar bone support should not be splinted
- Teeth with less than 1:1 crown root ratio and teeth which cannot be immobilised should not be used for splinting.

SHORT NOTES

Question 1

What is primary cast design?

Answer

- A primary cast is a prerequisite for the fabrication of the removable partial denture as it is used for designing the prosthesis
- In cases where pre-prosthetic procedures are not required, diagnostic cast is used as the primary cast
- However, in cases where pre-prosthetic procedures are needed to be carried out, primary cast is made from the primary impression taken after 6-week of any pre-prosthetic procedure
- This period is warranted for the complete healing of the surgical wounds
- The impression is made by using a stock tray and the most frequently used materials can be irreversible hydrocolloids or alginate, reversible hydrocolloid or agar, or elastomeric impression materials
- The cast is then poured with minimal expansion dendrite dental stone by two-pour technique.

Question 2

Name the various pre-prosthetic mouth preparation procedures prior to fabrication of removable partial denture.

Answer

The various procedures involved in pre-prosthetic mouth preparation are as follows:
- Oral surgical procedures
- Relief of pain and infection
- Conditioning of irritated and inflamed tissues
- Periodontal treatment
- Treatment of incorrect Occlusal Plane
- Endodontic therapy
- Support for periodontally weakened teeth
- Treatment of malaligned teeth.

Chapter 12 Diagnosis, Treatment Planning and Mouth Preparation

Question 3

What is an onlay?

Answer

An onlay is defined as a restoration, which covers more than two cusps of a tooth. Before placement of an onlay, the tooth should be reduced sufficiently so that the occlusal plane can be re-established by the onlay.

Indications

- Severely attrited teeth
- Grossly decayed abutment teeth
- Supra-erupted teeth
- Teeth with inadequate crown height.

Advantages

- Requires minimal tooth preparation in contrast to a full veneer crown
- Maintains natural contours of facial and lingual tooth surfaces as only occlusal surface is reduced.

Disadvantages

- Usually less retentive
- Unaesthetic appearance due to its metal composition
- The chrome alloy produces attrition of the opposing tooth.

Chapter 13: Major and Minor Connectors

LONG ESSAYS

Question 1

What is major connector? Describe the different types of maxillary major connectors.

Answer

Major Connector

- It is defined as a part of a removable partial denture which connects the components on one side of the arch to the components on the opposite side of the arch.
- It forms the basic framework and connects all the parts on one side of an arch to those on the opposite side
- They are basically categorised into:
  - Maxillary major connectors
  - Mandibular major connectors.

Ideal Requirements for Maxillary and Mandibular Major Connectors

- The various requirements that should be followed by all major connectors are listed below:
  - Should be non-flexible and rigid to allow the uniform distribution of occlusal forces acting on any portion of the prosthesis
  - Should offer opportunity for placing denture base where needed
  - Should acts as a means of indirect retention
  - Should be comfortable to the wearer
  - Should provide vertical support without causing impingement on the soft tissues
  - Should be self-cleansing and should not allow accumulation of food.

Types of Maxillary Major Connector

- Single posterior palatal bar
- Palatal strap
- Single broad palatal major connector or Palatal plate type major connector
- Double or antero-posterior palatal bar
- Horseshoe or U-shaped connector
- Closed Horseshoe or antero-posterior palatal strap
- Complete palate.

Single Posterior Palatal Bar

- It is narrow with half-oval cross section which runs across the palate **(Fig. 13.1)**
- Its special casting or pattern waxes are commercially available, which is fabricated by adapting the wax over the marked area on the cast.

Indication

This major connector is indicated for interim partial denture.

Disadvantages

- It has narrow antero-posterior width and hence, offers poor support from the hard palate
- It is not applicable in region anterior to premolar due to the hindrance from the tongue
- Owing to its poor vertical support, cannot be used in more than two teeth
- It cannot be used in Kennedy's classification I, II, IV, V or VI. Used in class III in cases where load bearing teeth should be present both anterior and posterior to the edentulous space.

Palatal Strap

- Palatal strap, the multipurpose used connector is comprised of a wide, thin band of metal plate running across the palate
- Though it should be at least 8 mm wide for sufficient rigidity, its width can be reduced on the basis of edentulous span

Chapter 13 Major and Minor Connectors

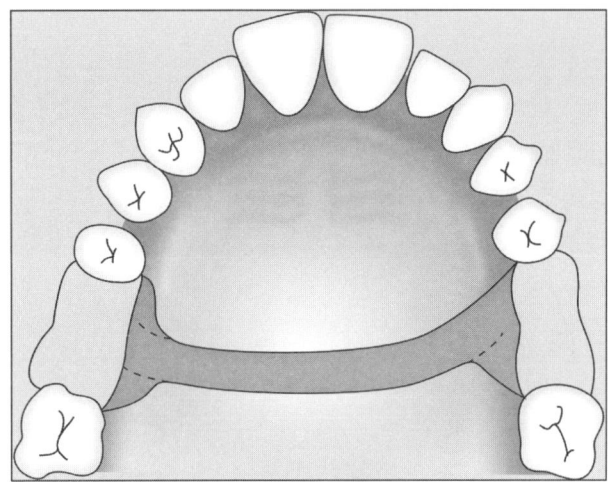

Fig. 13.1: Single posterior palatal bar major connector

Table 13.1: Various advantages and disadvantages of palatal strap

Advantages	Disadvantages
Adequate resistance is obtained with minimum volume of metal	Can lead to papillary hyperplasia
Exhibits indirect retention against dislodgment by gravity in an anterior direction or by sticky foods	Cannot be positioned across a protruded median suture
Due to its extension over three different planes, it offers excellent resistance against bending and twisting forces	Covers large part of palate
Greater retention due to increased adhesion and cohesion	Mandatory for posterior border to end before the intersection of hard and soft palate to prevent discomfort
Comfortable to the patient due to thin metal	

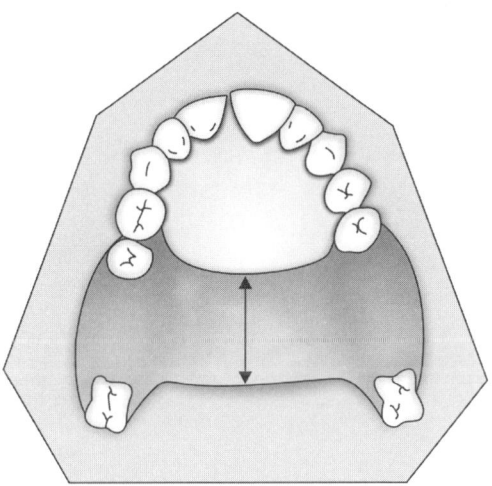

Fig. 13.2: Palatal strap major connector

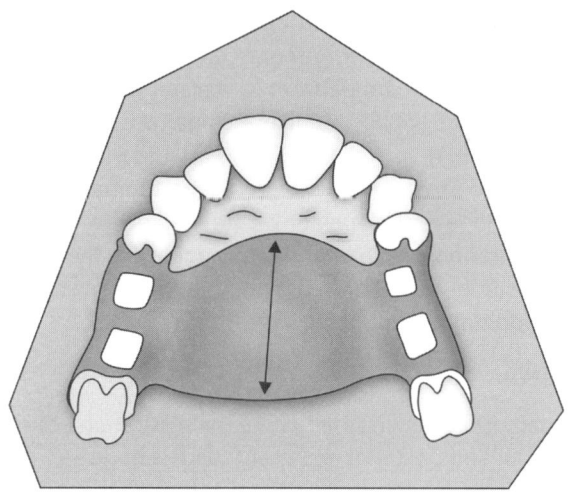

Fig. 13.3: Single broad palatal major connector

- This strap extends over three planes, namely; vault or horizontal plane, right and left lateral slopes of the palate. Its fabrication is similar to the palatal bar (Fig. 13.2).

Indications

- Usually indicated in unilateral distal extension partial denture
- Bilateral short span edentulous spaces in a tooth-supported prosthesis such as Kennedy's class III.

Various advantages and disadvantages are provided in **Table 13.1**.

Single Broad Palatal or Palatal Plate type Major Connector by Thompson

- It is also known as anatomic replica palatal major connector, which has a thin broad contoured palatal coverage
- Its fabrication is alike posterior palatal bar but is broader than a palatal strap (Fig. 13.3).

Indications

- It is indicated in Kennedy's class I cases with little vertical ridge resorption
- Patients with V or U shaped palate
- Patients with periodontally strong abutment teeth
- Patients with more than six remaining anterior teeth.

Its various advantages and disadvantages are given in **Table 13.2**.

Table 13.2: Various advantages and disadvantages of single broad palatal major connector

Advantages	Disadvantages
Offers good vertical support	Can lead to papillary hyperplasia
Owing to interfacial surface tension, it provides good retention	
Thin metal provides a natural feel to the patient due to its various surface corrugations	

Table 13.3: Various advantages and disadvantages of antero-posterior or double palatal bar

Advantages	Disadvantages
Has a limited coverage of soft tissues	Has inadequate support from palate
Has a strong design	Causes hindrance to the tongue
Has adequate rigidity	Is uncomfortable to the patient

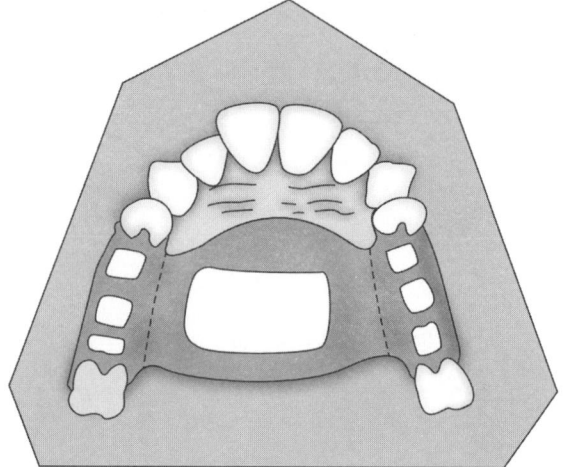

Fig. 13.4: Double or antero-posterior palatal bar major connector

Double or Antero-posterior Palatal Bar

- It is a combination of an anterior palatal strap and a posterior palatal bar. Among which, anterior strap is narrower in comparison to palatal strap whereas posterior bar is half-oval like a single posterior palatal bar **(Fig. 13.4)**
- These two are connected by two longitudinal elements along the lateral slopes of palate leading to a circular configuration, which in turn offers rigidity to the design
- In addition, support is provided from the remaining periodontally sound teeth.

Indications

- Usually indicated in cases where the separation between anterior and posterior abutment teeth is huge
- In patients having large palatal tori, which cannot be surgically excised
- Kennedy class IV
- In patients where complete palatal coverage has to be avoided
- Kennedy's class II modification 1.

Various advantages and disadvantages of antero-posterior or double palatal bar are listed in **Table 13.3**.

Horseshoe or U-shaped Connector

- It is a U shaped thin metal band running along the lingual surface of posterior teeth
- It acts like a thin plate in the anterior cingulum region of the teeth whereas posteriorly it extends upto 6–8 mm onto the palatal tissues **(Fig. 13.5)**.

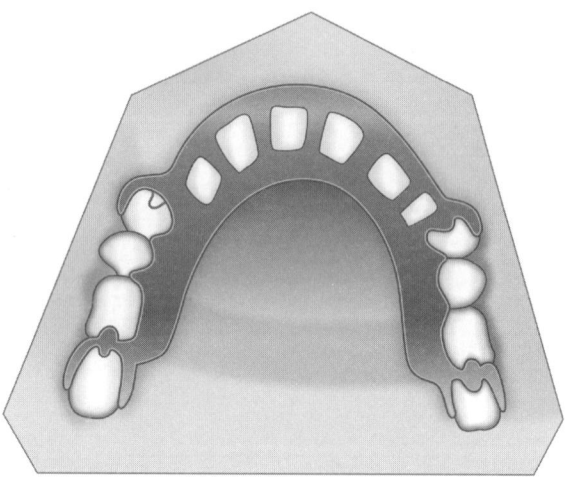

Fig. 13.5: Horseshoe or U-shaped major connector

Indications

- In cases with deep overbite of anterior teeth
- In patients, where the replacement of numerous anterior teeth are needed
- Used in patients with tori which extends upto the posterior border of hard palate
- Used in patients with a prominent median suture.

Various advantages and disadvantages of horseshoe or U-shaped connector are given in **Table 13.4**.

Closed Horseshoe or Antero-posterior Palatal Strap

- It poses similarity to the U shaped major connector
- The strap of uniform thickness of metal extends between the two open ends of the horseshoe while centre of the palate is left exposed **(Fig. 13.6)**

Chapter 13 Major and Minor Connectors

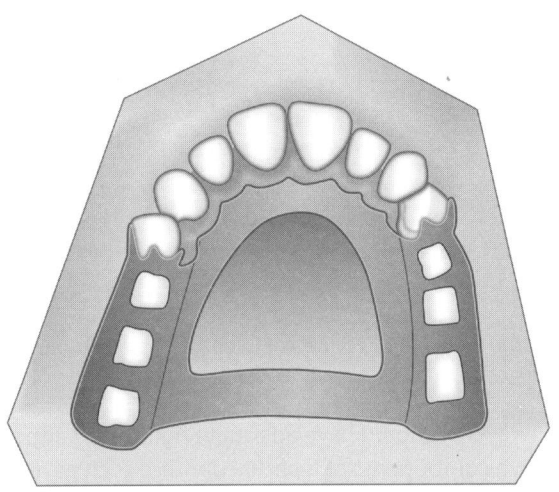

Fig. 13.6: Closed horseshoe or antero-posterior palatal strap major connector

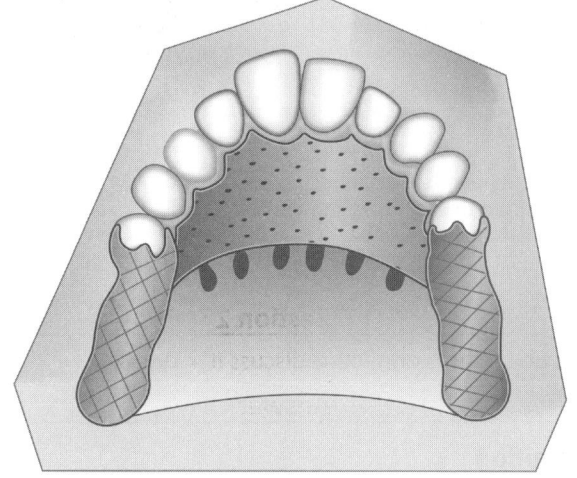

Fig. 13.7: Combination of metal and acrylic complete palate major connector

Table 13.4: Advantages and disadvantages of horseshoe or U-shaped connector

Advantages	Disadvantages
Moderate indirect retention	Greater bulk in design is required to prevent flexing
Comparatively stronger	Can cause discomfort to patient, if the thickness increases
Reasonable support	Cannot be used in cases of distal extension denture bases

Table 13.5: Advantages and disadvantages of closed horseshoe or antero-posterior palatal strap

Advantages	Disadvantages
Circular configuration provides rigidity	Causes hindrance with the tongue
Additional strength because of L-beam effect	Causes difficulty in speech
	Leads to discomfort of the patient

- The border should be kept 6 mm away from the gingival margin whereas the posterior strap, a thin plate should be placed in the most posterior position without touching the soft palate.

Indications

- In patients where various teeth are needed to be replaced
- In patients having the presence of torus
- Kennedy's Class I and Class II cases with anterior tooth replacement.

Various advantages and disadvantages are given in **Table 13.5**.

Complete Palate

- Its posterior border covers the entire palate while anterior border lies 6 mm away for the gingival margin or upto the cingulam region of the anterior teeth
- In addition, a minor peripheral seal should be given posteriorly in order to avoid the accumulation of food between the palate and the connector

- Usually constructed by using acrylic, combination of metal and acrylic, and all cast metals. Metal extends over the anterior half of the palate whereas the acrylic covers the posterior part of the palate **(Fig. 13.7)**.

Indications

- It is usually indicated in when several posterior teeth are needed to be replaced
- Also indicated in the replacement of anterior teeth along with a Kennedy's class I condition
- Used in patients with cleft palate and in cases with flat ridges and shallow vault
- In patients with excessive load and displacing forces due to well-developed muscles of mastication or presence of all mandibular teeth
- Can aid in accustoming patient to complete denture, thereby can act as a transitional partial denture
- In cases of cleft palate, for a narrow and steep vault.

Various advantages and disadvantages of complete palate are listed in **Table 13.6**.

Essential Quick Review: Prosthodontics

Table 13.6: Advantages and disadvantages of complete palate

Advantages	Disadvantages
Offers excellent rigidity and support	Can lead to inflammation and hyperplasia
Patients have better perception as all the temperature changes get transmitted through metal to the soft tissues	Causes difficulty in speech

Question 2

Describe minor connectors discuss it in detail.

Answer

Definition

According to GPT, it is defined as the connecting link between the major connector or base of a removable partial denture and other units of the prosthesis, such as clasps, indirect retainers and occlusal rests.

Role of Minor Connector

- It acts as a joining component connecting major connector to other parts like clasps, rest, indirect retainers and denture bases
- It transmits stresses homogeneously to all components to avoid concentration of load at any single point
- Moreover, it aids in transmitting forces from the prosthesis to the edentulous ridge and the existing teeth.

Classification of Minor Connectors

They are classified into four types:
1. Join the clasp assembly to major connector.
2. Join indirect retainer to the major connector.
3. Join denture base to the major connector.
4. Acts as approach arm in bar-type clasp.

Minor Connector which Join the Clasp Assembly to the Major Connector

- This connector with wide bucco-lingual and thin mesio-distal dimension joins the clasp assembly to the denture base
- Most of them that support clasp assemblies should be positioned on proximal surface of abutment teeth adjoining an edentulous area. If not, they should be located in the embrasure between abutments at its neighbouring tooth **(Fig. 13.8)**
- Nevertheless, it should not be located on the convex lingual surface of the tooth
- It is designed in a non-bulky manner, so that it does not cause any hindrance to the tongue

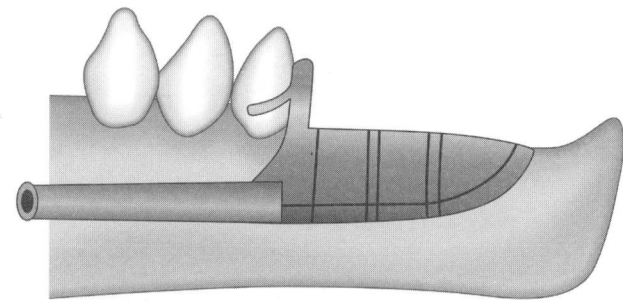

Fig. 13.8: Minor connector joining clasp assembly to major connector

- However, it should have adequate rigidity to support the active components of a partial denture such as retentive clasp etc.
- Due to its attachment to the rest of the clasp assembly, it impedes the vertical movement of the partial denture towards the tissue
- Moreover, it should exhibit a triangular cross section with the thickest portion near the lingual line angle of the tooth and the thinnest portion near the buccal line angle of the tooth for better arrangement of teeth.

Minor Connector that Join the Indirect Retainer to the Major Connector

- Minor connector, arises at right angles from the major connector, offers indirect retention and support to the denture **(Fig. 13.9)**
- It should be designed in such a way so that it fits well into the embrasure space
- Its surface which contact the tooth is the proximal plate whereas the surface of the tooth contacted by the proximal plate is called as guiding plane
- The area where minor connector is designed should not have any undercut
- Moreover, it should be parallel to the path of insertion.

Minor Connectors that Join the Denture Base with the Major Connector

- It should possess adequate rigidity to support and resist breakage of the denture base
- In cases of maxillary distal extension, minor connector should extend up to the maxillary tuberosity while in mandibular distal extension cases it should cover 2/3rd the length of edentulous ridge
- It should not hamper proper arrangement of natural teeth
- They are available in three forms namely; lattice work construction, meshwork construction and bead, wire or nail head minor connectors.

Chapter 13 Major and Minor Connectors

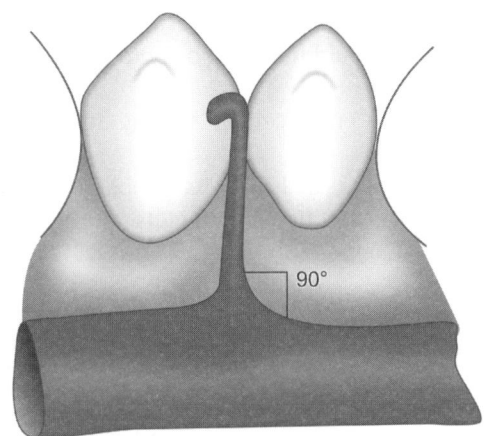

Fig. 13.9: Minor connector joining indirect retainer to major connector

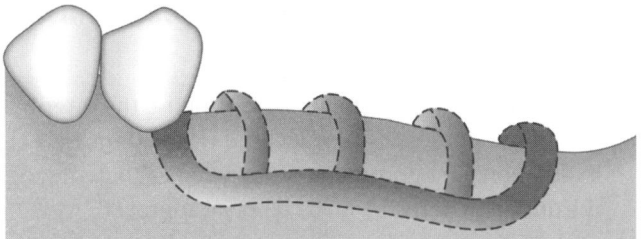

Fig. 13.10: Lattice work construction minor connector

Lattice work construction minor connector

- It comprises of two long struts of metal of 16 gauge located on the buccal and lingual slopes of the ridge with smaller struts of 12 gauge which runs over the crest of the ridge connecting the long struts
- The palatal strut is formed by the lateral border of major connector in the maxilla
- Longitudinal struts should cross the crest of residual ridge unlike transverse struts, but both should not interfere with the arrangement of teeth **(Fig. 13.10)**
- Intentional relief is provided between the struts and the ridge for acrylic to flow with the help of tissue stops.

Meshwork construction minor connector

- It is indicated in cases where multiple teeth are to be replaced
- It involves a sheet of metal positioned over the crest of residual ridge with small holes for retention of acrylic denture base **(Fig. 13.11)**
- However, its retention to the denture base is less due to the presence of smaller holes.

Bead, wire or nail head minor connector

- This is primarily indicated for tooth-supported dentures with well-healed ridges, which does not require regular relining and rebasing
- Usually, no relief is provided as the minor connector directly lines the edentulous ridge
- Therefore, various projections such as beads, nails, or pointing wires are required to enhance the retention of minor connector to the acrylic denture base

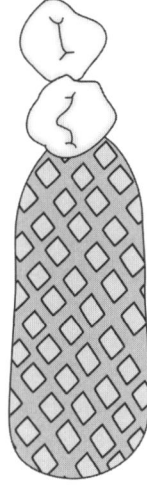

Fig. 13.11: Meshwork construction minor connector

- The preparation of beads is done by placing acrylic balls on the meshwork pattern, burnt-out and cast
- This construction provides an advantage of better soft tissue response to metal and is typically more hygienic
- However, procedure of relining of this construction is difficult.

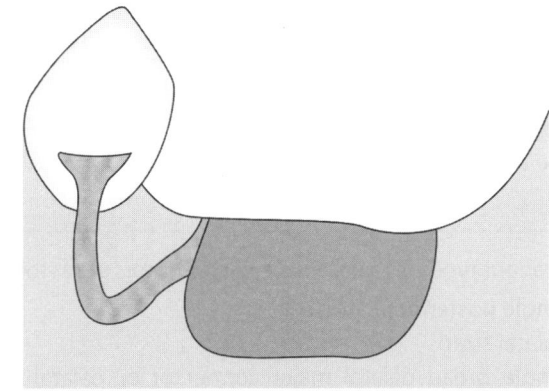

Fig. 13.12: Minor connector that acts as an approach arm for bar-type clasp

Minor Connector that Acts as an Approach Arm for Bar-type Clasp

- It serves as clasps and helps in positioning the retentive tips of the gingivally approaching clasps **(Fig. 13.12)**
- In addition, it supports the direct retainer that engages the undercut of the tooth by gingival approach
- It does not have to bear any load, therefore, it should not be rigid and should have flexibility to assist in insertion and removal
- Its retention is enhanced by springy action due to its flexibility
- Its disadvantage includes its inability to use this connector over soft tissue undercuts.

SHORT ESSAY

Question 1

Elaborate lingual plate major connector.

Answer

- This major connector poses similarity with lingual bar
- However, superior border of lingual plate runs up to the cingulum of the lingual surface of the teeth
- Moreover, scalloped shaped superior border lies in close contact with the teeth producing a knife edged margin
- However, in cases with large embrasures and spacing to avoid the visibility of the connector, the superior border is made to dip down
- It is usually made up of chrome metal due to its potential of high rigidity in thin dimensions
- If indirect retention is needed, the lingual plate should be supported by rests located on mesial fossa of the first premolars of either side, anteriorly
- The indications of lingual plate are as follows:
    - In patients with absence of most posterior teeth, where an additional indirect retention is required
    - In patients with periodontally weak existing teeth
    - In conditions where there is inadequate space for lingual bar
    - In patients with inoperable mandibular tori
    - In cases of bilateral distal extension edentulous areas and resorbed ridges
    - In cases where addition of anterior tooth is anticipated as additional teeth can be placed by attaching retention loops to it
    - In cases of Kennedy's class I, when there is excessive vertical ridge resorption to resist horizontal rotations
    - Also used to avoid over eruption in cases of retrognathic jaw.
- The various advantages and disadvantages are listed in **Table 13.7**.

Table 13.7: Advantages and disadvantages of lingual plate

Advantages	Disadvantages
It exhibits high rigidity and stability	Causes irritation of oral mucosa
Additional tooth can be easily placed	Causes food and plaque accumulation
Offers indirect retention	Can lead to decalcification of tooth

SHORT NOTES

Question 1

Name the different types of maxillary major connectors.

Answer

The various types of maxillary major connectors are as follows:
- Single posterior palatal bar
- Palatal strap
- Single broad palatal major connector or palatal plate type major connector
- Double or anteroposterior palatal bar
- Horseshoe or U-shaped connector
- Closed Horseshoe or anteroposterior palatal strap
- Complete palate.

Question 2

Write in detail about lingual bar major connector.

Answer

- Lingual bar, the most frequently used mandibular major connector is made from a thick, 6-gauge half pear-shaped wax pattern

- The minimum height of the lingual bar should be at least 5 mm
- A minimum of 8 mm vertical clearance from the floor of mouth and 3 mm clearance of upper border from the marginal gingiva should be provided to prevent any soft tissue injury
- Moreover, this major connector should be located in most inferior position to avoid hindrance to the movements of the tongue

Question 3

What are the ideal requirements for maxillary and mandibular major connectors?

Answer

The various requirements that should be followed by all major connectors are listed below:
- Should be non-flexible and rigid to allow the uniform distribution of occlusal forces acting on any portion of the prosthesis
- Should offer opportunity for placing denture base where needed
- Should acts as a means of indirect retention
- Should be comfortable to the wearer
- Should provide vertical support without causing impingement on the soft tissues
- Should be self-cleansing and should not allow accumulation of food.

Question 4

Write a short note on palatal strap major connector.

Answer

- Palatal strap, a multipurpose major connector is used in distal extension partial denture or in bilateral tooth supported prosthesis
- It is composed of a wide, thin band of metal plate running across the palate
- Its fabrication is similar to the palatal bar with width of 8 mm for adequate rigidity
- It has good resistance against bending and twisting forces with minimum volume of metal.

Question 5

Discuss briefly about complete palate.

Answer

- This major connector has full coverage over the palate with anterior border 6 mm away for the gingival margin or upto the cingula of the anterior teeth whereas the posterior border extends to the junction of the hard and soft palate
- In addition, a minor peripheral seal should be given posteriorly in order to avoid the accumulation of food between the palate and the connector
- Usually constructed by using acrylic, combination of metal and acrylic, and all cast metals
- It is usually indicated in when several posterior teeth are needed to be replaced
- Also indicated in the replacement of anterior teeth along with a Kennedy's class I condition
- Moreover, can be used in patients with cleft palate and in cases with flat ridges and shallow vault
- It has excellent rigidity and support.

Question 6

What are the design considerations for all major connectors?

Answer

- The borders of the major connector should lie parallel to the gingival margins
- The design of major connector should provide intentional relief to the highly vascular marginal gingiva, thereby its border should be 6 mm away from gingival margins in the maxillary arch
- However, the border of the major connector is placed 3 mm away from the marginal gingiva or extended across the marginal gingiva as a lingual plate in mandible
- The metal framework of the prosthesis should cross the gingival margin only at right angles and its part connecting the tooth surface should be hidden in the embrasures
- The borders of the major connector should not cause impingement to the soft tissues, thus, must have round edges
- In addition, bony prominences like tori should be either relieved or surgically excised
- The borders of maxillary connector should be symmetrical and should cross the palate in a straight line
- Moreover, anterior border of the maxillary major connector should end in the valley of the rugae. It is advisable to not extend or cover the rugae area, to prevent difficulty in speech.

Question 7

What are the design considerations for mandibular major connectors?

Answer

- The mandibular major connectors are longer and narrower as compared to the maxillary connectors due to the interference from the tongue

- The amount of relief provided in these connectors vary and is dependent on the type of major connector and amount of slope in the tissue, lingual to the anterior teeth
- In few cases like distal extension, additional relief is given to prevent the gingiva from trauma due to rotational movement of the denture base
- However, in cases where there is minimal rotation, e.g. Kennedy's class III cases, the relief given is less
- In patients where the lingual mucosa slopes towards the tongue, maximum relief is given whereas minimum relief is given when the lingual mucosa is vertical.

Chapter 14: Rests and Rest Seats

LONG ESSAY

Question 1
Explain prosthetic mouth preparation. Describe rest seat preparation.

Answer

Phase V of treatment involves prosthetic mouth preparation which is done to prepare the oral structures before placement of removable partial denture. It is classified into:
- Preparation of retentive undercuts
- Preparation of guiding planes
- Preparation of rest seats.

Preparation of Retentive Undercuts

- Retentive undercuts engage the retentive arm of the clasp and aid in providing retention
- Mostly, the tooth have convex surfaces with a undercut below the height of contour
- However, in few cases, artificial undercuts are prepared for retention of the prosthesis
- The frequently employed methods to prepare a retentive undercut are as follows:
  - Crowns
  - Cast restorations
  - Enameloplasty
  - Tilting the cast.

Crowns

- The tooth undergo reduction and full veneer crowns restore the contour of abraded, attrited and submerged teeth
- The wax pattern of the restoration is surveyed with an analysing rod to analyse guide planes, before casting
- Subsequent to the contouring of guide planes, determination of undercuts is done
- In absence of any favourable undercut, it is contoured directly on the wax pattern which is further invested and casted
- The final prosthesis having proper contour is then cemented to the tooth and further process of removable partial denture is carried out.

Cast Restorations

- Though, in cases of sufficient tooth structure, a cast restoration such as onlays is prepared instead of full veneer crowns, the procedure of fabrication poses similarity with the crowns
- A cast restoration is contoured in such a way so that the tooth surface below it becomes an undercut
- Retentive terminal engages the undercut on sound enamel instead of the cast restoration.

Dimpling (Enameloplasty)

- According to GPT, it is defined as the intentional alteration of the occlusal surface of the teeth to change their form
- The enameloplastic procedure that is done to form a retentive undercut is known as dimpling and prepared area of gentle depression on the enamel surface of the abutment is known as a dimple
- A dimple is at least 2 mm occluso-gingivally and 4 mm mesio-distally, and is prepared close to and parallel to gingival margin
- The process aids in providing retention for engaging clasps in an undercut
- It is indicated in small non-retentive undercuts requiring modification and in teeth with nearly vertical buccal and lingual surfaces.

Tilting the Cast

- The undercut on some areas of the tooth can only be viewed from a certain angle, therefore, in these conditions, cast is tilted on a surveyor so as to alter the path of insertion of the denture forming the new path of insertion in accordance with the undercuts

- The maximum angle upto which cast can be tilted is 10°, beyond which it will impart difficulty by excessive mouth opening during insertion and removal for the patient
- Usually, tilting the cast to obtain a retentive undercut is not a preferable procedure.

Guide Plane Preparation

- According to GPT, guiding planes or guide planes are defined as two or more vertically parallel surfaces of abutment teeth so oriented as to direct the path of placement and removal of removable partial dentures
- Guide planes are prepared by enameloplasty or by appropriate shaping of wax patterns of abutment teeth
- The guide preparation for various conditions are discussed in the following section.

Guide Plane Preparation For Abutment Teeth Adjoining Tooth-supported Segments

- A surveyed diagnostic cast is needed during preparation and preparation is carried out on abutment tooth with a cylindrical diamond point bur
- The same relationship of the primary cast should be carried out in the mouth
- A mild, sweeping stroke is made initially from the buccal line angle to the lingual line angle
- The preparation should be flat following the contour of the proximal surface with 2–4 mm height occluso-gingivally
- It should be finished and polished appropriately.

Guide Plane Preparation for Abutment Teeth Adjoining Distal Extension Edentulous Space

- The process of preparation is similar to the preparation done for abutment teeth adjoining tooth-supported segments
- However, the plane should be 1.5–2 mm high occluso-gingivally which in turn allow the rotation of the partial denture around the distal rest.

Guide Plane Preparation for Lingual Surfaces of the Abutment Teeth

- The preparation should be 2–4 mm in height and is done on the middle third of the crown
- It offers maximum resistance to lateral stress
- It also aid in the stabilization of the denture.

Guide Plane Preparation for Anterior Abutments

- The process is alike for the preparation of lingual surfaces of the abutment teeth

- The various advantages of this plane are as follows:
  - It increases retention and offers parallelism for stabilization
  - It decreases the space between the abutment tooth and the denture
  - It also diminishes the wedging action between the teeth
  - It enhances aesthetics of the prosthesis.

Rest Seat Preparation

- It is done before master impression making. The position and extent of the rest seat is measured using a surveyor on a diagnostic cast
- The various procedures for rest seat preparation on natural tooth surface and restorations are discussed in the following section.

Rest Seat Preparation On Enamel

- Depth orientation grooves followed by the removal of an island of enamel is done along the desired outline, which is confirmed with that marked on the primary cast
- Undercuts should be avoided and occlusal clearance is verified by using red beading wax or utility wax
  - The rest seat preparation must be highly polished and all the sharp line angle must be rounded with a No. 4 round steel bur.

Rest Seat Preparation On Gold Restorations

New gold restorations

- It involves the tooth preparation of the new gold restoration along with an additional depression as a rest seat
- The rest seat is prepared on the wax pattern of gold restoration after carving the guide planes
- It is done by using a no. 4 round steel bur in a slow speed hand piece with light pressure
- The rest seat preparation is then polished with the help of a small round finishing bur and further the pattern gets casted.

Existing gold restorations

- The rest seats are directly prepared on existing gold restorations which have good marginal integrity and occlusal harmony
- However, a new restoration is made if the restoration is not thick enough to accommodate the rest
- The procedure for preparation of rest seat poses similarity with that of enamel.

Rest Seat Preparation on Amalgam Restorations

- Generally, rest seat is not prepared on amalgam restoration as it has the tendency to creep or flow under constant pressure
- Moreover, to prevent risk of fracture, the junction between the proximal portion and isthmus of the restoration should not be made thin
- No. 4 round bur is used for preparing and its reverse motion is used for polishing
- The procedure followed for preparation has similarity to that of enamel.

Rest Seat Preparation for Embrasure Clasp

- Rest seat preparation for embrasure clasps which are made from two clasps fused at the body to fit into a single embrasure is done on the mesial and distal fossae of two adjacent posterior teeth
- The rest has the advantage of both marginal ridges which are reduced for better strength of the clasp
- The two occlusal rest seats are prepared concurrently following the procedure of rest seat preparation on enamel with the help of a small round or cylindrical diamond stone
- The contact point should not be broken and buccal and lingual extensions should extend to the buccal and lingual embrasures
- The preparation is finished and polished by using a No. 4 round steel bur
- After the procedure, adequate occlusal clearance is checked so that there is no highpoint between the opposing teeth and the clasp during occlusion.

Cingulum Rest Seat Preparation

The cingulum rest seat preparation differs according to the surface over which they are prepared.

Cingulum rest seat preparation in cast restorations

- Rests seats prepared on cast restorations are treatment of choice as compared to that of enamel
- They can be utilised for all maxillary and mandibular anteriors and the process is similar as occlusal rest seats preparation on new gold restorations.

Lingual rest seat preparation on enamel

- The preparation of a lingual rest seat is done on maxillary canines and few mandibular incisors
- The rest seat should be half-moon shaped, positioned above the cingulum area and gingival to the contact point with the adjacent teeth
- Generally, preparation is done with the help of a flat end, large diamond cylinder or safe-sided 1/4-inch diamond disc
- The disc should be positioned parallel or slightly labial to the path of insertion, but the flat end diamond cylinder should be tilted slightly gingival to the path of insertion
- The reduction of the tooth begins at marginal ridge from where the bur moves incisally above the cingulum and then gingivally to reach the opposite marginal ridge and finally, polishing and finishing of the rest seat is done.

Incisal Rest Seat Preparation

- The preparation is done on the distoincisal angle in case of Akers clasp or on the mesioincisal angle when a vertical projection clasp is used by the help of a small safe-sided diamond disc or knife edged stone
- A vertical cut about 1.5–2.0 mm deep and 2–3 mm away from the proximal angle along the incisal edge is made from the cutting instrument which should be placed parallel to the path of insertion
- The notches, unsupported enamel proximal to the notch and wall of enamel near the center of the tooth are rounded to eliminate stress concentration.

SHORT ESSAYS

Question 1

Define occlusal rest and elaborate the role and design of occlusal rest.

Answer

Occlusal Rest

According to GPT, an occlusal rest is defined as a rigid extension of a partial denture, which contacts the occlusal surface of the tooth.

Role of Occlusal Rest

- Offers resistance to lateral displacement and aids in the construction of occlusal plane of a tilted tooth
- It aids in distributing occlusal load by transmitting stress along the long axis of the tooth
- It secures the clasp in their appropriate position by preventing spreading of arms of clasp, which in turn avoid the displacement of clasp and the prosthesis
- It also impedes extrusion or supra-eruption of abutment teeth

- Also assist in providing indirect retention
- Used in cases where small spaces cannot be filled with tooth replacement
- Subsequently, avoids accumulation of food between the tooth and clasp.

Design of Occlusal Rest

- It is formed like a triangular-shaped depression, in which its base is at the marginal ridge and apex at the centre of the tooth
- Additionally, it should follow the contour of the mesial or distal marginal ridge and the triangular fossa
- Margins of the rest should be gently curved with smooth ends
- The size of the occlusal rest should be one-half of the bucco-lingual width between the cusp tips and one-third to one-half of the mesio-distal width of the tooth
- The angle between the floor of the rest seat and the line drawn along the proximal surface of the tooth should be less than 90°
- If the above-mentioned angle is more than 90°, the pro-sthesis will slip from the abutment tooth as the forces acting on the prosthesis gets transmitted along an inclined plane instead of along the long axis of the abutment tooth
- The greater angle can also lead to orthodontic movement of the abutment teeth resulting in pain and bone loss
- Moreover, the rest should be 0.5 mm thick at its thinnest portion and 1.0–1.5 mm thick where it crosses marginal ridge, non-adherence to these parameters can increases the risk of fracture
- The rest seat can also be constructed on restorations such as cast gold and amalgam
- Rest seats on amalgam can be used only for interim or temporary partial dentures whereas seat on cast gold restoration can be used to prepare seat for a permanent prosthesis.

Question 2

Define rests and rest seats. Also explain the points taken into consideration while preparing the rest seat.

Answer

Rest

Rest is defined as a rigid extension of a fixed or RPD, which contacts a remaining tooth or teeth to dissipate vertical or horizontal forces.

Rest Seat

That portion of a natural tooth or a cast restoration of a tooth selected or prepared to receive an occlusal, incisal, lingual, internal, or semi-precision rest.

Considerations during Rest Seat Preparation

- Rest seat serves as a vertical stop to avoid trauma to the soft tissues under partial denture
- Rest seat, a prepared surface of the tooth involves enamel
- Rests should be placed on the proximal surfaces of all the teeth adjoining the edentulous space
- The rest seat should be shallow and saucer-shaped
- The rest should be aligned to the crest of the edentulous ridge except in cases of rotated teeth
- The rest is designed in such a way that it should restore the tooth form which existed prior to the preparation of the rest seat
- A slight movement such as a ball and socket joint should be allowed to protect the abutment teeth by dissipating horizontal forces
- A rest and appropriately positioned minor connector can aid in reciprocation.

SHORT NOTES

Question 1

Write the classification of rest.

Answer

Rest can be classified into following types:

- On the basis of the relationship of the rest to the direct retainer
  - Primary rest
  - Secondary or auxiliary rest.
- On the basis of the position of the rest on the abutment teeth
  - Occlusal rest
  - Cingulum or lingual rest
  - Incisal rest.
- On the basis of the shape and structure of the rest
  - Triangular occlusal rest
  - Boomerang-shaped cingular rest
  - 'V' shaped incisal rest
  - Conservative circular cingular rest.

Question 2

Write a short note on primary and secondary rests.

Answer

Primary Rests

- Primary rests are the rest that are positioned along with the clasp assembly
- They provides vertical support and can be used for direct retention.

Secondary or Auxiliary Rests

- Rests that are positioned away from the clasp are known as secondary or auxiliary rests
- They are placed at the position where the perpendicular drawn from the mid-point of the terminal abutment axis meets the dentition
- A minor connector connects these rests with the major connector
- Thus, secondary rests in combination with minor connector provide indirect retention.

Question 3

What is rest? What are the indications of preparing the lingual rest?

Answer

Rest is defined as a rigid extension of a fixed or RPD, which contacts a remaining tooth or teeth to dissipate vertical or horizontal forces.

Indications of preparing the lingual rest are as follows:
- If the patients has good oral hygiene
- If caries index is low
- If the cingulum is prominent.

Question 4

Define occlusal rest and describe the general considerations while preparing occlusal rest.

Answer

An occlusal rest is defined as a rigid extension of a partial denture, which contacts the occlusal surface of the tooth.

Considerations in Preparing Occlusal Rest

- Ideally, an occlusal rest should measure 1/2 the width of the tooth bucco-lingually and 1/3 to 1/2 the width of the tooth mesio-distally
- Occlusal rest seat should be triangular in shape with its base at the marginal ridge and apex at the centre of the tooth
- Additionally, it should follow the contour of the mesial or distal marginal ridge and the triangular fossa
- Margins of the rest should be gently curved with smooth ends
- The angle between the floor of the rest seat and the line drawn along the proximal surface of the tooth should be less than 90°
- The thickness of the rest should be adequate at its junction with the minor connector
- It should be 0.5 mm thick at its thinnest portion and 1.0–1.5 mm thick where it crosses marginal ridge
- Inadequate rest-seat preparation may cause thinning of the rest-minor connector junction resulting in fracture of the same
- Rests which are closer to the axis of rotation will produce less torsional forces on the abutments.

Question 5

What are the advantages of guiding planes on anterior teeth?

Answer

Guide planes prepared on anterior teeth have the following advantages:
- It increases retention and offers parallelism for stabilization
- It decreases the space between the abutment tooth and the denture
- It also diminishes the wedging action between the teeth
- It enhances aesthetics of the prosthesis.

Chapter 15: Direct and Indirect Retainers

LONG ESSAYS

Question 1

Define and classify direct retainer. Also explain intra-coronal direct retainers.

Answer

Direct Retainer

- According to GPT, it is that component part of a removable partial denture that is used to retain and prevent dislodgement, consisting of a clasp assembly or precision attachment
- A direct retainer is the part of the fixed partial denture, which helps to prevent the displacement of the denture. The direct retainer functions based on certain principles. It is the most critical component for a removable partial denture.

Classification

- Extra-coronal direct retainers (clasps)
  - Manufactured retainers (Dalbo)
  - Custom-made retainers:
    - Occlusally approaching (circumferential or Aker's clasp)
    - Gingivally approaching (bar or Roach's clasp).
- Intra-coronal direct retainers (attachments)
  - Internal attachment
  - External attachment
  - Stud attachment
  - Bar attachment
  - Special attachments.

Intra-coronal Direct Retainers

In these types of retainers, a part or the whole of the retentive components are placed within the anatomical contour of the abutment teeth.

The following section discusses various types of intra-coronal retainer.

Internal Attachment

- It is defined by GPT as a retainer, used in removable partial denture construction, consisting of a metal receptacle and a closely fitting part: the former is usually contained within the normal or expanded contours of the crown of the abutment tooth and the latter is attached to a pontic or the denture frame work
- They are used in tissue-supported distal extension denture bases but are contraindicated in teeth with larger pulpal chamber as the depth of receptacle gets limited
- Most frequently used internal attachments are Ney-Chayes attachment, Stern Goldmith attachment and Baker attachment.

Advantages

- Causes removal of visible retentive components
- Also leads to eradication of visible vertical support element through a rest seat
- Its interim tent vertical massage induces underlying tissues
- Serves as horizontal stabilizer to some extent.

Disadvantages

- Causes difficulty in the placement within the circumference of the abutment tooth
- It is difficult to repair and replace
- It has lesser efficiency in teeth with small crowns
- The preparation requires abutments and castings
- The process of preparation is technique sensitive as it need clinical and lab procedures
- Its wear causes loss of frictional resistance.

Chapter 15 Direct and Indirect Retainers

External Attachment

This attachment is used for anterior prosthesis in young patients having large pulp chambers. The most commonly used retainer are ASC52, DALBO, CEKA and ERA.

Advantages

- It exhibits good aesthetics
- It is easy to insert this retainer
- The attachment is more resilient as compared to other retainer.

Disadvantages

- It has a tendency to break easily
- It is difficult to replace
- Owing to its bulky attachments, it require more space within the prosthesis.

Stud Attachment

It is indicated in overdenture abutments. It aid in directing the stress. For example: GERBER, DALLA BONA and ROTHERMAN.

Advantages

- It can also be utilised in patients with malaligned abutments
- It is easy to adjust and repair
- It has more versatility than other retainers
- It has reduced leverage.

Disadvantages

- It is complex in designing
- It is an expensive retainer
- It can not be used in insufficient space
- It has a tipping effect on the abutment teeth.

Bar Attachment

It is indicated in patients with alveolar bone loss around the abutment. For example: DOLDER, HADER.

Advantages

- It causes cross-arch stabilisation
- The retainer results in rigid splinting
- Can be used in combination with other attachments or implants for a combined fixed-removable prosthesis.

Disadvantages

- It requires soldering recurrent soldering
- It requires more space for placement
- With this retainer, it is difficult to maintain proper oral hygiene.

Special Attachment

- This retainer are categorised separately as it varies from both intra-coronal and extra-coronal retainers
- They are further classified into two types:
  1. Retention dependent on frictional resistance.
  2. Retention dependent on positioning of an element in the undercut.
- These types have both an intra-coronal as well as an extra-coronal locking device, which aid in the retention of retainer
- Most frequently used special attachments are namely; Neurohr spring-lock, Neurohr-Williams shoe, Dowel rest, Zest anchor device, intra-coronal magnets, Hannes Anchor or IC plunger, Servo Anchor SA or Ceka, Bona Ball, Rotherman, Long copings.

Advantages

- It aids in diminishing torque and tipping forces on the abutment
- It provides higher aesthetic due to the absence of the visible clasp components.

Question 2

What is extra-coronal direct retainer? Explain the components of clasps along with its basic principles and functional requisites.

Answer

According to GPT, extra-coronal retainer or clasp is defined as a part of a removable partial denture which acts as a direct retainer and/or stabilizer for the denture by partially encircling or contacting an abutment tooth.

Components of a Clasp

- The components of a clasp can be flexible or rigid. In a conventional design, only the tip of the retentive arm is flexible, which lies below the height of contour unlike rigid components which are placed above the height of contour
- The various components are described in the section below **(Fig. 15.1)**

Retentive Arm

- It is defined as a flexible segment of a removable partial denture which engages an undercut on an abutment and which is designed to retain the denture
- It comprises of a retentive arm and retentive terminal which is rigid and flexible, respectively.

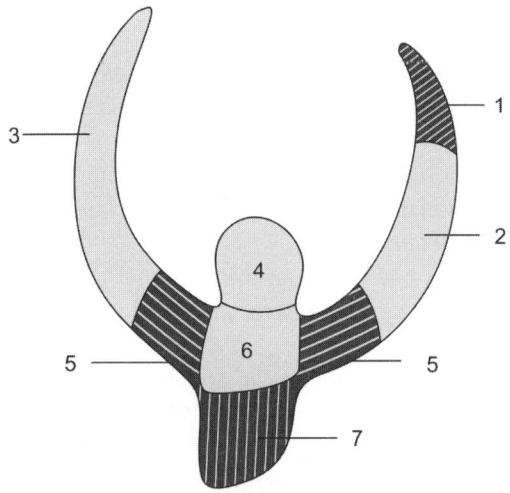

Fig. 15.1: 1- Retentive terminal; 2- Retentive clasp arm; 3- Reciprocal arm; 4- Occlusal rest; 5- Shoulder; 6- Body; 7- Minor connector

Reciprocal Arm

- It is defined as a clasp arm or other extension used on a removable partial denture to oppose the action of some other part or parts of the prosthesis
- It is located above the height of contour on the side of the tooth opposite to retentive arm
- It aids during insertion and removal of prosthesis by resisting the lateral forces exerted by the retentive arm
- Moreover, it can also serves as an indirect retainer as it prevents rocking of the denture.

Shoulder

- It acts as a connecting link between the body of the clasp to its terminals
- It stabilises the denture against horizontal displacements and lie above the height of contour.

Body

- It connects the rests and shoulders of the clasp to the minor connectors
- The design of the body contacts the guide plane of the abutment during insertion and removal of the prosthesis
- Moreover, the tissue surface of the body, which is closely associated with the guide planes, is called as a proximal plate of the direct retainer.

Rest

- A rest is a rigid (stabilizing) extension of a removable partial denture which contacts a remaining tooth or teeth to dissipate vertical or horizontal forces
- It lies on the occlusal or lingual or incisal edge or surfaces of the tooth and helps in resisting tissueward movement of the clasp by acting like a vertical stop.

Minor Connector

It is the connecting link between the major connector or base of a removable partial denture and other units of the prosthesis, such as clasps, indirect retainers and occlusal rests.

Principles of Designing a Clasp

- The basic principle includes encirclement so as to attain more than 180° of continuous contact for Aker's clasp and a minimum of 3-point contact for Roach clasps
- Occlusal rest should be fabricated so as to avoid the displacement of denture towards the tissue
- A reciprocal component should lie opposite to each retentive terminal
- A buccal retentive clasp should be present on both opposing sides to provide balanced retention
- The path of escapement should not be corresponding to the path of removal
- Minimal possible amount of retention should be used
- Tipping forces should not be applied on the abutment by primary abutment clasp of a distal extension denture base
- Reciprocal and retentive elements should be positioned at the height of contour and the below the height of contour, respectively.

Functional Requisites of a Clasp

The functional requisites of a clasp are as follows:

Retention

It is that quality inherent in the prosthesis which resists the force of gravity, the adhesiveness of foods and the forces associated with the opening of the jaws.

Stability

It is defined as the quality of a denture to be firm, steady, or constant, to resist displacement by functional stresses and not to be subject to change of position when forces are applied.

Support

It is defined as to hold up or serve as a foundation or prop for.

Reciprocation

It is defined as the means by which one part of a prosthesis is made to counter the effect created by another part.

Encirclement

It is the property of the clasp assembly to encompass more than 180° of the abutment tooth either by continuous or broken contact to prevent dislodgement during function.

Passivity

It is defined as the quality or condition of inactivity or rest assumed by the teeth, tissues, and denture when a removable partial denture is in place but not under masticatory pressure.

Question 3

What are circumferential clasps? Also write in detail about its various modifications.

Answer

Circumferential Clasps

These clasps are also known as Aker's clasps, and embrace more than half of the abutment tooth. A continuous or a limited three-point contact can also be seen with the tooth.

These clasps hold the abutment strongly and prevent the rotation of the denture.

Advantages

- It offers excellent support, bracing and retention
- It fabrication is easy along with its repair
- Leads to less accumulation of food.

Disadvantages

- Covers a large area on the tooth surface
- Causes decalcification of tooth
- Also causes trauma to the soft tissues due to lack of physiological stimulation
- It is difficult to adjust with pliers
- If the placement of clasp is high on tooth surface, it causes greater generation of occlusal forces.

Modifications of Circumferential Clasps

Simple Circlet Clasp

- They are best for tooth-supported partial dentures
- They are most commonly used
- It approaches the undercut from the edentulous space.
- They can only be engaged in one direction
- It engages the undercut, located away from the edentulous space.

Reverse Clasp

- They are used when the retentive undercut on the abutment tooth is located adjacent to the edentulous space
- These clasps clasp arises from the mesial side and ends on the distal undercut
- They are used are used in distal extension denture base to control the stresses acting on the terminal abutment teeth on the edentulous area.

Multiple Circlet Clasp

- They are made by joining two simple circlet clasps joined at the terminal end of the reciprocal arms
- They are used for splinting weakened teeth
- They are used in sharing the retention with additional teeth on the same side of the arch when the principal abutment tooth has poor periodontal support.

Embrasure Clasp

- It is prepared by joining two simple circlet clasps joined at the body
- It is used on that side of the arch where there is no edentulous space
- The clasp crosses the marginal ridges of two teeth to form the double occlusal rest
- The clasp is located on the facial surface and splits into two retentive arms
- The clasp may break if the metal is too thin.

Ring Clasp

- This clasp has a retentive arm extending all around the tooth from the distobuccal end to terminate in the distolingual undercut across the mesial side of the tooth
- This cusp is long and have additional support should be provided by adding an auxiliary bracing arm from the denture base minor connector to the center of the ring clasp on the buccal surface.
- Used mostly in lingually tipped molar abutments.

Hairpin Clasp

- They are used undercut is adjacent to edentulous area
- They can also be used in the presence of a soft tissue undercut
- It is used in conditions where the undercut is near the edentulous space
- The upper arm should be positioned above the height of contour in such a way that it does not interfere with occlusion.

Onlay Clasp

- It is an extension of a metal crown or onlay with buccal and lingual clasp arms
- They are used in occlusal surfaces of submerged abutment teeth
- Surfaces as this clasp covers a huge bulk of area. So it should be contraindicated in teeth caries resistant
- It can break the enamel surface
- Chrome alloy should be placed in the opposite tooth to protect from chromium alloy.

Back-Action Clasp

- It is a modification of the ring clasp
- Here the minor connector is connected to the end of the clasp arm and the occlusal rest is left unsupported.

Grasso's Clasp

- This clasp consists of a vertical reciprocal arm, an occlusal rest and a horizontal retentive arm each arising separately from the major connector
- It is a proposed concept which is hardly implemented.

SHORT NOTES

Question 1

Define onlay clasp.

Answer

- It is an extension of a metal crown or onlay with buccal and lingual clasp arms
- They are used in occlusal surfaces of submerged abutment teeth
- Surfaces as this clasp covers a huge bulk of area. So, it should be contraindicated in teeth caries resistant
- It can break the enamel surface.
- Chrome alloy should be placed in the opposite tooth to protect from chromium alloy.

Question 2

Define clasp.

Answer

A clasp is defined as a part of a removable partial denture which acts as a direct retainer and/or stabilizer for the denture by partially encircling or contacting an abutment tooth.

Question 3

What are fulcrum lines?

Answer

Fulcrum Line

Fulcrum line is defined as an imaginary line around which a partial denture tends to rotate.

Types

Fulcrum lines are of two types:
1. Retentive fulcrum line.
2. Stabilizing fulcrum line.

Retentive Fulcrum Line

It is defined as the imaginary line connecting the retentive points of the clasp arm, around which the denture tends to rotate when subjected to forces, such as pull of sticky foods.

Stabilizing Fulcrum Line

It is defined as an imaginary line connecting occlusal rest, around which the denture tends to rotate under masticatory forces.

Question 4

What are indirect retainers? Write the different types of indirect retainers.

Answer

Indirect Retainers

According to GPT, it is defined as a part of a removable partial denture which assists the direct retainers in preventing displacement of distal extension denture bases by functioning through lever action on the opposite side of the fulcrum line.

Types of Indirect Retainers

- Auxiliary occlusal rest
- Canine extension from the occlusal rest
- Canine rest
- Continuous bar retainers and linguoplates
- Modification areas
- Rugae support
- Direct indirect retention
- Indirect retention from major connectors.

Question 5

What are the functional requirements of a clasp?

Chapter 15 Direct and Indirect Retainers

Answer

The functional requirements of a clasp include:
- Retention
- Stability
- Support
- Reciprocation
- Encirclement
- Passivity.

Question 6

What are the various function of indirect retainers?

Answer

- Indirect retainers stabilise the denture by counteracting the lifting forces as it shifts the fulcrum line away from the point of application of force
- They provide support and stability to the denture by counteracting horizontal forces
- They can serve as an auxiliary rest to support major connector
- They can aid in splinting anterior teeth and thus, can protect them against lingual movement
- Their dislodgment indicates the need for relining of denture base.

CHAPTER 16

Surveying

LONG ESSAYS

Question 1

Define surveyor. Explain in detail the different parts and set up of surveying.

Answer

Surveyor

- According to GPT, surveyor is defined as an instrument used in the construction of a removable partial denture to locate and delineate the contours and relative positions of abutment teeth and associated structures
- It was first used by Dr. A. J. Fortunati in 1918
- The surveyor, a parallelometer is an instrument used to determine the relative parallelism of surfaces of teeth or other areas on a cast.

Types of Surveyors

The surveyors commonly used are:
- Ney surveyor
- Jelenko or Will's surveyor
- Willam's surveyor.

Parts of a Surveyor

Surveying platform

A metal plate forming the base of the surveyor lies parallel to the floor where a cast holder can be placed.

Cast holder table

It is a stand placed over the surveying platform and comprises of a base and a table to place a cast which can be locked in any position on the table by using a locking device.

Vertical arm

It arises vertically from the surveying platform and provides support to the horizontal arm and the surveying arm.

Horizontal arm

It extends horizontally from the top of the vertical arm and its free end is designed to support the surveying arm. It is fixed and revolve horizontally in Ney surveyor and Jelenko surveyor, respectively.

Surveying arm

It extends vertically from the free end of the horizontal arm and is parallel to the vertical arm. Tools used for surveying can be locked in the mandrel located at the lower end of this arm.

Surveying tools

The tools used for surveying are attached to the mandrel of the surveying arm. They are of different kinds such as analyzing rod, carbon marker, wax knife and undercut gauges.

- Analysing rod
  - It is a diagnostic tool and serves as a tangent to the convex surface of the object being surveyed.
- Carbon markers
  - They pose similarity with lead points and are circular in cross-section in Ney Surveyors whereas triangular in cross-section in Jelenko surveyors and resemble the lead points. They are used to draw the height of contour of the object being surveyed.
- Undercut gauges
  - A gauge, high precision instrument is used to measure the linear dimension of any structure. Moreover, undercut gauges are used to analyse the depth and location of the undercuts on the tooth in three dimensions.
- Wax knife
  - It can be attached to the mandrel of the surveying arm and directly trims the excess wax while surveying the wax patterns. It also eradicates and block out undesirable undercuts parallel to the path of insertion.

Set Up for Surveying

- It involves mounting the primary cast on a cast holder and locking it in place with zero degree tilt
- The cast holder is positioned on the surveying platform and correspondingly the surveying arm is positioned, further which the cast is analysed.

Mounting the cast

- The primary cast is mounted on the surveying table by fixing it tightly to the clamps on the surveying table
- The plane of occlusion of the existing teeth should be kept parallel to the base.

Placing the surveying arm

- After mounting the cast, the horizontal arm is positioned vertically and is locked to the vertical arm with the help of a thumbscrew
- It is adjusted so that the surveying arm can contact at least three different spaced out points on the cast.

Analysing the cast

- The analysing rod is attached to mandrel of the surveying arm and acts as the first surveying tool used during surveying
- The cast is rotated against the analysing rod to analyse the presence of undercuts
- Depending upon the favourable and unfavourable undercuts, the operator designs the prosthesis which will best suit the clinical conditions of the patient
- Favourable undercuts should be present on the abutment teeth to engage the retentive components of a clasp whereas unfavourable undercuts should be eliminated
- Soft tissues undercuts should be removed during pre-prosthetic mouth preparation
- If the undercuts are unilateral and deep, the cast is tilted and a different path of insertion is used for the prosthesis
- To attain this, the surveying table is tilted with the help of thumbscrew, until the undercut vanishes from the view
- However, the cast should not be tilted more than 10°
- Therefore, after completing the set up for surveying, the cast is surveyed.

Question 2

Elaborate the various uses of surveyor.

Answer

The various uses of a surveyor are as follows:
- To survey the diagnostic and primary casts
- For tripoding the cast
- To transfer the tripod marks to another cast
- To survey the master cast
- To contour crowns and cast restorations
- To perform mouth preparation directly on the cast to determine the outcome of treatment
- To survey the master cast
- To survey ceramic veneers before final glazing.

Surveying the Diagnostic and Primary Casts

- The diagnostic cast is surveyed before treatment planning while the primary cast is surveyed after pre-prosthetic mouth preparation
- Surveying of primary cast is done in order to determine the appropriate path of insertion of prosthesis
- With the help of surveying, proximal tooth surfaces where guide planes can be prepared can also be identified
- It can aid in locating various types of undercuts
- It also help in identifying height of contour
- It can also aid in assessing the required mouth preparations
- It includes the procedures namely; analysing the cast, surveying the teeth and surveying the soft tissues contours on the cast.

Tripoding the Cast

- Maintenance of the tilt for the primary cast maintains the angle of path of insertion
- Therefore, to attain this degree of tilt for the master cast, tripoding the primary cast is performed
- Tripoding, a procedure which records the spatial orientation of the cast and marks three different widely spaced out points of a single plane
- It helps in positioning the master cast and remounting the diagnostic casts on the surveying table.

Transferring the Tripod Marks to Another Cast

- The procedure orients the master cast with the help of the same angulation of the primary cast
- Subsequent to tripoding the primary cast, three additional reference points are marked, which are as follows:
  - Distal marginal ridge of the first premolar
  - Incisal edge of lateral incisor
  - Lingual cusp tip of the first premolar on the opposite side which lies opposite to the side where the other two points were marked.

Surveying the Master Cast

- The master cast is formed after prosthetic mouth preparation
- It is surveyed to check if the desired results have been replicated in mouth preparation

- The factors like parallelism of the guiding plane, depth of undercuts and retention, and height of contour are checked during the surveying procedure.

Contouring Crowns and Cast Restorations

- The wax pattern on the cast is mounted on the surveyor to acquire an ideal contour for preparing a cast restoration for an abutment tooth
- The process is done by using rotary instruments such as handpiece with a cylinder stone attached to the surveying arm which slowly moves over the sides of the restoration to trim the excess crown material
- While contouring, favourable undercuts are preserved to engage the retentive components.

Placing Internal Attachments and Rests

- Intra-coronal retainers, occlusal rests are prepared on wax pattern using a rotary handpiece
- The underlying mechanism of intra-coronal retainer is the frictional resistance obtained by the parallelism of its components, which is analysed by the surveyor.

Surveying Ceramic Veneers before Final Glazing

- The contour of the facial surface of the crown is formed in a surveyor in cases where a removable partial denture abutment is to be restored with a ceramic crown
- The ceramic restoration is positioned on the cast and the height of contour is checked prior to final glazing.

SHORT ESSAYS

Question 1
Write in detail about survey lines.

Answer

Surveying line is a line drawn on a tooth or teeth of a cast by means of a surveyor for the purpose of determining the positions of the various parts of a clasp or clasps.

Classification of Surveying Lines

- According to Blatterfein, survey lines are classified as:
  - High survey lines
  - Medium survey lines
  - Diagonal survey lines
  - Low survey lines.

High Survey Line

- High survey line passes from the occlusal third in the near zone to the occlusal third in the far zone **(Fig. 16.1A)**
- If a survey line lies higher in position, the undercut will be deep
- Therefore, a wrought wire clasp with more flexibility is used
- It is usually common in inclined teeth and in teeth with greater occlusal diameter than its cemento-enamel junction.

Medium Survey Line

- It passes from the occlusal third in the near zone to the middle third in the far zone **(Fig. 16.1B)**
- In teeth with medium survey line, either Aker's or Roach clasp is used

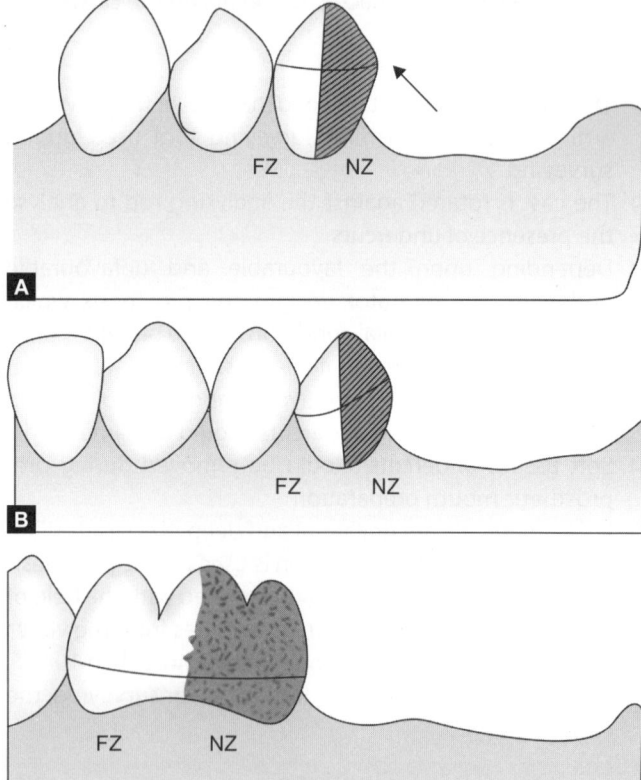

Abbreviations: FZ- Far zone; NZ- Near zone

Fig. 16.1: (A) High survey line; (B) Medium survey line and (C) Low survey line

- For acquiring maximum number of teeth with a medium survey line, the cast should be tilted during survey, .

Low Survey Line

- This survey line is closer to the cervical third of the tooth in both near and far zone **(Fig. 16.1C)**
- It is found in teeth with significant inclination when it is related to high survey line on the opposite side
- A modified T-clasp is used for teeth with low survey lines as a retentive clasp will lie very close to gingiva leading to food accumulation.

Question 2

Define surveyor. What are the objectives and uses of surveying?

Answer

Surveyor

A surveyor is defined as an instrument used in the construction of a removable partial denture to locate and delineate the contours and relative positions of abutment teeth and associated structures.

Types of Surveyor

- Ney surveyor
- Jelenko or Will's surveyor
- Willam's surveyor.

Objectives of Surveying

- It is done in order to achieve good retention and bracing by designing the rigid and flexible components of a removable prosthesis
- The process aids in marking the survey lines by determining the height of contour of hard or soft tissues areas above the undercut
- The other purpose it serves is deciding the path of insertion of a prosthesis
- Additionally, it can help in deciding the areas into which the prosthesis should not extend by determining the undesirable undercuts.

Uses of Surveyor

- To survey the diagnostic and primary casts
- For tripoding the cast
- To transfer the tripod marks to another cast
- To survey the master cast
- To contour crowns and cast restorations
- To perform mouth preparation directly on the cast to determine the outcome of treatment
- To survey the master cast
- To survey ceramic veneers before final glazing.

Question 3

Write a note on surveying tools.

Answer

Surveying Tools

- The tools used for surveying are attached to the mandrel of the surveying arm
- They are of different kinds such as analysing rod, carbon marker, wax knife and undercut gauges.

Analyzing Rod

It is a diagnostic tool and serves as a tangent to the convex surface of the object being surveyed.

Carbon Markers

- They pose similarity with lead points and are circular in cross-section in Ney Surveyors whereas triangular in cross-section in Jelenko surveyors and resemble the lead points
- They are used to draw the height of contour of the object being surveyed.

Undercut Gauges

- A gauge, high precision instrument is used to measure the linear dimension of any structure
- Moreover, undercut gauges are used to analyse the depth and location of the undercuts on the tooth in three dimensions.

Wax Knife

It can be attached to the mandrel of the surveying arm and directly trims the excess wax while surveying the wax patterns. It also eradicates and block out undesirable undercuts parallel to the path of insertion.

Question 4

Discuss briefly the various steps in surveying for removable partial denture fabrication.

Answer

Steps in Surveying

- Mounting the cast
- Positioning the surveying arm
- Analysing the cast.

Mounting the Cast

- The primary cast is mounted on the surveying table by fixing it tightly to the clamps on the surveying table
- The plane of occlusion of the existing teeth should be kept parallel to the base.

Placing the Surveying Arm

- After mounting the cast, the horizontal arm is positioned vertically and is locked to the vertical arm with the help of a thumbscrew
- It is adjusted so that the surveying arm can contact at least three different spaced out points on the cast.

Analysing the Cast

- The analysing rod is attached to mandrel of the surveying arm and acts as the first surveying tool used during surveying
- The cast is rotated against the analysing rod to analyse the presence of undercuts
- Depending upon the favourable and unfavourable undercuts, the operator designs the prosthesis which will best suit the clinical conditions of the patient
- Favourable undercuts should be present on the abutment teeth to engage the retentive components of a clasp whereas unfavourable undercuts should be eliminated
- Soft tissues undercuts should be removed during pre-prosthetic mouth preparation
- If the undercuts are unilateral and deep, the cast is tilted and a different path of insertion is used for the prosthesis
- To attain this, the surveying table is tilted with the help of thumbscrew, until the undercut vanishes from the view
- However, the cast should not be tilted more than 10o.
- Therefore, after completing the set up for surveying, the cast is surveyed.

SHORT NOTES

Question 1

What is the procedure of positioning an internal attachment?

Answer

The procedure of positioning internal attachment like intracoronal retainers is as follows:
- Firstly, the determination of the path of insertion with minimum interference is done
- Then, the teeth of the stone cast is cut to make place for a receptacle, which then holds a keyway of the attachment. The size of the recess is evaluated with the help of radiographs
- Subsequently, to receive the key of the internal attachment, a receptacle is carved in the wax pattern
- Then, the surveyor aids in placing the attachment with the receptacle wherein all the attachments of a single prosthesis lies parallel to one another.

Question 2

What is tripoding?

Answer

- Tripoding is a procedure where three different widely spaced-out points of a single plane are marked on the cast.
- These tripod points are used as a reference point and it should not be altered, until the treatment is completed.

Question 3

Define path of insertion and write various factors affecting it.

Answer

According to GPT, path of insertion is defined as the direction in which a prosthesis is placed upon and removed from the abutment teeth.

Various factors affecting path of insertion:
- Retentive undercuts
- Point of origin of the approach arm
- Guiding planes
- Interference
- Denture base
- Aesthetics
- Location of vertical minor connector.

Question 4

Write a short note on diagnostic cast and uses of surveying a diagnostic cast.

Answer

Diagnostic Cast

- A diagnostic cast is an exact replica of the hard and soft tissues of the mouth
- It provides important diagnostic data from which final diagnosis can be achieved

- In addition, it also aids in the formation of accurate treatment plan
- The diagnostic impressions required for making diagnostic casts are made using irreversible hydrocolloid (alginate)
- Surveying the diagnostic cast using a surveyor is one of the method by which a diagnostic cast can be evaluated

Surveying a Diagnostic Casts

- Surveying aids in evaluating the need for pre-prosthetic surgeries for elimination of any interferences like pathosis
- It helps in detecting and demarking the soft tissue undercuts, and severe undercuts found on the surface of the existing teeth
- It can be used in determining the path of insertion of prosthesis
  - It can aid in assessing proximal surfaces on which guiding plane can be made
  - It can analyse the retentive areas of the tooth
  - It helps in the determination of height of contour
  - It can also used as a record for future references.

Question 5

Define surveying.

Answer

According to GPT, surveying is defined as an analysis and comparison of the prominence of intraoral contours associated with the fabrication of a prosthesis.

Question 6

Write a note on undercut gauge.

Answer

- Undercut gauges, precision instruments are used to determine the depth and location of the undercuts on the analysed tooth in three dimensions
- According to Stewart, these are available in three sizes—0.010 inch, 0.020 inch and 0.030 inch
- All these gauges have different size of the tip or bead. However, the size of the shank remains same
- The gauges are mainly made up of standard sizes and the area of the tooth that is similar to the gauge is chosen as the undercut
- Ney surveyors exhibit a circular beaded whereas Jelenko surveyors have a fan-shaped beaded undercut gauge.

Question 7

State the examples of interferences that can influence the path of insertion?

Answer

- Various interference in the maxilla influencing the path of insertion are:
  - Bony exostoses
  - Buccally tipped teeth
  - Torus palatinus.
- Various interference in the mandible influencing the path of insertion are:
  - Bony exostoses
  - Lingual inclination of remaining teeth
  - Lingual tori.

Question 8

Define and classify survey lines.

Answer

Survey Line

According to GPT, a survey line can be defined as a line produced on a cast of a tooth by a surveyor or scriber marking the greatest height of contour in relation to the chosen path of insertion of a planned restoration.

There are four types of survey lines:

1. High survey line: It passes from the occlusal third in the near zone to the occlusal third in the far zone.
2. Medium survey line: It passes from the occlusal third in the near zone to the middle third in the far zone.
3. Low survey line: It runs closer to the cervical third of the tooth in both near and far zone.
4. Diagonal survey line: It runs from the occlusal third of the near zone to the cervical third of the far zone.

CHAPTER 17: Principles of Removable Partial Denture Design

LONG ESSAYS

Question 1

Elaborate the principles of design for removable partial denture.

Answer

The basic philosophy that underlies while designing a removable partial denture includes methods which can evenly disperse the forces acting on the denture across the hard and soft tissues of the oral cavity.

The four design approaches seen in stress distribution as principles of removable partial denture are as follows:
1. Stress directing concept.
2. Physiological basing.
3. Broad stress distribution.
4. Conventional rigid design.

Stress Directing Concept

- A stress breaker or a equaliser is defined as a device which relieves the abutment teeth of all or part of the occlusal forces
- A stress director is a device that allows movement between the denture base and the direct retainer which may be intra-coronal or extra-coronal
- When an occlusal load is applied in a tooth-supported denture, the denture has a proclivity to rock due to variation in the compressibility of the abutment teeth and the soft tissues
- This in turn also causes more stress on the abutment teeth. Therefore, stress breakers are included in the denture to protect abutment teeth from such conditions.

Types of Stress Breakers

Type I stress breaker

- In this type of stress breaker, a movable joint is placed between the direct retainer and denture base to permit the independent movement of the denture base
- In addition, it reduces the amount of force acting on the abutment
- The different kinds of joint can be:
  - A hinge
  - A ball and socket
  - A sleeve
  - A cylinder type.
- Various examples of hinge type of stress breakers are:
  - DALBO
  - CRISMANI
  - ASC 52 attachments.

Type II stress breaker

- In this type of stress breaker, a flexible connection is placed between the direct retainer and the denture base
- Wrought wire connector, split or divided major connectors or a movable joint between two major connectors can be used.

Advantages

- Reduces stress exerting on the abutment teeth and balances it with the residual ridge
- Restores alveolar support of the abutment teeth
- A massaging effect is generated on soft tissues by the movement of denture base
- Even without undergoing the process of relining, abutment teeth do not damaged
- Prevents the frequent requirement of relining and rebasing
- Splints the periodontally weak abutment teeth and protects them during the movement of the denture
- Needs minimum amount of direct retention.

Disadvantages

- It is prone to fracture due to weak structure
- Can be distorted due to rough handling
- Difficult to repair and cannot be relined appropriately

- Has complicated and expensive design
- Can cause ridge resorption due to inability to counteract lateral stress
- Exhibits lesser stability against horizontal forces
- Causes lodgement of food in case of split major connector.

Physiological basing

- The method employs fabrication of a denture base on the basis of on a functional record
- The functional record acquired by recording the tissues under occlusal load or by relining the denture under functional stress aids in distributing the stresses between the abutment teeth and the soft tissues
- It basically requires a rigid metal framework, functional occlusal rests, indirect retainers, broad coverage denture bases.

Advantages

- Transmits the occlusal load evenly to teeth and tissues
- Easy and economical in fabrication
- Minimum requirement of direct retention
- Denture base adaptation is good.

Disadvantages

- Excessive ridge resorption as denture compresses soft tissues even at rest
- At rest position, the denture has a tendency to lift leading to premature contacts
- Less stability due to reduced number of retentive components
- Reduces indirect retention.

Broad Stress distribution

- The aim of this concept is the distribution of occlusal load acting on the denture over a wider soft tissue area and maximum number of teeth
- Therefore, to attain the these objectives, number of direct retainers, indirect retainers, rests and the area of the denture base should be increased.

Advantages

- Simple and economical in fabrication
- Removable splinting is done with the help of multiple clasps
- Protects the abutment teeth by splinting.

Disadvantages

- Maintenance of oral hygiene is difficult
- Less comfortable to the patient.

Conventional Rigid Design

- The design of the denture is done with rigid components that acts like a raft foundation
- The design aids in distributing the forces evenly on the supporting tissues.

Advantages

- Construction is easy and economical
- Does not undergo distortion
- The load is distributed evenly between abutment and residual ridge
- Decreases the requirement of relining
- Indirect retainers aid in stabilising the denture by preventing rotational movements.

Disadvantages

- Difficult to construct
- Increases torqueing forces on the abutment teeth
- Damage to abutment teeth due to rigid continuous clasping
- It is difficult to reline
- Dovetail intra-coronal retainers cannot be used as tipping forces from the denture gets directed to the abutment teeth directly.

Question 2

What are the design considerations for a removable partial denture?

Answer

The factors that play a vital role in designing a removable partial denture for various Kennedy's classes are discussed in the section below.

In Kennedy's Class I and class II cases

Occlusion

- Occlusion of the denture should be in accordance with the existing teeth and should coincide with the centric relation of the patient
- The arrangement of the artificial teeth should be done in such a way so as to reduce the stresses
- Absence of any premature contact should also be taken into consideration.

Denture Base

- A selective pressure impression technique should be used
- A broad coverage denture base without any functional interference is preferred.

Direct Retention

- Close adaptation of the denture base, restoration of form and function and preservation of soft tissue play an important role during designing the prosthesis
- In addition, evaluation of the position of the undercut is significant for selecting the type of clasp.

Clasp

- The design of the clasp should be simple and accomplish all the essential prerequisites of a clasp
- In case of class I, two clasps on each terminal abutment are placed
- However, for class II cases, three retentive clasps are needed
- One clasp and two clasps are placed on the edentulous side and the dentulous side, respectively.

Rest

- The preparation of the rest seat should be done on the tooth surface to gain the maximum support
- It should have an ideal configuration and should be positioned near to the edentulous space.

Indirect Retention

- In class I cases, two indirect retainers are required and for a class II case one indirect retainer on the dentulous side is sufficient
- Lingual plate may be given.

Major Connector and Minor Connector

It should fulfil all the ideal requisites of major and minor connector for both classes.

In Kennedy's Class III case

Denture Base

For these cases, a functional impression is not essential but should fulfill all the ideal requirements of the denture base.

Direct Retention

The position of the undercut does not pose any importance in designing and the trauma to the abutment teeth is very less in comparison to other classes.

Clasp

- It should accomplish all the ideal requirements
- Usually, four clasps are placed to obtain a quadrilateral design.

Indirect Retention

Though indirect retention is not required, In cases where a clasp is not positioned on the posterior tooth, it should be provided alike class I and class II cases.

Rest, Major Connector, Minor Connector and Occlusion

It is similar to that of class I or II designs.

In Kennedy's Class IV case

- The positioning of the teeth can cause generation of tilting or lever forces against the abutment teeth
- Various factors that can reduce these forces are as follows:
  - Natural teeth as an intermediate abutment or as an over denture abutment
  - Tipping forces exerted become lesser if the edentulous area is shorter
  - Restoration of the labial alveolar bone.

Clasp

Usually, four clasps should be positioned to acquire a quadrilateral design.

Major Connector

The major connector should be rigid and should possess a broad coverage.

Indirect Retainer

The indirect retainer should be positioned posterior to the fulcrum line.

Denture Base

A functional impression is required for a large edentulous span.

Question 3

Elaborate the factors that are considered to reduce the impact of harmful forces on the abutment teeth.

Answer

The various factors that can reduce the negative impact of the forces on the abutment teeth are as discussed in the section below.

Length of the Edentulous Span

- The length of edentulous ridge influence the forces transmitted to the abutment teeth
- If the edentulous span is longer, longer will be the denture base

- This in turn, will produce greater amount of force
- Therefore, it is advisable to preserve the posterior teeth to limit the length of the edentulous area.

Quality of Support of the Ridge

- Large, well-formed ridges has potential of absorbing greater amounts of forces in contrast to small, thin, or knife edged ridges
- Moreover, Broad ridges with parallel sides also helps in stabilising the denture against lateral forces
- In addition to the ridges, 1 mm thick mucoperiosteum gives good support than a thin atrophic mucosa.

Response of Oral Structures to Previous Stress

Prognosis of the prosthesis can be affected by the previous stresses such as periodontal condition and amount of support of the existing teeth.

Qualities of a Clasp

A flexible retentive clasp arm can reduce the stress being transmitted to the abutment tooth.

Design of the Clasp

- The design of the clasp should be passive as it will exert less forces on the abutment teeth
- Moreover, a clasp should be designed such that the reciprocal arm contacting the tooth before the retentive tip passes over the greatest bulge of the tooth during insertion
- The reciprocal arm should be the last component to lose contact from the tooth during removal of the prosthesis.

Length of the Clasp

- The flexibility of a clasp is basically dependent on its length which is inversely proportional to the stresses on the abutment tooth
- If the length of the clasp gets double, the flexibility increases by five times.

Material Used in Clasp Construction

Owing to its greater rigidity, chrome alloy exerts more stress on the abutment tooth than a gold clasp.

Occlusal Relationship of the Existing Teeth and Orientation of the Occlusal Plane

Inappropriate occlusal relationship and a steep occlusal plane can increase the amount of force acting on the denture.

Tooth Surface of the Abutment

- More stress is exerted on the tooth with gold restoration in comparison to the tooth with intact enamel
- This is due to the more functional resistance offered by gold restoration to the movement of a clasp arm than enamel.

SHORT ESSAYS

Question 1

What are the armamentarium for designing the removable partial denture?

Answer

Armamentarium Required

- Surveyor and accessories
- Articulator (Galetti-Luongo type)
  - An excellent diagnostic tool does not utilize plaster instead uses clamps to hold the casts in position
  - The movement of the casts can be done independently in three dimensions, when the clamps are released.
- Pencils for colour coding
  - Red, blue, brown or green crayon and black lead pencil can be used for colour coding
- The most frequently utilised colour code key for laboratory design is as follows:
  - Red (solid) is used for rest seats
  - Red (outline only) is used for contoured and prepared tooth surfaces
  - Blue is used for acrylic resin portions
  - Brown or green can be used for metallic portions
  - Black is used for survey lines, tripod marks, soft tissue undercuts, type of tooth, use of wrought wire clasps.

Question 2

What are the principles of a removable partial denture?

Answer

A. H. Schmidt in 1956 gave the following five principles to be taken into consideration during the fabrication of a removable partial denture. They are as follows:

- The clinician should have exhaustive information about the forces exerting on the denture and soft tissues, along with the response of the denture to different forces. In addition, he or she should comprehend both the mechanical and biologic factors associated with removable partial denture design
- Planning of the treatment is dependent upon the complete examination and diagnosis of the individual patient, as their neglect can lead to the failure of the removable denture
- The clinician should consider all the significant factors like the current oral conditions of the patient, prior to the planning of treatment. Moreover, necessary modifications such as pre-prosthetic procedures, extractions, etc. should be performed before designing a removable partial denture
- A removable partial denture or prosthesis should maintain aesthetics along with the proper form and function without exerting negative impact on the health of surrounding soft tissues
- The patient should be properly followed-up for ensuring the success of the prosthesis, as a removable partial denture is a form of treatment and not a cure.

SHORT NOTES

Question 1

What are the factors that impact the magnitude of stresses transmitted to abutment teeth?

Answer

- Length of the edentulous span
- Quality of support of the ridge
- Response of oral structures to previous stress
- Qualities of a clasp
- Design of the clasp
- Length of the clasp
- Material used in clasp construction
- Occlusal relationship of the existing teeth and orientation of the occlusal plane
- Tooth surface of the abutment.

Question 2

What is L-bar or L-beam principle?

Answer

The L-beam or L-bar or linear beam theory states that the flexibility of a bar is directly proportional to the length of the bar and inversely proportional to its thickness.

Question 3

Define and classify lever.

Answer

- A lever is a long bar with a single support around which it rotates when a load is applied to any one of its ends
- It can be classified as:
  - Ist-order levers
    - In this lever the fulcrum is in the centre, resistance is at one end and effort (force) is at the other.
  - IInd-order levers
    - In this lever, the fulcrum is at one end, effort is at the opposite end and resistance or load is the centre.
  - IIIrd-order levers
    - In this lever, the fulcrum is at one end, resistance is at the opposite end and effort is at the centre.

Question 4

Define denture base and mention ideal requirements of denture base.

Answer

Denture Base

- It is defined as that part of a denture which rests on the oral mucosa and to which teeth are attached.
- The most frequently used types of denture base are:
  - Acrylic
  - Metal
  - Combination.

Ideal Requirements

- The denture base must possess thermal conductivity
- It should have adequate resistance against fractures or distortion
- It should be properly adapted to the tissues with minimal change in volume
- It should have weightlessness within the oral cavity with low specific gravity
- It should have potential to attain a good finish
- It should be easy to clean
- It should be economical
- It should be easy to reline, if necessary.

Chapter 17 Principles of Removable Partial Denture Design

Question 5

Describe the various principles involved in the functioning of a removable partial denture.

Answer

The various principles involved in the functioning of a removable partial denture are as follows:

- Different forces exerting on the denture inside the oral cavity
- Forces from the tongue
- Forces from the surrounding musculature such as lip and cheek muscles
- Response of the denture to various forces acting on it.

Chapter 18: Secondary Impressions for Removable Partial Denture

LONG ESSAYS

Question 1

What are dual impressions? Explain selective pressure functional dual impression technique.

Answer

Dual Impression Techniques

- In this technique, two master impressions are recorded, one portion in the functional form and the other in the anatomical form
- They are indicated in all tooth-tissue supported partial dentures
- They are basically divided into two, which are as follows:
  1. Physiological or functional dual impressions.
  2. Selective pressure functional dual impression technique.

Physiological or Functional Dual Impressions

- In this technique, one anatomical impression is made of the entire ridge whereas one physiological impression is made only on the edentulous portion
- The physiological impression displaces tissues and is made by exerting occlusal load on the impression tray during impression making
- Various types of functional impression are:
  - McLean's method
  - Hindel's method
  - Functional relining method
  - Fluid wax functional impression.

Selective Pressure Functional Dual Impression Technique

- The technique comprises of one anatomical impression and one selective pressure functional impression
- The master cast is fabricated from the anatomical impression which is further modified according to the selective pressure functional impression
- In this procedure, the tissue surface of the special tray lying over the relieving areas is reduced so as to prevent the occlusal load in those areas
- Therefore, while making the impression, tray contacts the tissues only over stress-bearing areas and record them in compressed state
- Henceforth, the method of employing pressure in selective areas during the making of functional impression defines selective pressure functional dual impression technique.

Procedure

- The master cast is fabricated from an anatomical impression above which a special tray without a wax spacer is made
- About 1 mm of acrylic along the tissue surface is trimmed along the crest of the ridge whereas the stress-bearing areas are left untouched
- The impression material such as zinc oxide eugenol is loaded on the special tray and inserted into mouth of the patient
- Finger pressure is used and only the stress-bearing areas are recorded in a compressed state.

Advantages

- Evenly distributes the stress between abutment teeth and soft tissues
- Rate of ridge resorption is reduced as the area which can not withstand stress are relieved.

Question 2

What are functional dual impressions in removable partial denture? Also describe techniques employed to record these impressions.

Answer

Functional Dual Impressions in Removable Partial Denture

- These impressions are also known as physiological dual impressions as the impression contains one anatomical impression made of the entire ridge and one physiological or functional impression made only on the edentulous portion
- In making functional impression, occlusal load is applied on the impression tray and tissues are recorded in displaced position
- The frequently employed impression techniques to record functional dual impressions are as follows:
  - McLean's technique
  - Hindle's modification of McLean's technique
  - Functional relining method
  - Fluid wax technique.

McLean's Technique

- In this technique, two impressions are made, i.e. a functional impression of the edentulous ridge and second impression over the functional impression recording the structures in their anatomic form
- The second impression is made by covering, and picking up the functional impression and is also known as the pick up impression
- However, the procedure can have errors as the supporting tissues may not be as compressed as they were while making the functional impression
- Moreover, inadequate alginate between the occlusal rim of the custom tray and the over-impression stock tray impedes the transfer of entire load from stock tray to the special tray.

Hindle's Modification of McLean's Technique

- To overcome the drawbacks of McLean's technique, Hindle modified it and suggested that a special tray with an occlusal rim and stoppers should be fabricated using the primary cast to record anatomical impression
- The stoppers are positioned on the tray extending over the stress-bearing areas so as to prevent excessive pressure on the tissues
- The over impression, a functional impression is taken by a special stock tray with large holes on which finger pressure is applied against edentulous ridge to provide a pseudo-functional stress
- Nevertheless, the tissues gets constantly compressed leading to excessive bone resorption.

Functional Relining Method

- This technique involves an anatomical master impression of all the oral structures
- The two casts are formed from this impression, one is master cast and the other one is refractory cast
- The framework of the prosthesis is fabricated using refractory cast and is further used to record functional impression
- Master cast fabricated from the anatomical impression is modified base upon the functional impression made on the tissue surface of the framework.

Fluid Wax Technique

- Fluid wax functional impression technique is an open mouth technique
- In this technique, fabrication of framework is done by using the anatomical impression, which is then converted into a special tray to record the functional impression
- This technique is used to reline the soft tissues of an existing removable prosthesis
- It can also be used to correct the distal extensions of the edentulous ridge of the original master cast
- It is advantageous as it can record non-stress-bearing areas in both anatomic form and functional form
- Moreover, it can achieve maximum extension of the peripheral borders of the denture.

SHORT NOTES

Question 1

What is physiological impression in removable partial denture?

Answer

- The functional impression or physiologic impression records the residual ridge under generalised compression
- This in turn prevents additional stress from the denture on the abutment teeth during functional loading
- The technique is advantageous as it evenly disperse the occlusal forces between abutment teeth and the soft tissues
- In addition, it avoids the concentration of harmful forces on the abutment teeth

- These impressions are needed only to edentulous saddles
- They are usually indicated in tooth-tissue supported partial denture cases.

Question 2

What is the impression technique used for relining the tissue surface of an existing removable partial denture?

Answer

- Fluid wax functional impression is the impression procedure used for relining the tissue surface of an existing removable partial denture
- Waxes used for this technique are namely; Iowa wax and Korecta wax No. 4
- In this technique, fabrication of framework is done by using the anatomical impression, which is then converted into a special tray to record the functional impression
- It is advantageous as it can record non-stress-bearing areas in both anatomic form and functional form.

Question 3

Name the methods of secondary impression procedures in removable partial denture.

Answer

Different Impression Techniques Employed in Removable Partial Denture

- Single pressure-free impression technique
- Selective pressure impression technique
- Physiologic or functional impression technique.
  - Mclean's impression technique
  - Hindel's impression technique
  - Fluid wax impression technique
  - Functional relining technique.

Question 4

What is fluid wax functional impression technique?

Answer

Fluid Wax Functional Impression Technique

- It is an open mouth technique
- In this technique, fabrication of framework is done by using the anatomical impression, which is then converted into a special tray to record the functional impression
- This technique is used to reline the soft tissues of an existing removable prosthesis
- It can also be used to correct the distal extensions of the edentulous ridge of the original master cast
- It is advantageous as it can record non-stress-bearing areas in both anatomic form and functional form
- Moreover, it can achieve maximum extension of the peripheral borders of the denture.

Question 5

Write a note on selective pressure functional dual impression technique.

Answer

Selective Pressure Functional Dual Impression Technique

- This technique comprises of both anatomical and selective pressure functional impression
- The master cast is made by taking the impression of compressed stress-bearing areas, therefore, the technique aids in directing forces to the areas of ridge having potential of bearing forces
- This impression technique is advantageous as it equalises the stress between the abutment teeth and the soft tissue
- Moreover, due to its capability of relieving the areas that cannot withstand forces, the rate of ridge resorption also gets reduced
- The least displacement is seen in the relief areas such as the crest of the ridge whereas maximum displacement is seen at the areas where the tray contacts.

Chapter 19: Laboratory Procedures for Removable Partial Denture Design

LONG ESSAY

Question 1

What are the ideal requirements of denture base? Also mention the different types of denture base materials used in removable partial denture.

Answer

Ideal Requirements for a Denture Base

- It should confer stability and retention of the prosthesis
- It should offer proper support for artificial teeth
- It should have appropriate extensions into functionally developed borders
- The base should counterbalance stresses produced by twisting and tilting during function
- It should possess the ability to transfer forces to both the abutments and residual ridges
- It should have close adaptation with the underlying mucosa
- It should exhibit other physical, mechanical and biological properties such as strength, rigidity, tarnish and corrosion resistance, biocompatibility, castability, etc.
- It should be comfortable to the wearer.

Types of Denture Bases

Denture bases can be broadly classified into:
- Metal
- Acrylic
- Metal-acrylic resin bases.

Metal

- The most frequently used partial denture alloys are base metal alloy, Ni-Cr, Co-Cr, Titanium (Pure Ti and Ti Alloy)
- These alloys have good castability, rigidity, tarnish and corrosion resistance and flexibility.

Indications

- In cases where aesthetics is not required
- In patients requiring thin base with reduced intermaxillary space
- In cases requiring deep-bites
- In patients who are allergic to acrylic.

Advantages

- It transmits the sensation of heat and cold
- It provides a natural feel to the patient
- It is more biocompatible than other types of denture bases
- It possesses good mechanical properties.

Disadvantages

- Appropriate extension cannot be obtained in buccal shelf area
- It is time taking procedure
- It cannot be used in patients allergic to metal.

Acrylic

Indications

- It is used in distal extension cases which require repeated relining
- In patients who are allergic to metal.

Advantages

- Its relining and rebasing are easy
- It is economical in comparison to other two types
- It is easy to repair.

Disadvantages

- It cannot be used as permanent prosthesis
- Its mechanical properties are inadequate.

Metal-acrylic Resin Base

Indications

- It is used in cases where both aesthetics and strength are taken into consideration
- Usually it can be used in most of the cases except in cases which can require relining.

Advantages

- It possess both the strength of the metal and the aesthetics of acrylic
- It is light in weight than all metal denture bases

Disadvantage

It cannot be used in cases which require relining.

SHORT ESSAYS

Question 1

Explain in detail about blockout or wax out procedure.

Answer

Blockout

- It is defined as elimination of undesirable under cut areas on the cast to be used in the fabrication of the removable partial denture
- In this process, the undesirable undercuts on the master cast are filled with wax and are eradicated in the refractory cast duplicated from the master cast
- On the basis of usage, it can be of three types:
  1. Parallel blockout
  2. Arbitrary blockout
  3. Formed blockout.

Parallel Blockout

- Undesirable undercuts should be blocked out or filled to avoid interference
- Block out is done using wax or block out material
- Usually block out is done in the master cast
- Undesirable undercuts should be eliminated below the height of contour for that path of insertion (height of contour will vary according to the path of insertion)
- The excess blockout material is trimmed to the height of contour using a surveying wax knife.

Arbitrary Blockout

- Blockout wax is filled in soft tissues and other unfavourable undercuts in the master cast
- The aim of the procedure is to eliminate the undesirable undercuts of ridge or soft tissue, which may cause hindrance in the path of insertion
- However in this type of blockout, the surface of the blockout wax may not be parallel to the path of insertion.

Shaped Blockout

- The procedure also known as formed blockout has a different purpose and is carried out in the undercut of the primary abutment along the lower border of the proposed retentive arm
- Instead of blockout wax to be trimmed to flush with the tooth surface, it is filled excessively, projecting from the surface of the teeth
- A ledge on the occlusal surface due to excess wax which follows the lower border of the proposed retentive arm
- The block out will then get reproduced as a ledge on the refractory cast, which further acts as a guide for the fabrication of the wax pattern for the retentive arm.

Question 2

Explain altered cast impression technique.

Answer

Altered Cast Impression Technique

- Alteration of master cast is done for functional reline, fluid wax and functional selective pressure dual impression techniques
- The altered cast technique is used to prevent the displaceability of the mucosa in free-end saddles, which have a tendency to get displaced under occlusal pressure
- Therefore, the technique is indicated in distal extension removable partial denture or cast partial denture
- The process involves altering of the master cast according to the functional impression which is primarily made by using the anatomical impression.

Procedure

- The edentulous area in the anatomical master cast is cut away with a saw and the cast is sliced using one bucco-lingual and one antero-posterior cut

Chapter 19 Laboratory Procedures for Removable Partial Denture Design

- The bucco-lingual cut is made 1 mm behind the terminal abutment across the edentulous ridge whereas the antero-posterior cut is made 1 mm lingual or medial to the lingual sulcus and these cuts are followed by the preparation of vertical grooves
- The framework together with the functional impression is placed over the cut anatomical master cast, in which edentulous areas is projecting in free space
- Softened modelling plastic is then used to seal the framework to the master cast
- The cast along with framework is further inverted and functional impression is projecting underneath the cut areas of the cast
- The impression in conjuction with the cast is beaded and boxed which is then soaked in slurry water for 10 minutes before pouring the impression by a low expansion dendrite stone
- The resultant master cast thus, have an altered ridge contour acquired from the functional impression.

SHORT NOTES

Question 1

What are the factors considered while selecting the mould of anterior teeth?

Answer

The factors considered while selecting the mould of the artificial teeth are as follows:
- It should be in accordance with the features of the patient
- The teeth should be in harmony with the natural teeth, even if the individual teeth are irregular
- The teeth adjacent and opposite to the edentulous space should be taken in to consideration
- Malocclusion relationships such as deep-bite, cross-bite should be considered
- Space regaining treatment procedures such as proximal slicing, fabricating crowns should be considered, if the edentulous space has been reduced due to migration of adjacent teeth or supra-eruption of opposing teeth.

Question 2

What are the reasons of the problems in framework during try-in procedure?

Answer

The reasons for the problems because of which the framework does not seat properly in to the patients mouth are:
- Improper impression
- Inaccurately poured cast
- Inappropriate alteration of the cast modified for dual impression
- Variation in the location of the natural teeth after making of the impression.

Question 3

Define investing.

Answer

According to GPT, it is defined as the process of covering or enveloping, wholly or in part, an object such as a denture, tooth, wax form, crown, etc. with a suitable investment material before processing, soldering or casting.

Question 4

What are the various steps of framework fabrication?

Answer

The various steps involved in the fabrication of framework are the following:
- Wax-up
- Duplication and preparation of refractory casts
- Waxing
- Investing
- Burn out
- Casting
- Finishing and polishing.

Chapter 20: Types of Removable Partial Denture and its, Correction and Repair

LONG ESSAY

Question
What are swing lock dentures? Also mention its steps of fabrication.

Answer

Swing Lock Dentures

- First described by Dr. Joe J. Simmons in 1963, the design of the denture includes a labial bar and a lingual major connector
- Among which, the labial bar is used to support the periodontally weak teeth
- The labial bar can be unlocked during insertion and locked after insertion
- The labial bar is attached to the remaining parts of the denture by a hinge on one side and a lock on the other
- Since, the labial bar moves around a hinge joint these dentures are called swing lock dentures.

Indications

- The swing lock denture uses the remaining teeth to derive support, retention and stability, therefore, it can be used in cases where the key abutments are missing
- It can be used in patients, where the teeth have questionable prognosis
- It retains the prosthesis for patients who have lost large segments of teeth and have resorbed alveolar ridge
- It can be used when retention and stability of a maxillofacial prosthesis is required
- It is indicated when few remaining teeth exist
- It is used when the placement of natural teeth is not conducive for a conventional design
- It is used in patients with undesirable tooth contours like excessive inclination and unfavourable soft tissue contours like soft tissue undercuts.

Contraindications

- It has shallow vestibule
- Oral hygiene maintenance is poor
- In patients with high frenal attachment.

Advantages

- The prosthesis is economical and uses most of the existing teeth for achieving retention and stability
- An artificial tooth can be easily added to the existing prosthesis, in case where further extraction is required.

Disadvantages

- In cases of distal extension partial denture, tipping of abutment teeth can occur due to the leverage forces produced by the movement of the denture base towards the tissue
- It imparts poor aesthetics, particularly in patients with short or extremely mobile lips.

Steps of Fabrication

Selection of metal

- Chrome alloy is preferred for the fabrication of these dentures in place of gold alloy
- This is due to the reason that gold alloy after a short period of usage tends to wear
- Moreover, large quantity of metal needs to be incorporated with gold alloy into the framework for adequate rigidity and strength.

Surveying and design

- The cast is mounted on a surveyor with the occlusal plane parallel to the base and surveyed, accordingly
- The path of insertion is from a lingual direction with the labial arm open

Chapter 20 Types of Removable Partial Denture and its, Correction and Repair

- Various design considerations required are as follows:
  - Lingual plate
    - It is designed to end above the survey line so as to inhibit the displacement of the denture towards tissues.
  - Occlusal rest
    - It is designed according to the ideal requirements in order to prevent tissueward displacement of the denture.
  - Major connector
    - Lingual plate is the desired mandibular major connector in these dentures which lies above the survey line with scallops extending up to contact points
    - For maxillary major connector, complete palate or a closed horseshoe with borders extending up to or above the survey line is preferred.
  - Labial arm
    - The vertical projections of the labial bar impede occlusal movement by contacting the teeth below the height of contour
    - Two different types of labial arm design are as follows:
      1. Conventional design.
      2. Acrylic resin retention loops.

Selection of impression material

- The impression material should tear in the interproximal areas, without causing damage to teeth, for easy removal as wide gingival embrasures are usually present in these cases
- Therefore, heavy-bodied alginate is the choice of material used for these dentures.

Tray selection

- A custom tray is required to record maximum labial and buccal vestibular depths and secondary impression is recorded while placing a spacer of thickness of about 5–6 mm
- In addition, holes should be made in the tray to retain the alginate.

Impression making

- The procedure for impression making has similarity to that of conventional dentures
- In cases of distal extension, dual impression technique can be used.

Fabrication of the framework

- A master cast poured from the secondary impression is waxed and undercuts are blocked out prior to its duplication to form the refractory cast
- The design also gets transferred to the refractory cast over which the wax pattern is fabricated. The refractory cast is then invested, burned out and casting is performed
- The framework formed is further trimmed, finished and polished.

Framework try-in

- A framework is tried in the patient prior to the arrangement of the artificial teeth
- Furthermore, fit of the labial bar and the rest of the framework are checked separately.

Jaw relations

- Occlusal rims are fabricated over the temporary denture base which is made by using the try-in framework
- This denture base is inserted into the patient's mouth and all the three jaw relations are recorded
- The recorded jaw relation along with the cast are mounted in an articulator.

Arrangement of artificial teeth

- Artificial teeth are arranged according to the appropriate occlusion, in which there is no exertion of lateral forces on the prosthesis
- Simultaneous contact between artificial and natural teeth should be present
- After the arrangement, contouring and polishing of the modelling wax that is to form the denture base is done
- Subsequently, the trial denture is flasked and acrylized.

Insertion of the denture

- A lingual path of insertion is followed and pressure indicator paste is utilised to detect pressure areas
- Occlusion is also assessed in centric and eccentric relations
- However, in case of distal extension prosthesis, the vertical projections are bent away from the teeth using two prong pliers in order to prevent the tipping of anterior teeth lingually by the labial bar under occlusal load.

Post-insertion care

- Instructions for the maintenance of oral hygiene should be given to the patient
- Loosened lock mechanisms should be tightened
- In distal extension cases, relining should be done frequently
- Moreover, if further extraction is required, teeth can be added to the framework at later stages.

SHORT ESSAY

Question 1

Write in brief about rebasing of removable partial dentures.

Answer

Rebasing

- It is defined as a process of refitting a denture by the replacement of the denture-base material
- The technique is similar to relining in which the bulk of denture base material and the impression material is removed and replaced by new resin.

Indications

- It is used in cases when the denture borders do not extend to cover all the supporting tissues
- It is also used in patients whose denture is stained or discoloured
- It is indicated in fractured denture base cases.

Procedure

- Relieving and trimming of the tissue surface of the denture base is done which serves as a space for re-adaptation of borders with modelling plastic
- Border moulding is performed followed by the making of final impression with the help of framework
- A cast is poured against the rebase impression and modelling plastic and final impression material is scrapped away from the denture base
- Trimming of the denture base extending over the area to be rebased is done except 2–3 mm area adjacent to the base of the teeth
- In cases where anterior teeth are included, the junction of the new resin and the existing denture base is kept in an area which is invisible when the patient smiles
- The borders of the resin should be at 90° to the external surface to reduce the line of junction
- However in cases, where aesthetics is not crucial, the junction is rounded to decrease the stress concentration and increase the strength
- Small amounts of base plate wax is added to provide a finished contour to the processed rebase which in turn also decreases the finishing time
- Flasking is performed in which a boil-out procedure is done to soften the wax and modelling plastic
- Then the trimming of tissue surface of denture resin is done to accommodate new resin
- The process of acrylization and processing is done subsequent to which the denture is de-flasked using a lab knife or pneumatic blade and a shell blaster
- Final step includes finishing and polishing.

SHORT NOTES

Question 1

Describe metal repair.

Answer

- Metal repair of retentive clasp arm is most frequently performed among all metal repairs
- In this procedure, a repair cast is made on which the design of the replacement clasp is drawn on the abutment tooth
- In the laboratory, the replacement clasp is embedded in the resin of the denture base or its electro-soldering to the framework is done
- Both infra-bulge clasps and circumferential clasps are used
- They may be cast or made of wrought metal.

Question 2

Define temporary partial dentures and classify them.

Answer

Temporary Partial Dentures

According to GPT, it is defined as a dental prosthesis to be used for a short interval of time for aesthetics, mastication, occlusal support or convenience or to condition the patient to the acceptance of an artificial substitute for missing natural teeth until more definitive prosthetic therapy can be provided.

These are classified in to three types:

1. Transitional partial denture.
2. Interim partial denture.
3. Treatment partial denture.

Chapter 20 Types of Removable Partial Denture and its, Correction and Repair

Transitional Partial Denture

A removable partial denture serving as a temporary prosthesis to which artificial teeth will be added as natural teeth are lost and which will be replaced after post-extraction tissue changes have occurred.

Interim Partial Denture

A transitional denture may become an interim denture when all of the natural teeth have been removed from the dental arch.

Treatment Partial Denture

A dental prosthesis used for the purpose of treating or conditioning the tissues which are called upon to support and retain a denture base.

Question 3

Define and classify immediate partial denture. Also mention its advantages.

Answer

Immediate Partial Denture

It is defined as a removable partial denture constructed for insertion immediately following the removal of natural teeth.

Classification

There are two types of immediate dentures:
1. Temporary Immediate denture.
2. Permanent Immediate denture.

Advantages

- It acts as a splint over the surgical site and aids in the management of haemorrhage and oedema
- It provides psychological benefit to the patient by improving its aesthetics
- It also impedes supra-eruption of the opposing teeth
- Moreover, it prevents drifting of the adjacent teeth.

Question 4

What are the indications of swing lock partial denture prosthesis?

Answer

- The swing lock denture uses the remaining teeth to derive support, retention and stability, therefore, it can be used in cases where the key abutments are missing
- It can be used in patients, where the teeth have questionable prognosis
- It retains the prosthesis for patients who have lost large segments of teeth and have resorbed alveolar ridge
- It can be used when retention and stability of a maxillofacial prosthesis is required
- It is indicated when few remaining teeth exist
- It is used when the placement of natural teeth is not conducive for a conventional design
- It is used in patients with undesirable tooth contours like excessive inclination and unfavourable soft tissue contours like soft tissue undercuts.

Question 5

Write a note on every denture.

Answer

Every Denture

- First described by Every are also termed as precision plastic base dentures
- They are widely used in maxilla and are indicated in Kennedy's class III cases with modifications
- The denture is designed on the basis of broad palatal coverage, which aids to withstand the vertical load whereas the palatal tissues and anterior teeth help to withstand the lateral load.

Advantage

The fabrication of the denture is economical.

Disadvantage

The denture has inadequate strength and is too flexible.

Question 6

What are claspless dentures?

Answer

Claspless Dentures

- These dentures were developed to overcome the shortcomings of using clasps
- They do not cause discomfort to the patient and are aesthetic in appearance
- These dentures are designed with spring-loaded nipples, which engages the proximal undercut of the primary abutment such as ZA anchor system
- This ZA system has a nipple and a casing, the nipple is spring loaded and is made of nylon or metal whereas casing is a hollow cylinder with external threading which can be screwed into the acrylic denture base
- The nipple fits into the casing which should be placed parallel to the ridge near the undercut

- It then engages the proximal undercut during insertion of the prosthesis.

Advantage

The attachment is small, therefore can be used in a single tooth removable partial denture.

Disadvantages

- Requires repeated replacement
- Metal nipple can abrade the tooth
- Nylon nipple can wear out in a short time.

Question 7

Describe two-part denture.

Answer

Two-part Dentures

- This was first described by Lee and was designed to correct the technical difficulties in using the proximal undercuts in unilateral dentures
- The denture us fabricated in two parts, which have different paths of insertion but both these parts are designed so as to engage the mesial and distal undercut of a single abutment tooth
- For example in a Kennedy's class III without any modification, this unilateral bounded saddle will obtain support from both mesial and distal abutments.

Advantages

The labial and buccal clasps are not used as the denture fill the undercuts.

Disadvantages

The design of construction the prosthesis is complex and technique sensitive.

Question 8

Write in brief about disjunct denture.

Answer

Disjunct Denture

- This is Kennedy's class I denture with special stress breakers between the tooth-supported part and the tissue-supported part of the denture
- The stress breaker in the denture is a bar and slot unlike a conventional hinge and this bar of the stress breaker is termed as a disjunct bar
- It is used when the existing teeth have less periodontal support
- The denture has two parts connected by a stress breaker and the two parts are called on the basis of the supporting structures, which can be either tooth borne part or mucosa or tissue born part.

Advantage

The teeth which are periodontally weak can be restored by these dentures.

Disadvantages

- The design of the denture is difficult and technique sensitive in construction
- Movement of both parts individually can cause discomfort to the wearer.

SECTION 3

FIXED PARTIAL DENTURES AND IMPLANTS

Chapter 21: Introduction to Fixed Partial Dentures

LONG ESSAYS

Question 1

Define and classify fixed partial denture.

Answer

A fixed partial denture (FPD) is defined as a partial denture that is cemented to natural teeth or roots which furnish the primary support to the prosthesis.

Classification of Fixed Partial Dentures

FPDs are grouped into categories which is based on factors such as components, abutments, length of the span, etc.

The classification should fulfill the following criteria:
- It should allow differentiation between tooth support and tooth tissue supported partial denture
- It should serve as a guide for the type of design that is to be used
- It should include codes for the designs that are in common use
- It should be universally accepted
- Visualisation of the type of partially edentulous arch being considered is allowed

There are three major classes of FPDs and these classes are divided into three divisions and than there divisions are divided into four more subdivisions. So, overall there can be 12 designs possible in each single class.

Class

A class identifies the location of the edentulous space.
- Class I: Posterior edentulous spaces. One or more of the posterior teeth (premolars and molars) are missing
- Class II: Anterior edentulous spaces. One or more of the anterior teeth (incisors and canines) are missing
- Class III: Antero-posterior edentulous spaces. Edentulous spaces involving both the anterior and posterior regions, i.e. some anterior and posterior teeth are missing.

Division

A division gives information about the teeth present adjacent to the edentulous space that are capable of taking support.
- Division I: Cantilever FPDs. Abutments present only on one side of the edentulous space are capable of taking support
- Division II: Conventional FPDs. Abutments that are capable of taking up occlusal load are present on both sides of the edentulous space
- Division III: Pier Abutments. A single tooth is surrounded by an edentulous space on either side. Two division II FPDs separated by a single tooth, which is capable of providing support is a division III FPD. Such cases are treated with a single prosthesis.

Sub-division

A sub-division denotes the status of the tooth that is to be used as an abutment.
- Sub-division I: Ideal abutments. Healthy teeth, which provide good support
- Sub-division II: Tilted abutments. Either the design of the prosthesis should be modified or the tilt of the abutment should be corrected
- Sub-division III: Periodontally weak abutment. This abutment cannot take up occlusal load as effectively as healthy abutment
- Sub-division IV: Extensively damaged abutment. The abutment has good bone support but require extensive restoration, e.g. inlay, onlay, dowel core. The status of the abutment crown determines the type of attachment required for the FPD
- Sub-division V: Implant abutment. The abutment is an implant and the design of the prosthesis should be modified accordingly.

- Each sub-division can be further grouped into A and B:
  - A: Denotes that the support for one side of the edentulous space is taken from a single abutment
  - B: Denotes that the support for one side of the edentulous space is taken from more than one abutment tooth.

Objectives of Classification

It aids in visualising the following factors:
- Edentulous space location
- Occlusal load that is expected on the prosthesis
- Design of the prosthesis
- Detail of the design
- Status of the abutment teeth.

For Examples

Class I, Division I, Sub-division I-B

- In a case with missing first and second premolar, when there is healthy posterior teeth and periodontically compromised teeth it is a class I case as it involves the replacement of posterior teeth
- In this case, anterior teeth are periodontically compromised the posterior teeth provide the support
- So, it is a cantilever design which is grouped under division I
- The abutment that is used for support is healthy and falls under subdivision I
- A single molar cannot support two missing premolars in this case a second molar is used as an abutment
- So, in this case the support is taken from two abutment teeth on the same side of edentulous space so it is considered as sub-division I-B.

Class I, Division II, Sub-division IV-A

- In this case there are teeth present on either side of the edentulous space which are capable of providing support, additional support from adjacent teeth is not required
- In some cases both abutments are extremely damaged which requires special designs like inlay, only, precision attachment or a dowel core.

Class I, Division III, Sub-division I-A

- It is a more than one posterior edentulous space sharing a single abutment
- In this case all other abutment are healthy and they can provide support independently.

Question 2

Write about diagnosis and treatment planning of fixed partial denture.

Answer

Diagnosis

- Diagnosis and treatment planning are very important in the success of any prosthetic treatment
- The factors like dental caries, periodontal diseases affect the health of abutment leading to failure of the treatment
- The factors which help in proper diagnosis are history of the patient, clinical examination, diagnostic cast preparation
- The success of FPD depends on the healthy abutment teeth.

History

- A patient's history should include all necessary information concerning the reasons for seeking treatment along with any personal details and past medical and dental experiences that are pertinent. A screening questionnaire is useful for history taking
- Medical History: An accurate and current general medical history should include any medication the patient is taking as well as all relevant medical conditions
- Dental History: Primarily and significantly patient's periodontal, restorative and endodontic history should be noted. Orthodontic history should be an integral part of the assessment of a prosthodontic rehabilitation.

Clinical Examination

Clinical examination can be grouped as:
- Systemic examination
- Local examination.
  - Extra-oral examination
  - Intra-oral examination.

Systemic examination

Although the history has been taken the check up should be done to rule out if there is any systemic disease.

Local examination

- Extra-oral examination [temporomandibular joint (TMJ) evaluation]
  - The TMJ is palpated bilaterally just anterior to the auricular tragic
  - The maximum jaw opening which is less than 40 mm indicates jaw restrictions, it is because the average opening is more than 50 mm
  - When examining the mandibular movement clicking, crepitus or any alteration of the joint is noted

- ○ If there is any deviation from the midline it is recorded
- ○ Maximum lateral movement is measured which is normally 12 mm.
- ❑ Intra-oral examination
  - ○ Intra-oral examination is the hard tissue and soft tissue examination
  - ○ The following are the steps for checking it intra-orally:
    - ‣ It begins with patients oral hygiene
    - ‣ It should be examined if there is presence of attached gingiva or pressure of other occlusal disharmony
    - ‣ Other things include dental caries and periodontitis
    - ‣ Occlusion is also examined.

Diagnostic casts

- ❑ Diagnostic casts that are articulated are very important in the planning of fixed prosthodontics treatment
- ❑ They provide information which are static and dynamic in relation to the teeth
- ❑ It can be examined without interference from any protective neuromuscular reflexes
- ❑ Diagnostic casts also reveal those aspects of occlusion which are not detected within the confines at the tie of mouth examination
- ❑ Moreover, mounted diagnostic casts helps in analysing the dimensions of the edentulous space
- ❑ It can also determine the height, rotations, inclination of the abutment teeth
- ❑ The number, size and position of wear facets can be observed
- ❑ It also guides in analysing the amount of occlusal load from the opposing teeth.

Radiographic examination

Radiographs helps in providing the information to correlate the facts that have been collected during diagnosis, clinical examination or by evaluating the diagnostic casts.

Radiographs helps in:
- ❑ To calculate the crown root ratio
- ❑ The length, direction and configuration of its roots
- ❑ To determine the widening of periodontal ligament
- ❑ The level of alveolar bone
- ❑ If the previous restorations are good
- ❑ The size, number and location of caries
- ❑ Presence of any root stumps
- ❑ Soft tissue thickness.

Treatment Planning

The treatment should be done by evaluation of design of partial denture and based on the denture that best suits the patient.

Treatment planning depends on:
- ❑ Patients need
- ❑ The occlusion with the opposite tooth
- ❑ Identify the material that best suits the patients
- ❑ Appropriate prosthesis
- ❑ Residual ridge examination and examining the ridge defects which are corrected or to be corrected before prosthesis
- ❑ Selection of appropriate prosthesis
- ❑ Partial denture depends on the following factors:
  - ○ Periodontal and soft tissue factors
  - ○ Aesthetics
  - ○ Biomechanical factors.

Conventional Tooth Supported Fixed Partial Dentures

It is indicated for the following cases:
- ❑ There is absence of any soft tissue defect
- ❑ There is no systemic disorder related to salivation
- ❑ If there is xerostomia it is advised to use fluoride application
- ❑ Patients with no periodontal issues and healthy periodontal ligament
- ❑ Short and straight edentulous span.

Resin Bonded Fixed Partial Denture

They are given in patients with:
- ❑ When there is single missing anterior tooth or a premolar
- ❑ There is no presence of defect in abutment
- ❑ When axial inclination in the abutment is less that 15°
- ❑ With one missing molar which has least occlusal load
- ❑ When there is no deep vertical overlap
- ❑ Patients that are young and don't have any risk of caries and large pulp chambers.

Implant Supported Fixed Partial Denture

They are implemented when:
- ❑ There is high caries risk
- ❑ When abutment are missing for long span of time in edentulous areas
- ❑ Young adults with single tooth replacements
- ❑ When distal abutment is absent and there is good density in the bone is present.

SHORT ESSAY

Question 1

What are the indications and contraindications for fixed partial denture?

Answer

Indications

- It is indicated in patients that have low chances of dental caries and have good oral hygiene
- Its also indicated in cases where the abutment teeth are periodontically sound
- They are indicated if the retainers and abutments are very well designed
- Indicated when there is missing teeth or loss of tooth
- When there is fracture, discolouration and malformation of teeth
- When the edentulous span is straight and short.

Contraindications

- It is contraindicated in long span bridge
- When there is no support for prosthesis
- When there is presence of secure malocclusion
- With patients below 18 years old
- When the previous prosthesis done showed unfavourable response and there was reaction of the mucous membrane
- When there is lack of resilience of periodontal ligament, also known as aged mouth
- When root surface of tooth is greater than abutment tooth which is to be replaced.

SHORT NOTES

Question 1

Define onlay.

Answer

Onlay only incorporates a replacement for a tooth cusp by covering the area in which the missing cusp would be present. It is a inlay supplemented with occlusal veneer to restore large lesions.

Question 2

Define abutment.

Answer

Abutment is a natural tooth or implanted tooth substitute which is used to support or anchor a fixed or removable dental prosthesis or bridge.

Question 3

Define connectors.

Answer

- It is a part of partial denture that unites its components
- They are found between pontic and retainer
- They are movable as well as non movable
- The rigid connectors are immovable while non rigid connectors can be moved.

Question 4

Define pontic.

Answer

- It is an artificial tooth on a FPD
- It replaces the lost natural tooth and restore its functions which are usually occupy the space which has been previously occupied by natural crown
- Pontic are usually attached to the retainers in which the forces acting on it are transferred to the abutment through retainers.

Chapter 22: Treatment Planning and Mouth Preparation

LONG ESSAYS

Question 1

Classify pontic. Discuss in detail the various pontics used in fixed partial dentures.

Answer

Pontic

- It is defined as an artificial tooth on a fixed partial dentures (FPD) that replaces a missing tooth, restores its function and usually fills the space previously filled by a natural crown
- A pontic in which a concave gingival surface that overlaps the ridge buccally and lingually is called a saddle
- There are some short-term results, thats why it is not widely accepted
- The adaptation of pontic to the ridge is not acceptable
- They are difficult to maintain and there is accumulation of food debris which cannot be avoided
- Only the buccal and lingual ends of the gingival surface will contact the tissue there is no continuous contact between gingival surface and the saddle pontic
- If there is close contact and adaptation between mucosa and pontic there will be less chances of food accumulation
- There is difficulty in maintenance thats why its important to floss the teeth and the same instructions are given to the patient.

Classification of Pontics

Pontics are classified according to three types, which are as follows:
- On the basis of amount of mucosal contact
  - With mucosal contact
    - Saddle pontic
    - Ridge lap pontic
    - Modified ridge lap pontic
    - Ovate pontic.
  - Without mucosal contact.
    - Bullet pontic
    - Hygienic or sanitary pontic.
- On the basis of the type of material used
  - Metal and porcelain veneered pontic
  - Metal and resin veneered pontic
  - All metal pontic
  - All ceramic pontic.
- On the basis of method of fabrication.
  - Custom made pontic
  - Prefabricated pontic.
    - Trupontic
    - Inter-changeable facing
    - Sanitary pontic
    - Pin-facing pontic
    - Modified pin-facing pontic
    - Reverse pin-facing pontic
    - Harmony pontic
    - Porcelain Fused to metal pontic.
  - Prefabricated custom modified pontic.

Ovate Pontics

- They are evolved from root extended or root tipped pontics
- In cases, where the residual ridge has defects and is not completely healed
- The pontic is designed in such a way that the cervical end is extended
- They are also used in broad and flat ridges
- They are used into the defect of edentulous ridge.

Bullet-shaped Pontics

- They are used where aesthetics are of importance for the replacement of mandibular posterior teeth
- If there is presence of wide embrasures, it will lead to poor aesthetics
- The surface of this pontic is convex

- It helps in contacting tissue at one single point without pressure
- These pontics can be easily cleaned and maintained.

Sanitary or Hygienic Pontics

- In sanitary pontic the high occluso-gingival height should be at least 3 mm
- These pontics have zero tissue contact
- They are highly unaesthetic and easy to maintain
- They are mostly used in the posterior teeth
- There are more designs that can be fabricated in sanitary pontics.

Bar sanitary pontics

They have a flat gingival surface with adequate gingival clearance.

Conventional sanitary or fish belly pontic

- They are also called fish belly pontic due to their appearance
- The gingival surface is convex both on bucco-lingual and mesio-distal surface
- Its disadvantages are:
  - Decreased size of connectors
  - Lesser strength
  - It is difficult to maintain mesial and distal contours of the pontic.

Modified sanitary or perel pontic

- The arch shape helps the connectors to increase their size which further aids in better cleaning and maintaining of the pontic
- The gingival surface is concave mesio-distally
- The gingival surface is convex bucco-lingually
- Hyperparaboloid design is provided on the gingival surface of the pontic
- No fish belly limitations can be fulfilled.

Custom-made Pontics

- Wax pattern is prepared and cast to prepare pontic
- Most commonly used type of pontic
- Superior aesthetics and flexibility is offered.

Pre-fabricated Pontic Facings

- Commercially available as porcelain pontics
- They are adjusted according to individual requirement
- They are finally reglazed and fit to metal backing.

True Pontic

- It consist of a large gingival bulk, which can be adapted to ridge
- It is indicated in cases with limited inter arch distance.

Inter-changeable Facing

It consists of vertical slot in its flat lingual surface. The major disadvantage is its complex designing which leads to accumulation of plaque and gingival inflammation.

Sanitary Pontic

- They have slots on proximal surface to fit into metal projections made in FPD
- The facing has a flat occlusal surface which is customized as needed.

Pin Facing Pontic

- Lingual surface of this facing is flat and consist of pins for retention
- It is indicated in cases with reduced occluso-gingival height.

Modified Pin Facing Pontic

Here, the flat lingual surface of pin facing is modified by adding additional porcelain onto gingival portion of its lingual surface.

Reverse Pin Facing

- The pins in porcelain tooth are ground off and the tooth is altered and customized according to ridge
- Precision drill holes are made on lingual surface of facing and these acts as source of retention
- It is indicated for cases with deep overbite where short pins are required.

Harmony Pontic

- This consists of flat lingual surface with two retentive pins
- They are not indicated for cases with decrease occluso-gingival height.

Porcelain Fused to Metal Pontic

- It consist of metal core over which porcelain is fused to closely resemble the contour of a natural tooth
- It is more aesthetic and is indicated for anterior teeth.

Question 2

Write in brief about connectors.

Answer

Connector in a fixed partial denture can be defined as the portion of a fixed partial denture that unites the retainer(s) and pontic(s).

Connectors can be broadly classified as:
- Rigid connectors

- Non-rigid connectors.
  - Tenon-Mortise connectors
  - Loop connectors
  - Split pontic connectors
  - Cross pin and wing connectors.

Rigid Connectors

- Retainers and pontics are united with the help of rigid connectors in fixed partial dentures
- The entire load on the pontic can be transferred directly to the abutments rigid connectors are used.

Non-rigid Connectors

- When a there are non-parallel abutments and when a single path of insertion cannot be achieved these connectors are indicated
- There is a very limited movement between pontics and retainer.

Tenon Mortise Connector/Dovetail Connector

- They are with a male and female component
- The nonrigid connector consist of a mortise (female) prepared within a contours of retainer and a tenon (male) attached to pontic
- The alignment of dove tail connector is critical it must be parallel to the path of withdrawal of other retainer
- Paralleling is accomplished by dental surveyor
- The female component may be prepared free hand in wax pattern or with precision milling machine
- The female component is refined as necessary, the male key is fabricated with auto-polymerising resin and attached to pontic.

Loop Connectors

- The palatal connector seen in a spring cantilever fixed partial denture is a type of loop connector
- The connector consists of a loop on the lingual aspect of the prosthesis that connects adjacent retainers and/or pontics
- The loop may be cast from a platinum-gold palladium alloy wire
- Loop connectors are used when an existing diastema is to be maintained in a planned fixed prosthesis
- The loop should be carefully designed such that it is easy to maintain.

Split Pontic Connectors

- The distal segment is fabricated with a keyway to fit over the shoe
- Here the connector is incorporated within the pontic
- The pontic is split into mesial and distal segments
- They are used only in cases with a pier abutment
- Each of these segments are attached to their respective retainers
- The mesial segment is fabricated with a shoe/key
- The two components are designed by aligning in a surveyor.

Cross Pin and Wing Connector

- It is used for tilted abutments
- A wing is attached to distal retainer
- The wing along with distal retainer is termed as retainer using component
- The pontic is attached to mesial retainer and is designed to fit to wing in retainer wing component
- The pontic along with mesial retainer is turned as retainer point component
- After fabricating retainer wing and retainer pontic components, they are aligned on working cast and a 0.7 mm pinhole is drilled across wing and pontic using toward drill
- A rigid pin of 0.7 mm diameter is fabricated using same alloy
- The pin should be seated within pinhole created on wing and pontic and adjusted to its exact length
- After cementing the components, the pin is seated into the hole using punch and mallet.

SHORT ESSAY

Question 1

What are sanitary pontic?

Answer

Sanitary Pontics

- In sanitary pontic, the high occluso-gingival height should be at least 3 mm
- These pontics have zero tissue contact
- They are highly unaesthetic and easy to maintain
- They are mostly used in the posterior teeth
- There are more designs that can be fabricated in sanitary pontics.

Bar Sanitary Pontics

They have a flat gingival surface with adequate gingival clearance.

Conventional Sanitary or Fish Belly Pontic

- They are also called fish belly pontic due to their appearance
- The gingival surface is convex both on bucco-lingual and mesio-distal surface
- Its disadvantages are:
  - Decreased size of connectors
  - Lesser strength
  - It is difficult to maintain mesial and distal contours of the pontic.

Modified Sanitary or Perel Pontic

- The arch shape helps the connectors to increase their size which further aids in better cleaning and maintaining of the pontic
- The gingival surface is concave mesio-distally
- The gingival surface is convex bucco-lingually
- Hyperparaboloid design is provided on the gingival surface of the pontic
- No fish belly limitations can be fulfilled.

SHORT NOTES

Question 1

What are connectors in fixed partial dentures?

Answer

Rigid Connectors

- Retainers and pontics are united with the help of rigid connectors in fixed partial dentures
- The entire load on the pontic can be transferred directly to the abutments rigid connectors are used.

Non-rigid Connectors

- When a there are non-parallel abutments and when a single path of insertion cannot be achieved these connectors are indicated
- There is a very limited movement between pontics and retainer.

Question 2

What are tenon mortise connectors?

Answer

Tenon mortise connectors with a male and female component or dovetail connectors:

- The position of dovetail should be parallel to the path of withdrawal of the other retainer as this connection is very sensitive
- It consists of mortise prepared with the contours of the retainer and tenon which is attached to the pontic
- By using a dental surveyor paralleling can be attained in it
- The female component (mortise) is prepared using the milling machine using free hand in wax pattern
- Mortise is refined and tenon is fabricated with autopolymerising resin which is then attached to the pontic
- On other hand, special mandrel is embedded in the wax pattern and abutment retainer is cast
- Also a prefabricated plastic component for the mortise and tenon of a non connector is used as a additional method.

Question 3

What are split pontic connectors?

Answer

- Split pontic connectors are fabricated with the distal segment and keyway which fit over the shoe
- The connector is along the pontic
- Mesial and distal segments in the pontics are split
- On the pier abutment they are used
- Individual segments are attached to their respective retainers
- The fabrication with shoe/key is done in the medial segment.

Question 4

What are reverse pin facing?

Answer

- Nylon bristles are aligned to the drill holes and incorporated into the wax pattern of the backing
- The pins in the porcelain tooth are ground off and the tooth is altered and customized according to the ridge
- Precision drill holes are made on the lingual surface of the facing and these act as source of retention
- Commercially available porcelain denture teeth with pins can be altered to obtain this facing
- It is indicated for cases with deep overbite where short pins are required.

Question 5

What are loop connectors?

Answer

- The palatal connector seen in a spring cantilever fixed partial denture is a type of loop connector
- The adjacent retainer or pontics are connected by loop on the lingual aspect of the prosthesis
- The loop of the cast can be made from platinum-gold palladium alloy wire
- When an existing diastema has to be kept loop connectors in planned fixed prosthesis
- The loop should be easy to maintain.

Chapter 23

Occlusion

LONG ESSAYS

Question 1

Describe factors affecting mandibular movements and various concepts of occlusion in fixed partial dentures.

Answer

The following factors are said to have a direct influence over mandibular movement:
- Temporomandibular joint (TMJ)
- Occlusion
- Neuromuscular coordination
- Hinge axis
- Muscles and ligaments that are attached to it.

Determinants of Mandibular Movement

- The anatomic structures that allow and limit the movement of the mandible are known as its determinants
- They are of two types:
  1. Anterior determinants
  2. Posterior determinants.

Anterior Determinants

- It is also known as anterior controlling factors of mandibular movement
- Anterior teeth determine how anterior portion moves
- When the mandible protudes or moves laterally, the incisal edge of the mandibular teeth occlude with lingual surface of maxillary anterior teeth
- There is very little vertical guidance when it comes to mandibular teeth
- Anterior guidance is altered by pathologic conditions like caries or oral habits.

Posterior Determinants

- They are also called posterior controlling factors
- The angle at which the condyle moves away from the horizontal plane is called condylar guidance plane
- It is provided by temporomandibular joint (TMJ) for posterior portion of the mandible
- It is unalterable in healthy patients but they are altered under conditions such as trauma, surgical procedures or pathosis.

Vertical Determinants of Occlusal Morphology

- The vertical determinants of occlusal morphology are factors influenced by height of the cusp and the depth of fossae
- It is determined by three factors:
  1. The posterior controlling factors of mandibular movement (condylar guidance)
  2. The anterior controlling factor (anterior guidance)
  3. The nearness of the cusp to these controlling factors.

Horizontal Determinants

- Horizontal determinants are the relationships which influence the direction of ridges and grooves on the occlusal surface
- The anatomy of the occlusal surface is influenced by the relationships between tooth passing across it and its movement.

Theories and Concepts

The various theories and concepts of occlusal are discussed in the following section:
1. Bonwill theory of occlusion
2. Conical theory of occlusion
3. Spherical theory of occlusion.

1. Bonwill theory of occlusion in 1858

- Bonwill developed the theory of equilateral triangle, in which there was a 4-inch distance between the condyles

Chapter 23 Occlusion

and between each condyle and incisor point. This theory proposed that teeth move in relation to each other as guided by the condylar controls and the incisal point
- In 1950's–60's, another group of researchers headed by Mc Collum believed that if the rotational centres in the condyles could be located and if the border movements of these rotational centres were recorded and reproduced on a sophisticated three-dimensional articulator, then all functional movements for the patient could also be reproduced by that instrument which are:
  - Establishing the hinge axis (location of the rotational centres of condyles)
  - Using a pantographic tracing to record the three-dimensional envelope of motion
  - Centric relation (CR) = Centric occlusion (CO) or intercuspal position (ICP)
  - Bilateral balance with eccentric jaw movements.

2. **Conical theory of occlusion by R.E. Hall (1915)**
- Theory proposed that the lower teeth move over the surfaces of the upper teeth as over the surfaces of a cone with a generating angle of 45 degree and with a central axis of the cone tipped at a 45 degree angle to the occlusal plane
- The Hall automatic articulator designed by R.E. Hall is an example of such a theory.

3. **Spherical theory of occlusion by G.S. Monson in 1918.**
- This theory was based on the observations of natural teeth and skulls made by Von Spee. This form of occlusion is sometimes referred to as having Monson's Curve
- The spherical theory shows the lower teeth moving over the surface of the upper teeth as over the surface of a sphere of a diameter 8 inches (20 cms)
- The center of the sphere is located in the region of the glabella and surface of the sphere passes through the glenoid fossa along the articulating eminences or concentric with them.

Mutually Protected System

- The *Cuspid Protection Theory* was proposed by two researchers; Stalled and Stuart (1960)
- This theory states that the balancing contents during eccentric jaw movements were eliminated by making the canines on the working side disocclude the posterior teeth
- This theory developed into mutually protected system, i.e., CR = CO. During lateral or protusive excursions, there is no posterior occlusal contacts
- The fabrication of the two piece custom built metal clutches are done for accurate impression.

Rationale
- Anterior teeth have an advantage over posterior teeth when it comes to mechanical properties
- As the forces generated by muscles of mastication is comparatively lesser when the tooth contact occurs more anteriorly
- The class III lever arm at the anterior teeth exerts lesser pressure, therefore, the forces by the musculature are less effective at the anteriors and in turn also results in lesser load on them.

Features
- When condyles are in their most superior position uniform contact of all the teeth happens
- With functional jaw movement, the anterior tooth contact is harmonised
- At the lateral or protusive movement, there is no contact of the posterior teeth
- CR = CO or ICP.

Optimum Occlusion

- When there is optimum occlusion the load exerted on the dentition should be distributed equally. When there is any restorative procedure to be implemented, it will affect the occlusal stability which in turn affects the timing and the intensity of the elevator muscle activity
- However, horizontal forces on any tooth should be avoided and also the loading should be parallel to the long axis of the teeth. In addition, the cusps of the posterior teeth should have sufficient height to improve mastication.

Biological Occlusion

A flexible concept of occlusion has the concept to achieve an occlusion that functions to restore health. Though this occlusion may involve malposed teeth, evidence of wear, missing teeth and CR = CO, do not need occlusal therapy.

Goals
- There should be no interference between CR and CO
- There should be minimum of one contact per tooth
- There should be no balancing contact
- There should be cusp to fossa relationship
- Remove the possibility of the functional mobility of teeth
- There should be no posterior contact with protusion
- The occlusal contacts are eliminated on inclined planes
- A cusp to fossa occlusal arrangement should be made
- Elimination of occlusal contacts on inclined planes to increase the stability of teeth.

Myocentric Occlusion

Myomonitor produces relaxation of the mandibular muscles, which then initiates controlled isotonic muscle contraction. This then propels mandible from the rest position to a neuromuscularly oriented occlusal position in space.

Pathologic Occlusion

When sufficient disharmony exists between the teeth and TMJ, which leads to symptoms that require intervention.

Question 2

What is occlusal rehabilitation? Also describe in detail the remounting procedure.

Answer

Occlusal Rehabilitation

- It is defined as the intentional alteration of the occlusal surfaces of teeth to change their form
- It is a diagnostic procedure that is done before the fabrication of fixed partial dentures
- The procedure should be done ideally with all the patients. When fixed dentures are constructed against complete dentures and removable partial dentures, this process of occlusal rehabilitation becomes more important.

Correction of Occlusal Errors in Complete Dentures Opposing Fixed Partial Dentures

The process of selective grinding is performed to correct the minor processing errors that occur during fabrication of the denture. The process of checking occlusal errors involves the following steps:

- The patient is guided to his centric position manually and the mandible is guided to its posterior most position
- The patient is instructed to slowly close his mouth and asked to indicate when he feels feather touch contact between the teeth
- Patient should be instructed not to move the mandible anteriorly during this process
- After the feather touch contact is made between the natural dentition, the patient is asked to close his mouth tightly
- It should be noted that if the patient slides his mandible to obtain a tight closure, if he does, it denotes that there are discrepancies in the occlusion.

Remounting the Dentures

- It can be defined as any method used to relate restorations to an articulator for the analysis and/or to assist in the development of a plan for occlusal equilibration or reshaping
- The occlusal errors are checked and the remounting should be done to correct these errors
- Remount procedure is used to accurately relocate the correction of the errors
- Remounting is done in laboratory or clinically by the means of using inter-occlusal records
- The advantages of lab remounting over clinical remounting are the following:
  - As the patient can not remain in the same position for uncertain period of time during clinical remounting, therefore, lab procedure is preferred as time dislocation
  - Shifting of the denture to a desired place for convenience is possible in lab remounting
  - Eccentric closure of the mandible.

Laboratory Remount Procedures

- These procedures are used to used to correct only processing errors such as mild displacement of the tooth
- It cannot be used to correct errors that are made during impression making or during jaw relation
- The technique to re-establish occlusion during these procedures is as follows:
  - Firstly, all the movements are carried out in the articulator and then the identification of occlusal interference is done using an articulating paper
  - It should be noted that the denture should not be separated from the cast after processing
  - Occlusal grinding is done after identified contacts are ground in relation to the opposing teeth. The denture is then removed from its casts and is polished
  - If new dentures are planned, new centric and eccentric records are need to be obtained
  - Same articulator is used for teeth arrangement and remounting is done
  - Reattachment of upper and lower cast to the articulator is done.

Clinical Remount Procedures

- The procedure is done using inter-occlusal records
- These records are made in the centric and eccentric positions
- The process is a part of finishing the fixed prosthesis
- It should be performed prior cementing the fixed partial denture.

Clinical remounting by making inter-occlusal record in centric position

- The wax is sealed to the denture using a warm spatula

- A bowl with hot water at temperature of 54° is used for wax to be dipped which softens the wax
- Maxillary denture is lubricated using a vaseline, the occlusal surface is lubricated before the insertion
- After the denture is removed, the mandibular partial denture is kept in cold water which hardens the wax and record is then taken
- The mandible is guided to the centric position and the patient is asked to close his mouth
- This is done so that the maxillary teeth penetrates about 1–1.5 mm deep into the wax
- There should be 1 mm deep occlusal imprints in the wax without any perforation
- Two layers of Alu wax is placed over the posterior teeth
- The process is repeated with complete closure of mouth
- There should be no torquing and tilted force.

Remounting using centric record

- Using centric record against articulated maxillary denture, mandibular denture is positioned and articulated
- The maxillary denture is remounted with remount cast on the articulator
- The centric element should be against the centric stop when articulator is placed.

Remounting using eccentric relation record

- After centric relation, record the eccentric record
- The process of eccentric record hold similarity with that of centric relation record
- Inspection of he centric relationship should be done prior the proceeding to eccentric relations
- Re-articulating the dentures is contraindicated.

Transferring the eccentric records to the articulator

- The dentures are positioned on the articulated remount casts
- For the upper compartment of the articulator to move posteriorly, the protrusive inter-occlusal record is placed on the mandibular teeth and the condylar guidance is modified till the maxillary denture teeth fit perfectly in to the protrusive record
- The values of horizontal condylar guidance should be recorded and noted on the nearby mounting plaster
- Using the horizontal condylar guidance value (H), lateral condylar guidance (L) can be calculated using the formula $L = (H/8) + 12$
- Selective grinding can now be done as the programmed articulator with remounted casts and dentures are ready.

Question 3

Elaborate the process of selective grinding.

Answer

- Selective grinding is defined as the intentional alteration of the occlusal surfaces of teeth to change their form
- The process of selective grinding different from one teeth to other
- The selective grinding procedures in relation to anatomic and non-anatomic teeth are discussed in the following section.

Correcting the Identified Occlusal Errors in Anatomic Teeth

Selective grinding procedures to correct identified occlusal interferences in the centric relation are carried out followed by the correction of the errors in the eccentric relation.

Selective Grinding in Anatomic Teeth in Centric Relation

- The process is performed in laboratory and is done on remounted casts
- Between the occlusal surface of opposing teeth articulating paper with minimal thickness is placed
- Without sliding against the teeth, the articulator is opened and articulating paper is removed
- On the occlusal surface the deflective contacts can be seen where the articulating paper was positioned
- Using a Chayes stone No. 16, 11 and 5, the grinding is done to relieve the contacts
- It should be remembered that grinding is not done on the cusps or cuspal inclines. It is always done on the fossa.

Selective Grinding in Anatomic Teeth in Eccentric Relation

- Subsequent to occlusal reshaping in centric position, the articulating paper is positioned between the teeth and the articulator is moved to lateral position
- If the incisal pin rises away from the incisal table during laterotrusion, selective grinding is required on the working side
- Contacts between the maxillary buccal and mandibular lingual cusps appears on the non-working side
- Selective grinding on the working side should follow the BULL rule (buccal cusps of upper and lingual cusps of lower teeth) and it should be repeated till the incisal pin contacts the incisal table during lateral movement
- On the balancing side, markings will appear on the maxillary palatal cusps and mandibular lingual cusps and

the reduction should be done on the lingual slope of the buccal cusps
- Similarly, protrusive interferences should also be corrected by selective grinding.

Correcting the Identified Occlusal Errors in Non-anatomic Teeth

- Selective grinding after identifying the deflective contacts with an articulating paper is done on the occlusal surface of tipped or elongated teeth
- Grinding is contraindicated on the disto-buccal portion of the mandibular second molar during eccentric movements
- The lingual portion of the occlusal surface of maxillary second molar is grinded for removing interferences on the balancing side
- Eccentric movements are made on the upper member of the articulator by placing milling the teeth by placing abrasive paste between them
- Moreover, spot grinding can be done to correct minor interferences in centric relation after grinding with abrasive paste.

SHORT NOTES

Question 1
What are the indications for full mouth rehabilitation?

Answer
- It is indicated if there is a change in vertical dimension
- If the remaining teeth have altered occlusal plane such as supra-erupted teeth
- If a combination of removable and fixed partial dentures needs to be inserted for a patient
- In cases where replacement of both anterior and posterior teeth is required
- In conditions, where maxillary single complete dentures are to oppose a mandibular distal extension denture base.

Question 2
Mention the uses of a pantograph.

Answer
- It is an extra-oral tracing device which aids in designing the harmonious relationship between the occlusal surfaces of the restoration and mandibular movements
- It has six sets of styli and flags, which is used to record the mandibular movements
- It is used to record the envelop of motion
- It produces canine protective occlusion, where CR = CO
- It is used in developing eccentric relation of cusps
- It also directs the forces on a restoration along the long axis of the tooth.

Question 3
What is selective grinding?

Answer
- According to GPT, selective grinding is defined as the intentional alteration of the occlusal surfaces of teeth to change their form
- The process of selective grinding different from one teeth to other
- These procedures to correct identified occlusal interferences in the centric relation are carried out followed by the correction of the errors in the eccentric relation.

Question 4
What are the types of occlusion in fixed partial denture?

Answer

Types of Occlusion in Fixed Partial Denture
The types of occlusion infixed partial denture are as follows:
- Canine-guided/protected occlusion
- Bilateral balance
- Unilateral balanced occlusion
- Optimum occlusion
- Mutually protected occlusion
- Centric occlusion
- Biological occlusion.

CHAPTER 24

Abutments

LONG ESSAYS

Question 1

What is abutment? Explain cantilever, pier and tilted abutments.

Answer

Abutment

- An abutment is defined as a tooth, a portion of a tooth, or that portion of a dental implant that serves to support and/or retain a prosthesis.
- An ideal abutment should have the following characteristics:
  - It should have proper gingival contour
  - There should be no periodontal diseases
  - The crown root ratio should be ideal
  - The thickness of enamel and dentine should be proper
  - There should be adequate bone support.

Cantilever Abutments

- Cantilever fixed partial dentures are defined as having one or more abutments at one end of the prosthesis while the other end is unsupported (Fig. 24.1)
- The reason why cantilever abutment becomes more and more important is the fact that the prosthesis involved are going to withstand forces that are more than the normal forces
- The requisites for a cantilever abutment are:
  - They should have good periodontal attachment (covering maximum rot surface)
  - It should have good alveolar support
  - There should be favourable root length, shape, and crown length
  - There should be favourable arch-to-arch relationship favourable tooth-to-tooth relationship
  - The final retainer should be more retentive there should be sufficient amount of tooth structure that needs to be present

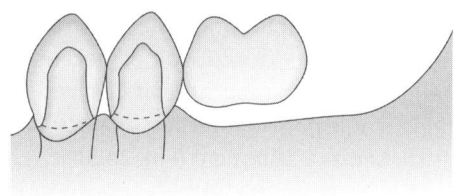

Fig. 24.1: Cantilever Abutments

- In required situations it should replace the lateral incisor with canine support also the first premolar with second premolar and first molar support
- The teeth with excessive crown damage are contraindicated
- Teeth that have very short roots are contraindicated.

Pier Abutments

- A pier abutment is a single tooth adjoining two edentulous spaces on either side (Fig. 24.2)
- Though, the single tooth acts like an abutment for both the edentulous spaces, it creates unbalanced forces leading to trauma of the periodontium
- The forces exerting on one end of the prosthesis will have the tendency to lift the other end such as a lever using the abutment as a fulcrum and in turn will reduce the life span of the retainer
- Therefore, to overcome these difficulties, a stress breaker, a non-rigid connector with a key in a keyway is provided near the pier abutment.

Tilted Abutments

- The difficulty that occurs with some frequency is the mandibular molar abutment that has tilted mesially into the space formerly occupied by the lost natural teeth anterior to it
- It is not possible to prepare the abutment teeth for a fixed partial denture along the long axes of the respective teeth and achieve a common path of insertion

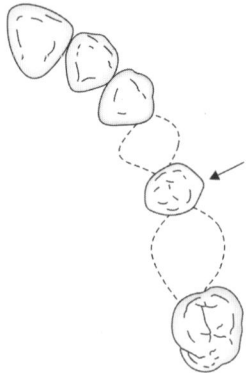

Fig. 24.2: Pier Abutments

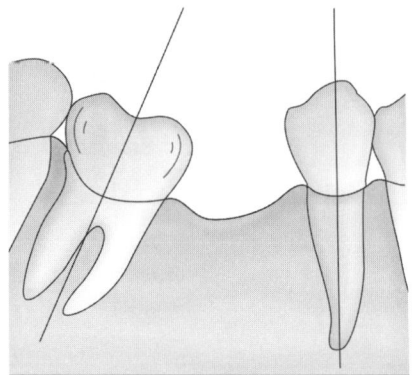

Fig. 24.3: Tilted Abutments

- There is a further complication if the third molar is present
- Tilted abutments are usually avoided because they have complex design when fabrication is involved
- To obtain a single path of insertion is difficult when tilted tooth is chosen as a abutment (**Fig. 24.3**).

Mesial reduction of third molar

- In this type of abutment, medial surface of the mandibular molar is reduced to the point where it becomes parallel to the long axis of the other abutment
- This process makes the insertion of the crown over the second molar abutment easy.

Non-rigid connector

- They are also called as key-keyway connectors
- They are prepared parallel to the long axis of the tilted second molar
- This is done so that the fixed partial denture is inserted along the long axis of the second molar to slide into the keyway of the anterior abutment.

Telescopic crown

- The telescopic bridge or prosthesis is a dual supported (teeth and gums) removable coverage restoration designed to fit over your natural teeth and gum areas in order to replace missing teeth
- The telescopic denture consists of:
  - The primary crowns or caps made of precious or non precious dental alloys that will be cemented on the prepped teeth
  - The secondary crowns (dental alloys) that are slipping over the primary caps and thus maintaining the bridge through sliding friction tight on the teeth
  - The secondary crowns have facings (surfaces) of acrylic resin with ceramic fillers
  - The framework made out of non precious dental alloy is embedded in plastic (acrylic resin) and supports the acrylic teeth which will replace the own missing teeth
  - In this process, the tooth is reduced and a coping or retainer is fabricated over the tooth that the contour of the crown is altered to receive a second crown which is a telescopic crown the fabrication is done with vertical slots in the vertical direction.

Question 2

Write in detail about prier abutments.

Answer

- A pier abutment is a single tooth adjoining two edentulous spaces on either side
- Though, the single tooth acts like an abutment for both the edentulous spaces, it creates unbalanced forces leading to trauma of the periodontium
- The forces exerting on one end of the prosthesis will have the tendency to lift the other end such as a lever using the abutment as a fulcrum and in turn will reduce the life span of the retainer
- Therefore, to overcome these difficulties, a stress breaker, a non-rigid connector with a key in a keyway is provided near the pier abutment
- The keyway of the stress breaker is positioned on the distal surface of the pier abutment whereas the key is attached to the mesial surface of the mesial pontic of the distal edentulous space
- In normal situation, excessive stress is transferred through the connector to the pier abutment
- However, forces acting on the distal end of the distal edentulous space in pier abutment disengages the connector and prevent excessive stress
- In case where the pier abutment is mobile or the posterior abutment opposes an edentulous space or a removable partial denture, a non-rigid connector is contraindicated and a rigid connector is used.

Chapter 24 Abutments

SHORT ESSAYS

Question 1

Describe implant surgery.

Answer

It involves the surgical placement of the implant. The procedure can either be done in one or two stages.

Surgical Guide Template

- They are the appliances which act as guide which helps in the placing the implant during implant surgery
- They are used to delineate the embrasures that can occur between two adjacent implants
- They are used to locate the implants on the ridge
- They are used to identify level of cement-enamel junction and also tooth emergency profile of the implant
- They are used to align the implants along the long axis of the completed restorations.

Single Stage Surgery

In this process the process of the surgically accessing and the placement of the implants is done in a single procedure.

Two Stage Surgery

- It is done in two phases
- In the first phase the surgery is proceed with exposure of the surgical site and the implant is placed and the osseo-integration is allowed
- The second phase starts in six months time. The surgical site is exposed one again and a super structure is placed.

Question 2

Describe about complications of implant abutments.

Answer

Bone Loss

The bone loss around the implant is treated as the most complicated situation happening with dental implants the bone loss that exceeds 0.2 mm is considered as the cause for worry.

Factors Associated with Bone Loss

- Unsuccessful osseo-integration
- Instability of the implant
- Excessive occlusal forces
- Presence of periimplantitis
- Tobacco chewing smoking,diabetes
- Technical complications that involve implant body/fixture fracture
- Abutment screw fracture
- Gaps between implants part which allows bacterial colonisation
- Trauma during healing phase
- Abutment fracture
- Inadequate fit of prosthesis
- Fractured prosthesis.

SHORT NOTES

Question 1

What is pier abutment?

Answer

- A pier abutment is a single tooth adjoining two edentulous spaces on either side
- In pier abutment a single tooth act as an abutment for both the edentulous spaces.

Question 2

What are the ideal characteristics of an abutment?

Answer

An ideal abutment should have the following characteristics:
- Ideal crown root ratio
- Adequate thickness of enamel and dentin
- Adequate bone support
- Absence of periodontal disease
- Proper gingival contour.

Question 3

What are telescopic crown?

Answer

- Here, the tooth is reduced considerably
- A coping or retainer is fabricated over the tooth so that it alters the contour of the crown
- This crown should be fabricated with vertical slots so that it can receive a second crown (telescopic crown) in a vertical direction.

Question 4

What are the indications for implant placement?

Answer

- In a partially edentulous patient who is unable to wear a removable partial denture or complete denture
- For long-span fixed partial dentures with poor prognosis
- Unfavourable number and location of potential tooth abutments
- Single tooth loss that would necessitate preparation of undamaged teeth for a fixed prosthesis, e.g. missing single lateral incisors.

Chapter 25: Tooth Preparations

LONG ESSAYS

Question 1

Write in brief about tooth preparation and its principles in fixed prosthesis.

Answer

Tooth Preparation

The process of removal of disease and/or healthy enamel and dentine and cementum to shape a tooth to receive a restoration.

Principles

According to Shillingburg:
- Preservation of tooth structure
- Retention and resistance form
- Structural durability
- Marginal integrity
- Preservation of the periodontium.

Preservation of Tooth Structure

- While replacing a lost tooth structure, a restoration must preserve the remaining tooth structure as much as possible
- Tooth structure is conserved by using the following guidelines:
  - Use of partial coverage rather than complete coverage restorations
  - Preparation of teeth with minimum practical convergence angle (taper) between axial walls
  - Preparation of the occlusal surface so reduction follows the anatomic planes to give uniform thickness in the restoration
  - Preparation of the axial surfaces so that the tooth structure is removed evenly, if necessary, teeth should be orthodontically repositioned
  - Selection of a conservative margin compatible with the other principles of tooth preparation
  - Avoidance of unnecessary apical extension of the preparation.

Retention and Resistance Form

- Post retention refers to the ability of post to resist vertical dislodging forces
- Post resistance refers to the ability of the post and the tooth to withstand the lateral and rotational forces.

Preservation of tooth structure

- One should try to preserve maximum of the coronal and radicular tooth structure whenever possible
- Minimal removal of additional radicular dentin for post space preparation should be the criteria
- Further enlargement of posts only weakens the tooth
- Minimal enlargement of post space means a post must be made of a strong material than can withstand functional and parafunctional forces.

Ferrule effect

- Ferrule is defined as band of metal which encircles the external surface of residual tooth
- It is formed by walls and margins of the tooth
- If artificial crown extends apical to margins of the core, and encircles sound tooth structure for 360 degree, the crown serves as reinforcing ring
- In this way ferrule helps to protect the root from vertical fracture
- It has been seen that a ferrule with 1–2 mm of vertical tooth structure doubles the resistance to fracture than in teeth without any ferrule effect
- This is called as crown ferrule.

Mode of Failure

- All post systems show some percentage of failure but with variable range
- Post failures are higher in cases of non-restorable teeth.

Retrievability

- Ideally, a post system selected should be such that endodontic treatment fails, or failure of post and core occurs, it should be retrievable
- Metal posts especially the cast post and core system is difficult to remove
- Fiber posts are easy to retrieve whereas zirconium and ceramic posts are difficult to remove
- Posts can be removed by:
  - Use of rotary instruments and solvents
  - Use of ultrasonic
  - Using special kits like Messeran kit, post removal system and endodontic extractors.

Taper

- The axial walls of the preparation must taper slightly to permit the restoration to seat
- A slight convergence, or taper is necessary when preparing a tooth
- The sum of the degree of taper is called as degree of convergence
- The relationship of one wall of a preparation to the long axis of that preparation is the inclination of that wall
- Theoretically maximum retention is obtained when a tooth preparation is having parallel walls, but slight taper is required to avoid undercuts and complete seating of restoration
- Recommended convergence between opposing walls is 6 degree
- A tapered diamond bur will impart an inclination of 2–3 degrees to any surface it cuts, if the shank of the instrument is held parallel to the intended path of insertion of the preparation
- Two opposing surfaces, each with, a 3 degree inclination, would give the preparation –6 degree taper
- Tooth preparation taper should be kept minimal because of its adverse effects on retention
- The degree of taper is inversely proportional to the retention form
- Resistance area decreases as taper increases.

Freedom of displacement

- Retention is improved by geometrically limiting the numbers of paths along which a restoration can be removed from the tooth preparation
- Maximum retention is achieved when there is only one path
- Limiting the freedom of displacement from torquing or twisting forces in a horizontal plane increases the resistance of a restoration.

Length

- Occluso-gingival length is an important factor in both retention and resistance
- Longer preparations will have more surface area and therefore will be more retentive
- The length must be great enough to interfere with the arc of casting pivoting about a point on the margin on the opposite side of the restoration
- The walls of shorter preparations should have little taper, if possible to increase the resistance.

Substitution of internal features

- The basic unit of retention for a cemented restoration is two opposing axial walls with a minimal taper
- It may not be possible always to use opposing walls for retention
- Therefore, internal features such as the groove, the box form and the pin hole can be substituted for an axial wall or for each other.

Path of insertion

- The path of insertion is an imaginary line along which the restoration will be placed onto or removed from the preparation
- If the center of the occlusal surface of a preparation is viewed with one eye from a distance of approximately 30 cm (12 inches), it is possible to sight down the axial walls of a preparation with a minimum taper
- However, it is possible to sight down the axial walls, of a preparation with a reverse (i.e., undercut) taper of 8 degrees when both eyes are open
- The path of insertion must be considered in two dimensions namely; facio-lingually and mesio-distally
- The facio-lingual orientation of the path can affect the aesthetics of metal-ceramic or partial veneer crowns
- The mesiodistal inclination of the path must parallel the contact areas of adjacent teeth
- If the path is inclined mesially or distally, the restoration will be held up at the proximal contact areas and be locked out.

Structural Durability

- A restoration must contain a bulk of material that is adequate to withstand the forces of occlusion

- The bulk must be confined to the space created by the tooth preparation.

Occlusal reduction

- Most important feature for providing adequate bulk of metal and strength to restoration
- Amount of occlusal reduction:
  - For gold alloys: 1.5 mm (functional cusp), 1.0 mm (non-functional cusp)
  - For porcelain fused to metal: 1.5–2.0 mm (functional cusp), 1.0–1.5 mm (nonfunctional cusp)
  - For all ceramic crowns: 2.0 mm
- Occlusal reduction should reproduce basic inclined planes rather than being cut as one flat plane
- Functional cusp bevel: It is an integral part of the occlusal reduction
  - A wide bevel on the lingual inclines of the maxillary lingual cusps and the buccal inclines of the mandibular buccal cusps provides space for an adequate bulk of metal in an area of heavy occlusal contact
  - If a wide bevel is not placed on the functional cusp, several problems may occur:
    - If the crown is waxed and cast to normal contour it can cause a thin area or perforation in the casting
    - To prevent this crown may be waxed to optimal thickness resulting in over contouring and poor occlusion
    - If an attempt is made to obtain space for an adequate bulk in a normally contoured casting without a bevel, it will result in over inclination of the buccal surface which will destroy excessive tooth structure while lessening retention.

Axial reduction

- It plays an important role in securing space for an adequate thickness of restorative material
- Inadequate axial reduction can cause thin walls and a weak restoration subjected to distortion or a bulbous, over contoured restoration which will strengthen the restoration but may have a disastrous effect on periodontium
- There are other features that serve to provide space for metal that will improve the rigidity and durability of the restoration
  - Offset
  - Occlusal shoulder
  - Isthmus
  - Proximal groove
  - Box.

Marginal Integrity

The restoration can survive in the biological environment of the oral cavity only if the margins are closely adapted to the cavo surface finish line of the preparation.

Margin placement

- Whenever possible the margin of the preparation should be supra-gingival
- Advantages of supra-gingival margins are:
  - They can be easily finished
  - They are more easily kept clean
  - Easy to make impressions with less damage to soft tissue
  - Restorations are easily evaluated at recall.
- Subgingival margins of cemented restorations are a major factor in periodontal disease
- A subgingival margin is justified if any of the following pertains
- Dental caries, cervical erosion extend subgingivally
- Proximal contact area extends to the gingival crest
- Additional retention is needed
- Margin of a metal-ceramic crown is to be hidden behind the labiogingival crest
- Root sensitivity not controlled by more, conservative means like the application of dentin bonding agents
- Modification of axial contour is indicated.

Margin adaptation

- The junction between a cemented restoration and the tooth is always a potential site for recurrent caries because of the dissolution of luting agent and inherent roughness
- The more accurately the restoration is adapted to the tooth, the lesser the chance of recurrent caries or periodontal disease.

Finish line requirements

- The point at which a preparation terminates on the tooth is called the finish line. It is also defined as the peripheral extension of a tooth preparation
- The finish line serves the following functions:
  - During visual evaluation of the tooth preparation, it is a measure of the amount of tooth structure already removed. It also delineates the extent of the cut in an apical direction. The more distinct it is, the better it serves these purposes
  - The finish line is one of the features that can be used to evaluate the accuracy of the impression made for indirect procedures

Essential Quick Review: Prosthodontics

- In the die, a distinct finish line helps to evaluate the quality of the die and helps in accurate die trimming
- The correct marginal adaptation of the wax pattern depends on an obvious finish line
- The evaluation of the restoration is also aided by a proper finish line
- At cementation, a sharp finish line aids in determining whether the restoration is fully seated.

Question 2

Discuss in brief about preparation of all-ceramic crowns.

Answer

Crown

An artificial crown is a fixed restoration of the entire coronal part of a natural tooth that restores anatomy, function and esthetics, usually of metal, porcelain, synthetic resin, or combinations.

All-ceramic Restorations/Porcelain Jacket Crown

Armamentarium

- Mouth Mirror
- Periodontal probe
- Explorer
- Chisels and hatchets
- High- and low-speed handpiece
- Thin tapering fissure diamonds
- Narrow round tipped tapered diamonds regular and coarse grit
- Flat-end tapered diamond regular grit
- Football shaped diamond
- Finishing stones and carbides.

Tooth Preparation Steps for All-ceramic Restorations on Upper Central Incisor

- Placement of depth orientation grooves
- Incisal reduction
- Facial reduction
- Lingual reduction
- Axial reduction
- Lingual axial reduction
- Marginal development and refinement.

Placing of depth orientation grooves

- Three depth orientation grooves, 1.0 mm deep, are placed. One in the middle of the facial wall and one each in the mesio-facial and disto-facial transitional line angles in the incisal edge
- Two more depth orientation grooves of 2.0 mm depth are placed on the incisal half
- 2 mm deep grooves are placed on the incisal edge for incisal reduction.

Incisal reduction

- Instrument used is flat-end tapered diamond
- The completed incisal reduction should provide 1.5-2 mm clearance for porcelain in all excursive movements of the mandible.

Facial reduction

This is done in two stages:

1. Reduction of incisal half of facial surface
   - A coarse, flat-ended diamond or No. 700 carbide bur is used to plane away tooth structure between the depth orientation grooves, on the incisal half, at a 450 angle to the long axis of the tooth in a normal occlusal relationship
   - The reduction is done parallel to the original contour of the tooth to provide uniform porcelain thickness and good aesthetics.

2. Reduction of gingival portion of facial surface.
   - Gingival portion of the labial surface is reduced with a flat-end tapered diamond in a flat plane perpendicular to the long axis of the tooth to a depth of 1.0 mm
   - The reduction is carried out with cervical component parallel to the proposed path of withdrawal
   - This reduction extends till the labio-proximal line angles
   - The reduction is done on half of the facial surface at a time.

Lingual reduction

- Depth orientation grooves of 0.8 mm depth are placed
- Football-shaped diamond/small wheel diamond is used for lingual reduction
- Reduction is carried out until a clearance of 1 mm in mandibular excursive movements are obtained.

Axial reduction

- A thin tapered fissure diamond is used to break the point with the adjacent tooth. While breaking the contact the adjacent tooth should not be abraded
- The mesial and distal areas are first reduced to a 20 to 50 taper without establishing a shoulder at this time.

Lingual axial reduction

- Instrument used for tooth preparation is flat-end tapered diamond
- The same path of withdrawal as that of the facial preparation is followed with lingual axial reduction

- A depth groove is placed in the middle of the cingulum wall
- The preparation of 2–5 degree taper is done from the centre of the cingulum wall until the lingual shoulder meets the facial shoulder
- A 0.75 mm cingulum shoulder is placed with a flat-ended tapered diamond.

Instrument used for marginal development and refinement

- An end-cutting bur held perpendicular to the shoulder can be used for lowering margin
- A sharp chisel is used to remove undermined enamel and finishing the shoulder
- The axial walls are smoothed and all the sharp line angles and point angles are rounded
- An acceptable emergence profile needs to be created for good aesthetics.

Variation in Margin Preparation

- Instead of shoulder preparation heavy chamfer can also prepared
- For sub gingival margin placement, a gingival retraction is done before the preparation for good access and less trauma to gingival tissue
- Initial preparation is followed by refinement with chisels
- The completed shoulder should be 1 mm wide, smooth continuous and without any irregularities.

Indication

In cases with high aesthetic requirement with sound tooth structure.

Contraindications

- Where a more conservative restoration can be used
- Not recommended for molar teeth
- Where increased occlusal load are present
- When adequate support cannot be provided
- When an even shoulder width cannot be prepared.

Advantages

- A similar shade for luting agent can be selected
- It has good biocompatibility
- It has superior aesthetics
- It is very translucent as that of natural tooth.

Disadvantages

- It is of very low strength if metal reinforcing substructure is not included
- It is very difficult to get a well-fitting margin
- In comparison to metal ceramic they are less conservative
- Proper preparation designed leads successful restoration
- In long duration of fixed partial denture they cannot be used as retainers
- Large cross-sectional dimension connectors need to be incorporated for all-ceramic restorations to have bulk of material
- Due to large connectors, impingement on the interdental papilla can lead to periodontal failure
- Wear on the functional surfaces of opposing natural teeth.

Full Metal Crowns/Full Cast

Armamentarium

- High and low-speed contra-angles
- Tapered carbide bur used for occlusal guiding grooves, additional retentive features
- Round-end tapered diamond regular (0.8 mm) used for occlusal reduction, axial reduction and chamfer preparation
- Round-end tapered diamond fine grit for finishing
- Utility wax and wax caliper for verification of occlusal clearance.

Tooth Preparation Steps for a Full Metal Crown on Mandibular First Molar

- Placement of occlusal guiding grooves
- Occlusal reduction
- Placement of functional cusp bevel
- Placement of axial alignment grooves
- Axial reduction
- Margin placement
- Finishing of preparation.
- Metals that can be used are as follows:
  - Gold alloys
  - Base metal alloys.

Placement of occlusal guiding grooves

- A tapered carbide bur is used to place the guiding grooves of approximately 1 mm depth in the central, mesial, and distal fossae
- Guiding grooves are also placed in the buccal and lingual grooves and in each triangular ridge extending from the cusp tip to the centre of its base.

Occlusal reduction

- The occlusal reduction follows the depth orientation grooves

- Functional cusps (buccal cusps) on mandibular molars are reduced with minimum clearance of 1.5 mm
- For non-functional cusp a minimum of 0.6–1 mm reduction is required
- Reduce the inclined planes between the depth guides in the developmental grooves and those along the triangular ridges
- Reduce the marginal ridge by 1.5 mm
- Evaluate occlusal clearance with wax bite and measure with wax gauge.

Placement of functional cusp bevel

- A functional cusp bevel is placed to protect tooth during function by ensuring adequate thickness of metal, as this area contacts with the opposing tooth
- Functional cusp bevel ensures ideal restoration contour, maximum durability and conservation of tooth structure
- A functional cusp bevel is placed 45 degrees to the long axis of teeth on the functional palatal cusp for maxillary molar and buccal cusp for mandibular molar.

Placement of axial alignment grooves

- Three depth orientation grooves are placed:
  1. On each buccal and lingual wall with round-end tapered diamond
  2. In the centre of the wall
  3. On each mesial and distal transitional line angles.
- A round end tapered diamond with a taper of 6 degrees forms an identical taper on the preparation wall
- Gingivally: Only one-half of the tip of diamond should penetrate
- Facial and lingual reduction:
  - The facial and lingual surface reduction is done with taper of 2–5 degrees. For maxillary molar, a two-plane reduction is common on the facial surface
  - During the facial and lingual reduction, the taper established is in relation to the path of insertion
  - The sharp line angles created after the proximal, facial, and lingual surfaces are rounded
  - Vertical seating grooves on the buccal cusp fossa for mandibular and palatal cusp fossa for maxillary to improve retention.

Axial reduction

- Break the contact points with a thin tapering fissure bur without abrading the adjacent tooth
- In tight contact point areas, a metal matrix band can be placed
- Axial reduction forms the retention and resistance form
- The islands of tooth structure between the alignment grooves are removed while the chamfer margin is placed with a round-end tapered diamond
- The preparation is done on one-half at a time
- A 5 degrees convergence on the mesial surface of the tooth is required
- Gingival finish line is not made at this time
- The distal surface is prepared next.

Margin placement

- The width of the chamfer margin should be 0.5 mm
- Chamfer margin must be smooth and continuous mesiodistally and ideally located supra-gingivally
- Unsupported enamel should be removed with chisel
- The tip of the bur should not exceed the depth of one-half the diameter of the bur.

Finishing the preparation

- Finish the preparation by refining the line angles and point angles
- Smoothen sharp angles or surface irregularities with the diamond and finally with a cuttle fish disc.

Indications

- For restored posterior tooth in non-aesthetic zone unable to withstand normal occlusal loads
- For a retainer requiring maximum retention
- For short clinical crowns
- For extensively damaged or fractured teeth
- Complete gold veneer crowns can be prepared on both vital and pulp less teeth
- Ideal retainer for long-span fixed partial denture
- For endodontically treated teeth
- Retainers for removable partial denture.

Advantages

- Good strength
- Better retention
- Conservative tooth preparation
- Less chance of pulpal injury
- Can easily modify axial tooth contour
- Convenient development of contact areas
- Can be given for caries damaged tooth after core built up
- Can be given for endodontically treated teeth
- Ideal retainer for restoring craniofacial anomalies
- Can withstand occlusal loads
- Occlusal plane modifications are easily facilitated with supra erupted teeth

Chapter 25 Tooth Preparations

- Ideal retainer for long span fixed partial denture and short clinical crowns.

Disadvantages

- Not aesthetic
- Cannot be used as anterior retainers
- Not as biocompatible as ceramic restorations
- Chances of over contouring the restoration (Over contouring can result in periodontal problems)
- Distortion of metal margins is common
- Uniform gingival finish lines are difficult to achieve
- Post cementation gingival caries is difficult to detect.

SHORT ESSAY

Question 1

Write in detail brief about partial veneer crowns.

Answer

Partial Veneer Crown

- It is an extra coronal metal restoration that covers only part of the clinical crown
- Partial veneer crowns include all tooth surfaces except the buccal or labial wall in the preparation.

Types of Partial Veneer Crowns

There are of three types:
1. Reverse three quarter crown.
2. Seven eight partial veneer crown.
3. Mesial half crown.

Indications

- Intact or minimally restored teeth with intact buccal wall
- To re-establish anterior guidance
- Used as retainers for a fixed partial denture when alteration of the occlusal plane is needed
- To splint teeth
- Can be prepared on teeth with average crown length
- Prepared when teeth have normal anatomic crown form
- Anterior teeth need to have adequate labio-lingual thickness.

Contraindications

- High caries rate (more for partial veneers where both the unveneered surface and the margin to finish line interface are susceptible to decay)
- Teeth with extensive core restorations
- Deep cervical abrasion
- Short teeth
- Teeth that are severely constricted at the cervical require more axial reduction to provide adequate groove length

Tooth Preparation Steps of Partial Veneer Crowns

- Incisal reduction
- Lingual reduction
- Interproximal reduction
- Proximal box or groove placement
- Incisal offset placement
- Facial bevel
- Finishing the preparation.

Armamentarium

- High and low speed contra-angle handpieces
- Utility wax and wax gauge to evaluate lingual reduction.

Incisal reduction

Round ended tapered diamond used. Reduce the incisal edge 1 mm at 45° angle to the long axis of the tooth. Remove 1.0–1.5 mm following the facial contour of the tooth.

Lingual reduction

It is done in two steps:

1. Lingual surface reduction
- A football-shaped diamond is used to reduce the lingual surface in two planes, with a slight ridge along the centre of the lingual surface inciso-gingivally. A clearance of at least 0.7–1 mm is required with the opposing tooth.

2. Lingual gingival reduction
- A round-ended tapered diamond is used to achieve a chamfer of 0.5 mm deep at the cervical finish line. The chamfer is extended to include the lingual line angles.

Interproximal reduction

- It is done in three steps:
  ○ The proximal surface is reduced with a 169L carbide bur from the lingual to the facial surface with the contact point intact. The facial line angles must remain intact for good aesthetic results

- A light chamfer finish line is made on the proximal surface with a narrow chamfer diamond
- This chamfer should merge with the lingual chamfer
- The contact with adjacent tooth is broken with a hatchet instrument from the facial surface, to form labial proximal extensions
- The flare of proximal extensions is finished with a flame-shaped diamond.

Proximal grooves

- A 167 carbide bur is used for groove placement at the proper alignment
- The proximal grooves are placed parallel to the incisal two-thirds of the facial surface (169L carbide bur)
- These grooves resist lingual displacement and should be a minimum of 3 mm long with 0.5 mm of the gingival finish line
- The facial and lingual walls of the grooves should have a 2–5 degree incisal divergence
- The lingual wall of the proximal grooves should have a 2–5 degree incisal convergence with the lingual gingival wall
- The facial wall of the groove should be continuous with the proximal flare to add bulk to the facial margin.

Incisal groove

- Inverted cone carbide bur is used
- A 0.5–1 mm groove is prepared within the dentin and is made parallel to the dentino-enamel junction connecting the proximal grooves. The groove is not placed at the expense of the incisal edge.

Facial bevel

- Fine, flame-shaped diamond bur is used
- A narrow bevel <0.5 mm is prepared on the labio-incisal finish line at right angles to the incisal two-thirds of the facial surface.

Finishing the preparation

- A carbide finishing bur is used
- All the sharp and point angles are rounded to ensure continuity of all finish lines.

Cingulum modification for additional retention

- A ledge in prepared in the coagulum after paralleling a 170 bur to the long axis on the proximal grooves
- A pilot hole is cut in the ledge with a No. 1/2 round bur.

SHORT NOTES

Question 1
What is proximal flare?

Answer
- Flare is a flat plane on the facial wall of a groove
- The facial wall of the proximal groove should be extended such that it forms a line angle with the facial surface
- This produces a proximal flare.

Question 2
What is the armamentarium used in crowns preparation?

Answer
- Handpiece
- Small wheel diamond
- Small round diamond
- Long needle diamond
- Torpedo diamond
- Torpedo bur
- No. 169L bur
- No. 170L bur
- Flame diamond
- Flame bur
- Enamel hatchet.

Question 3
What is a pin modified three-quarter crown?

Answer
- This is an aesthetic modification of the classic three-quarter crown
- It is used as a retainer on sound abutments for short span fixed partial denture in aesthetically critical areas
- This restoration extends over the lingual and a single proximal surface
- The labial and the other proximal surface are spared Retentive pins are used to compensate for the educed tooth coverage
- It does not affect the periodontal health
- It has better aesthetics due to minimal metal display.

Question 4
What is a metal-ceramic full veneer crown?

Answer
- It is also known as porcelain fused to metal restoration
- It has a thin metal coping with a facial ceramic layer
- This crown has the strength and accurate fit of a metal crown and aesthetics of a ceramic crown

- Metal ceramic crowns are stronger than all ceramic crowns and can be used as a fixed partial denture retainer.

Question 5

Define path of insertion.

Answer

- It is an imaginary line along which the restoration will be placed onto or removed from the preparation
- It should be accurately determined using a surveyor as minor undercuts in the preparation tend to be hidden by the human binocular vision.

Question 6

Define primary retention and secondary retention.

Answer

- Primary Retention:
  - Sleeve retention provided by the opposing vertical surfaces of the tooth preparation
  - Wedge type retention seen in intra-coronal restorations.
- Secondary Retention:
  - Retention obtained by retentive features like pins, boxes and grooves, etc. is known as secondary retention.

Chapter 26: Types of Fixed Partial Dentures

LONG ESSAYS

Question 1
Write in brief about various types of fixed partial dentures.

Answer

Conventional Fixed Partial Dentures
- They are the most commonly used fixed partial dentures
- It takes support from the abutments on either side of edentulous space.

Cantilever Fixed Partial Dentures
- It is used when support can be only from one side of edentulous space
- The support of there partial dentures is not satisfactory
- In this process, to obtain the support more than one teeth or the same side of the edentulous space is required.

Advantages
- When a single abutment is involved there is a very conservative design
- Parallel preparations are easily obtained when secondary abutment are used, this is because of the reason that the abutments are adjacent to each other
- They are very easy to fabricate.

Disadvantages
- In case of long duration edentulous spaces they can't be restored
- They produce torquing forces on the abutment
- Even if there is a minor error in design of the abutment it will effect largely on its success.

Spring Cantilever Fixed Partial Dentures
- This can only support a single pontic
- Posterior abutments are used for obtaining the support
- To connect the posterior retainer to anterior pontic long resilient bar connector is used.

Advantages
- To replace the missing incisors, metal crown retainers which require minimal tooth preparation are used in posterior teeth
- They are also used in diastema cases.

Disadvantages
- There are chances of tissue hyperplasia as there can be food lodging under he connector bar
- There are chances that the connector bar interfere with the speech and mastication
- There can be coronal displacement of the pontic when connector bar is deformed.

Fixed-Fixed Partial Dentures
- They are the rapid connectors at both ends of the pontic
- They are very convenient
- They have rigid abutment teeth which are splinted together
- They are prepared parallel to each other which is 3 units and can be cemented in one piece
- As the property of being rigid there is no movement between the connector components.

Procedure
- The fabrication of rigid connector is fabricated by casting or soldering
- Using a single unit pattern while casting, the poetics and retainers are fabricated
- They are then joined together and soldering is done using a different soldering alloy
- The cast technique is preferred because there is no galvanic corrosion

Chapter 26 Types of Fixed Partial Dentures

- The soldered connectors should be flat, parallel and uniform because the solder alloy flow is very easily controlled.

Advantages

- They are very easy to fabricate
- They have very good strength
- They are very easy to maintain
- They are used to splint the mobile abutments
- They have very economical design
- The design robust gives maximum retention and strength
- It is used in periodontically weak abutments
- It is used in long bridges.

Disadvantages

- The forces are directly transferred to the abutment as the connectors are very rigid causing stress and cover forces, which produces serious damage
- To obtain a single path of placement excessive tooth preparation is required
- In case where multiple abutments are present it is difficult to cement
- They can be used in pier abutments.

Fixed Movable Partial Dentures

It is defined as, a fixed partial denture having one or more non-rigid connectors. These dentures have the qualities of both the fixed partial denture and removable partial dentures.

Advantages

- While transmitting unwanted leverage forces they act as stress breakers
- They help in the improvement of the abutment health
- The cementation of different parts can be done separately
- The tooth preparation may or may not be parallel to each other
- Each abutment tooth can be prepared differently as required
- There are minor movement between the components of the prosthesis.

Disadvantages

- The design is very complex
- It has very difficult temporisation
- Very hard to maintain
- The laboratory procedure is very technical
- Very expensive prefabrication connectors
- They are contraindicated in long span bridges.

Fixed Removable Partial Dentures/Removable Bridges

- Defined as a fixed partial denture having one or more non-rigid connectors–GPT
- A non-rigid connector is used
- They are designed to have any one of the non-rigid connectors.

Design

- In the process the cementation over the abutment is done by individual cast gold coping
- There are threaded sleeves that are incorporated into the copings
- Over the coping the bridge is retained and is done by screws or weak cements.

Modified Fixed Removable Partial Dentures

- They are indicated for edentulous ridges with severe vertical deficit
- Prosthesis consist of a removable and fixed component.

Fixed Component

- Full metal is used for the fixed components when they are fabricated completely
- They are connected by a load bearing bar with two copings
- On the prepared abutment the two copings are cemented on both sides of edentulous ridge.

Biomechanics

- The bar is rectangular when seen in cross section
- The height of bar is more than the width
- The concept of simple bridge is followed in which the strength of the bridge is determined by distance between the action of compressive and tensile forces
- It should be noted that height of the bar is more important than its bulk.

Removable Component

- They consist of artificial teeth and a denture flange which is designed to fit or clasp the bar
- The teeth arise from the denture base so they give very natural appearance rather than in other cases where teeth are suspended freely
- Vertical ridge is also hidden by the denture base
- It provides a comfortable experience to the patient and also easier to maintain

- In few cases when there are less teeth left, the coping is done on the remaining teeth and the component is designed over those copings.

All Metal Fixed Partial Dentures

- They are not used when aesthetics is of importance
- They possess very high strength and durability
- It is used for replacing maxillary and mandibular posterior teeth.

Metal-ceramic Fixed Partial Dentures

- Metal is used to fabricate the core of the prosthesis and external surface is fabricated using ceramic.
- They are of 2 types:
  1. Metal is surrounded by porcelain on all surfaces.
  2. Lingual and occlusal surface is formed by metal and labial and gingival surface is formed by porcelain.

Advantages

- They are very aesthetically accepted
- They are able to hold with the internal and external strains
- They have very strong metal structure.

Disadvantages

- Tooth preparation that is required is very specific and not conservative
- Sub-gingival placement of facial margins are done on the anterior restoration to achieve aesthetics which in turn results in gingival destruction
- Ceramics are better substitutes when it comes to aesthetics
- At the metal ceramic junction there can be brittle fracture that can happen at the time of failure in he process
- It is expensive than ceramics.

All Ceramic Fixed Partial Dentures

They are less fracture resistant and do not render as good retainers.

Advantages

- They are superior when it comes to aesthetics
- They require more facial surface preparation
- They possess good translucency
- The appearance can be altered and modified by selecting the luting agent.

Disadvantages

- They have less reinforcement with metals, so it causes decreased strength
- Ceramic edges can chip off easily that is the reason the finished margins cannot be prepared
- The crown fails to support restorations thats why they are not used in severely damaged teeth
- They increase the chance of periodontal diseases as large connects are used because porcelain is brittle in nature which impingements the inter-dental papilla
- They cause wear and tear of opposite natural teeth.

All Acrylic Fixed Partial Denture

- Indicated for long term temporary or interim prosthesis
- Exhibits poor wear resistance
- Has good aesthetics
- Is easy to fabricate.

Other Types

- Short span bridges
- Long span bridges
- Fixed partial denture splints
- Fibre reinforced composite resin bridges
- Resin bonded fixed partial dentures.

Question 2

Write in brief about fixed partial denture splints.

Answer

Splints

- A fixed partial denture usually requires the splinting of additional abutments to overcome the loss of bone support of an abutment
- It has been contended that splinting of abutments increases their resistance to applied force of teeth and supporting structure.

Principle of Splinting

- Splinting is needed on both sides and even one single side for the adjustment to the periodontically involved teeth and its treatment
- When splinting is done in more teeth which are single rooted it transforms them into single multicoated unit.

Purpose of Splinting

- The main purpose of splint is to distribute and direct the functional forces that brings them within the tolerance of the supporting structures and tissues that are remained
- It also serve the purpose to eliminate any mobility present
- Splints also serve the purpose of stabilising and reorientation of the forces.

Chapter 26 Types of Fixed Partial Dentures

Secondary Purpose of Splinting

- They improve the function and the form of the teeth
- Occlusal contact patterns can be modified
- Masticatory efficacy is can be bettered
- Jaw relations are adjusted.

Classification of Splints

- Based on the extent of the prosthesis across the midline, fixed partial denture splints can be classified as:
  - Unilateral splints
  - Bilateral or cross-arch splints.
- Based on the duration of use, fixed partial denture splints can be classified into:
  - Temporary or provisional splints
  - Permanent splints.

Unilateral splints

- Unilateral splints is the joining of two or more teeth in one plane of an arch segment
- Unilateral splints are very resistant to the mesio-distal forces.

Bilateral splints

- They are also called as cross-arch splints
- These splints cross midline
- The splinting action is resistive to forces that comes from all the direction
- They can either involve two or more segments or the entire arch.

Temporary or provisional or healing splints

- These are the splints that are used of a shorter span of time
- Fabrication:
  - Tooth preparation is done as a conventional fixed partial denture and is fabricated in heat-cured tooth coloured acrylic resin and is cemented with zinc oxide eugenol cement
  - Generally, they are utilised for a period of few weeks to few months.

Permanent splints

- They help in the prevention of further progress of periodontal diseases
- They are the constant adjuncts to the maintenance of periodontal diseases
- The following prosthesis can be used as permanent splints:
  - Resin-bonded retainers or Maryland bridges
  - Fiber reinforced composite resin bridges.

Telescopic Copings in Fixed Partial Denture Splints

- Peeso introduced telescopic crowns as abutment retainers in 1916
- In this type of coping, the teeth that are included in the splints are first reduced and than covered with thin gold copings
- These copings are than permanently cemented in that place
- There is a space for retainers which is already designed that is telescopes into them
- Before the tooth preparation, place an acrylic tooth in place of the missing tooth and make an alginate impression index
- Patient's teeth are prepared in the regular manner
- Lubrication of the teeth is done and also the lubrication of the adjacent gingival margins is done with a petroleum jelly and is reseated the index or the alginate impression with the restorative material
- The restoration is removed and reset still it sets
- Finally finishing and polishing and cementing the restoration is done.

Advantages

- With minimum tooth preparation a common, parallel path of insertion is achieved
- Fabrication of full arch splints with multiple smaller segments is possible
- Permanent cementing by metal coping prevents the teeth
- Teeth that are severely tipped or widely spaced are brought together in single design
- The crown structure can be converted to pontics when the abutment is extracted which makes it very flexible in function
- Pin grooves can be given between coping and superstructure which can be used as a additional retention.

Disadvantages

- When there are narrow embrasures it is contraindicated for short abutment
- There is large bulk on the embrasures giving it a very unaesthetic appearance
- The complex treatments are required like orthodontic moments and also the root sectioning so that the oral hygiene is maintained
- It has a very complex design
- It is very expensive.

SHORT ESSAY

Question 1

Discuss fibre reinforced composite resin bridges.

Answer

Fibre Reinforced Composite Resin Bridges

These bridges are reinforced by a bar of glass fibres over which indirect posterior composites are built.

Materials Used

They are divided into two parts:
- Reinforcing constituents which provides strength and stiffness
- Surrounding matrix which supports the reinforcement and provides workability
- Available polymer are:
  - Polymers reinforced with glass
  - Polyethylene or carbon fibres
  - Reinforcing fibres are unidirectional, woven and braided.

Classification

Fibre reinforced composites can be classified into:
- Pre-impregnated: The manufacturer impregnates them with the resin
- Impregnation required: Fibre impregnation has to be done by the dentist.

Contraindications
- In cases where fluid control is not possible it is contraindicated
- In long span bridges it is not used
- It is contraindicated when used opposite to the unglazed porcelain teeth
- Patient's with parafunctional habits are contraindicated.

Advantages
- It does not contain metal
- Exhibits optimum aesthetics
- It causes less wear of opposing teeth.

SHORT NOTES

Question 1

What are short span bridges?

Answer

- These type of simple fixed partial dentures replace one or two teeth, and the teeth on either side are ideal abutments
- Their main advantage is the minimum torquing forces
- For example, first molar replacement.

Question 2

What are the indications of long term temporary bridges?

Answer

These restorations may be given for the following conditions:
- During the interim period of treatment when the patient is undergoing extensive occlusal rehabilitation. (e.g. intruding a supra-erupted tooth)
- In patients undergoing periodontal therapy these restorations may be inserted to act as splints.

Question 3

Write the classification of splints.

Answer

Classification of splints is as follows:
- Based on the extent of the prosthesis across the midline:
  - Unilateral splints
  - Bilateral or cross-arch splints.
- Based on the duration of use:
  - Temporary or provisional splints
  - Permanent splints.

Question 4

What are the advantages and disadvantages of cantilever fixed partial dentures?

Chapter 26 Types of Fixed Partial Dentures

Answer

Advantages

- In case of single abutment the design very conservative
- As the abutment are adjacent to each other in secondary abutment a parallel preparation can be easily made
- They are very easy to fabricate.

Disadvantages

- It produces torquing forces on the abutment
- To restore long span edentulous spaces there are not indicated
- If there are minor design errors they can affect the abutments in a big way.

Chapter 27: Impression Making

LONG ESSAYS

Question 1

Write in detail about impression techniques.

Answer

Impression Techniques

- According to the type of impression trays
  - Stock tray/putty-wash impression
    - Double mix
    - Single mix.
  - Custom tray impression
    - Single mix technique.
- Closed bite double arch method or triple tray technique.
- Copper tube impressions.
- Segmental impression technique.
- Post space impressions.

Stock Tray/Putty-wash Technique

- In this technique, primary impression is made using a stock tray and a final impression is made using the preliminary impression as the custom tray
- It is indicated in cases where combination of medium to heavy bodied elastomer and light bodied elastomer is warranted
- The two different methods of making putty wash impression are single mix putty-wash technique and double mix putty-wash technique.

Single mix putty-wash technique

- The technique involves concomitant use of both light body and putty
- Impression of the full mouth is made using the loaded stock tray
- The light body material is syringed around the tooth preparation whereas putty material is loaded into the stock tray.

Double mix putty-wash technique

- A suitable stock tray is selected and uniformly applied with tray adhesive
- Then, the putty impression material is mixed and made into a rope and loaded onto the tray followed by placing of spacer over the loaded putty material and a full mouth impression is made
- Subsequent to the removing of the impression, spacer made of polythene is carefully peeled away
- Additional relief is provided by scraping the areas, which recorded the tooth preparation
- Then the light body material is syringed over the putty impression and the tooth preparation to record the accurate details.

Advantages

- Metal trays exhibit rigidity and avoid distortion
- Stock trays are easily available.

Disadvantages

- The trays are required to be sterilised
- More impression material is needed in this technique.

Custom Tray Impression Technique

The technique involves fabrication of a custom tray over the primary cast, made using a primary impression.

Technique

- An acrylic special tray is fabricated over the cast with two sheets of thin foil spacer to offer adequate for the impression material
- Tray adhesive is applied over the acrylic special tray and medium viscosity elastomer is loaded on the tray
- The light body elastomer is syringed around the tooth preparation and the tray with the impression material is seated over it to record the accurate details.

Advantages

- The tray do not require sterilisation as it is used for a single patient
- Uniform thickness of impression material reduces the chances of distortion
- Lesser amount of impression material is needed.

Disadvantages

- Needs more time for fabrication
- The tray can not be used in patients who are allergic to acrylic.

Closed Bite Double Arch Method or Triple Tray Technique

- It is also known as dual quad tray or accu-bite technique. It is indicated in cases where adequate inter-digitation between the natural teeth is present
- Moreover, in conditions where vertical dimensions are maintained. The other conditions requiring this technique include cases where there is sufficient space available distal to the existing teeth.

Technique

- The syringe material is injected into the area to be recorded with high viscosity material mixed and positioned in excess on both the arches
- Tray is placed in between the arches and the patient is asked to bite slowly on it
- The patient is instructed to open his mouth slowly following the making of the impression, the tray will be seen adhered to one arch
- Uniform pressure should be applied bilaterally to remove the tray
- Then the impression of the tooth preparation is poured with the die stone and the impressions are boxed and casts of both arches are poured
- Articulation of these casts is done on a hinge articulator with an incisal pin to maintain vertical dimension.

Advantages

- Requires less impression material as the impression area recorded is limited to only one part of the arch
- The technique takes lesser time as both the arches are recorded simultaneously
- It can help in recording maximum intercuspation position accurately.

Disadvantages

- Due to flexibility of the tray, impression can get distorted
- Non-homogenous distribution of impression material can take place during impression making
- The tray cannot be used for more than one casting per quadrant.

Copper Band Impression Technique

- The impression technique is employed for single tooth impression wherein a copper band is placed around the prepared tooth and the impression material is loaded into the band to record the impression
- Therefore, it is indicated in the impression of a single tooth. Moreover, the technique is used for the impression of one or two preparations in case of multiple preparations, which have been recorded accurately.

Procedure

- A copperband or tube is customised according to the patient, which should be well-adapted to the tooth
- An orientation hole is made on the facial surface of the tube
- To prevent the compound from sticking, fingers are coated with a thin layer of petroleum jelly
- The green stick compound is heated over an open flame
- Then the softened mass is then placed into the copper band and filled to one-third of the tube through the open end of the tube, which is then placed onto the tooth preparation to record the occlusal surfaces
- Light bodied material is then syringed over the prepared tooth
- The surface of the compound is coated with adhesive and seated over the syringed material to record fine details.

Advantages

- An accurate finish line can be acquired
- It is less time consuming as the entire impression is not required to be repeated.

Disadvantages

- It need additional impressions
- Attaining proper orientation of the die with the dies of adjacent or opposite teeth is technique sensitive.

Segmental Impression Technique

Indications

- In cases where simultaneous impression is made of multiple teeth
- In patients where moisture control is difficult.

Technique

- Impression of the arch with multiple prepared teeth is made in segments
- Individualized custom trays are fabricated for each segment with acrylic resin over the diagnostic cast
- All the segmented trays should be able to seat on the cast simultaneously
- Tray adhesive is applied on each segmented tray on the internal surface
- Automix polyvinyl siloxane is loaded onto the tray and seated on the segment of the arch
- Once the material is set, the tray is not removed and another segment is loaded and seated over that segment
- Procedure is repeated till impression of all segments is made
- Then an oversized stock tray is used to make a pick up impression with appropriate material
- The completed impression is evaluated and poured. Post space impressions for endodontically treated teeth or Impression for pin retained restoration.

Direct Technique

- Pattern is fabricated directly in the patients mouth using pattern resin or inlay wax
- Canal is lubricated and plastic dowel is extended to the apical end of the prepared canal
- Resin is incrementally added onto the plastic dowel and placed and removed several times into the canal
- Resin should not be allowed to harden to the prepared canal
- This step is repeated until properly fitting resin-coated dowel is polymerized
- Pattern post is rechecked for its fit and ease of removability.

Indirect Technique

- Separating medium is applied on pin holes and post spaces
- Light bodied secondary impression material is injected over the pin hole or post space
- Lentulospiral is used to move the impression material in pin-hole or post space
- Orthodontic wires (preferred) or elastomeric bristles can be used to stabilize the impression material within the pin hole or post space
- A tray adhesive (methyl cellulose) should be applied on the stabilizing bristle or wire. Before the syringe material gels, the tray material is loaded with medium or heavy body irreversible hydrocolloid and an even impression is made
- The syringe and tray materials are allowed to gel together as a single unit
- The whole assembly is removed carefully.

Question 2

What are the methods to control fluid? Write about soft tissue management.

Answer

Fluid Control

- Successful restorative procedures demand dry operating field and clear visibility
- For that fluid control is essential. Fluid control provides the following:
  - A dry clear operative field
  - Improves accessibility and visibility
  - Comfortable for both operator and patient
  - Aids in impression making.

Methods

There are essentially two methods of fluid control, namely mechanical and chemical methods.

1. Mechanical methods
   - Rubber dam
   - High volume suction
   - Saliva ejector
   - Svedopter.
2. Chemical methods
   - Antisialagogues
   - Local anaesthetics (adrenaline).

Rubber dam

- It was introduced by SC Barnum
- This is the most effective isolation method
- It is used during tooth preparation of inlays and onlays, post and core fabrication cementation and pin-retained amalgam
- It should not be used with polyvinyl siloxane impression material because it inhibits polymerization.

High volume suction

- It is very useful during crown preparation
- It is used effectively by assistant
- It is an excellent lip retractor
- It is not used during impression making or cementation procedure.

Saliva ejector

- It is most useful when used as an adjunct to high-volume evacuation

- It can be used alone for maxillary arch during impression making and cementation
- It is placed at the corner of mouth, opposite to the quadrant being treated and head of patient is tilted towards it.

Svedopter

- It is used for isolation of the mandibular arch
- It consists of metal saliva ejector with attached tongue deflector
- Cotton rolls can be used along with it during cementation or impression making
- It is most effective when the patient is upright
- Drawbacks:
  - Accessibility to lingual surface of lower teeth is limited
  - Should not be used in patient with mandibular tori.
  - Metal component may injure the soft tissues in the floor of the mouth.

Anti-sialagogues

- These drugs are helpful in controlling the salivary flow
- They are gastrointestinal anticholinergics which act on the smooth muscles of the GI tract, urinary or biliary tract and produces dry mouth as side effect
- Contraindications:
  - Hypersensitivity to this drug, glaucoma, asthma, congestive heart failure, patient on corticosteroids.

SHORT ESSAYS

Question 1

Write about the procedure of impression making using a stock tray.

Answer

Stock Tray/Putty-wash Technique

In this technique, primary impression is made using a stock tray and a final impression is made using the preliminary impression as the custom tray. It is indicated in cases where combination of medium to heavy bodied elastomer and light bodied elastomer is warranted. The two different methods of making putty wash impression are single mix putty-wash technique and double mix putty-wash technique.

Single Mix Putty-wash Technique

- The technique involves concomitant use of both light body and putty
- Impression of the full mouth is made using the loaded stock tray
- The light body material is syringed around the tooth preparation whereas putty material is loaded into the stock tray.

Double Mix Putty-wash Technique

- A suitable stock tray is selected and uniformly applied with tray adhesive
- Then, the putty impression material is mixed and made into a rope and loaded onto the tray followed by placing of spacer over the loaded putty material and a full mouth impression is made
- Subsequent to the removing of the impression, spacer made of polythene is carefully peeled away
- Additional relief is provided by scraping the areas, which recorded the tooth preparation
- Then the light body material is syringed over the putty impression and the tooth preparation to record the accurate details.

Advantages

- Metal trays exhibit rigidity and avoid distortion
- Stock trays are easily available.

Disadvantages

- The trays are required to be sterilised
- More impression material is needed in this technique.

Question 2

Discuss impression making for pin-retained restoration for endodontically treated teeth.

Answer

Procedure

- Irreversible hydrocolloid impression material is used for making impression for both pin-holes or post space
- A separating medium followed by light bodied secondary impression material is injected over the pin-hole or post space

- A lentulospiral in slow speed, clockwise rotation is utilised to move the impression material into the pinhole post space
- Impression material within the pin hole or post space is stabilised with the help of orthodontic wires or elastomeric bristles which should also be coated with a tray adhesive
- The over impression is made by loading the tray material with medium or heavy bodied irreversible hydrocolloid, before the syringe material gels
- In this technique, the syringe and tray materials serve as a single unit to gel together
- The whole assembly is removed carefully after the setting of the impression.

SHORT NOTES

Question 1

Write a short note on svedopter.

Answer

- Svedopter, a metal saliva ejector is used for isolating the mandibular teeth
- Usually, it is attached with a tongue deflector and can be placed when the patient is in a near upright position
- However, it causes difficulty in accessing the lingual surface of mandibular teeth
- Moreover, it needs to be carefully used so as to avoid any trauma to the floor of the mouth
- It can not be used in presence of mandibular tori.

Question 2

What is electrosurgical unit (ESU)?

Answer

- The electrosurgical unit is specially designed electrodes used for gingival reduction
- The unit has knobs to modify the frequency and the flow of current
- Two electrodes can be attached to each unit, among which one is the surgical electrode and the other is the ground electrode or ground plate.
- This unit can be used in following procedures:
  - Enlargement of gingival sulcus
  - Crown lengthening procedure
  - Removal of edentulous cuff.

Question 3

Describe ground electrode.

Answer

- The ground plate is also known as ground plate, indifferent plate, indifferent electrode, neutral electrode, dispersive electrode, passive electrode, or patient return
- It aids in completing the electrical circuit so as to prevent electrical accidents by the use of a single electrode
- It should be placed under the thigh or the back of the patient and helps in stabilising the electrical flow within the body of the patient
- However, the ground plate should not be positioned close to bony tubercles as it has the potential to produce electricity sufficient to cause a burn.

Chapter 28: Provisional Restorations and Laboratory Procedures

LONG ESSAYS

Question 1

Elaborate the different kinds of provisional restorations.

Answer

Provisional restoration, a temporary prosthesis is used after the tooth preparation as a protective or functional restoration until the fabrication of final prosthesis. These restorations are classified according to the following procedures:
- Technique used for fabrication
- Process of fabrication
- Type of material used in fabrication
- Duration of usage.

Technique

According to technique used for fabrication, provisional restorations can be categorised into three types:
1. Direct technique-fabricated provisional restorations.
2. Indirect technique-fabricated provisional restorations.
3. Direct-indirect technique-fabricated provisional restorations.

Direct Technique-fabricated Provisional Restorations

This procedure involves alteration, adaptation and cementation of a preformed crown over a tooth preparation.

Metal provisional restoration on a posterior tooth using direct technique

Various steps that are required in the fabrication of the restoration, are as follows:
- Vernier caliper is used to determine the mesio-distal diameter of the prepared tooth
- Then, a stretching block is used to flare the gingival margins of the preformed crown for the desired size
- The crown then should be placed and checked for the discrepancy between the height of the marginal ridge and the adjacent teeth
- If the discrepancy exists, it denotes excessive length of the crown which should be trimmed gingivally
- Approximated crown length is then removed from the gingival margin
- After the removal, the gingival margin is smoothed
- Subsequently, contouring of axial surfaces with pliers is done for better fitting of the crown
- The prosthesis is finally seated over the prepared tooth surface and is checked for correct occlusion with help of articulating paper
- The crown is then cemented with the help of zinc oxide-eugenol cement
- The margins of the crown are burnished
- A dental floss is further used to remove all the excess cement from the inter-proximal region
- Excessive cement needs to be removed from the crevice with the help of an explorer.

Composite provisional restoration using direct technique

This technique uses bis-acryl composites for the fabrication of the provisional restoration as it exhibits less heat and polymerisation shrinkage. The various steps followed are:
- The preparation of the tooth is followed by making an over impression with the help of addition silicone
- The base and catalyst of the bis-acryl composite is mixed and is loaded over the over impression
- This composite-filled over impression is then re-seated over the petrolatum coated tooth preparation in the patient's mouth
- Provide a period of 10 mins for the composite to polymerise intra-orally
- The over impression is then removed from the mouth
- The polymerised composite restoration is then carefully teased out from the over impression

- If the restoration shows the presence of voids, it can be repaired by filling additional composite
- After repairing, the crown is polished and thus, cemented over the prepared tooth.

Indirect Technique-fabricated Provisional Restorations

Fabrication of the provisional restoration is entirely a laboratory procedure in indirect technique, unlike direct technique. The various steps followed in fabrication of an acrylic provisional restoration on posterior tooth are:
- Firstly, impression of the unprepared tooth is recorded and its cast is poured
- An over impression is prepared from the diagnostic cast and the thin edges of the gingival margin should be scrapped off
- Subsequently, the tooth preparation should be carried out
- Then an impression of the prepared tooth is taken by using an alginate impression, after which a cast is poured
- The cast is further trimmed and is tried in the over impression before processing a provisional restoration
- A layer of separating medium is placed on the plaster cast
- Acrylic resin is placed into the over impression, which then is firmly placed over the cast and tied with a rubber band
- The cast is then broken to remove the acrylic restoration and any plaster remaining in the cast should be removed
- Excessive resin is removed with the help of carborundum disc while a sandpaper disc is applied for smoothening out the ginigval margins
- The crown is seated in the mouth and is checked for occlusion with articulating paper
- Any occlusal prematurity should be removed and further checked in patient's mouth
- The crown with correct occlusion is then polished and seated onto the prepared tooth with the help of zinc-oxide eugenol cement, which is often mixed with a small amount of petrolatum
- The excessive cement from the gingival cervices, after crown insertion is then removed with the help of an explorer.

Direct-indirect technique-fabricated provisional restorations

- In this technique, external finish and fit of the preformed crown is checked in the patient's mouth
- However, the tissue surface of the preformed crown is processed in the laboratory
- The crown is customised for each patient by placing it on the cast made by pouring the impression of the prepared tooth
- It is formed by altering the contours of the preformed crown with the help of resins.

Process of Fabrication

On the basis of the process of fabrication, it can be divided into two types:
1. Preformed provisional restorations.
2. Custom made provisional restorations.

Preformed Provisional Restorations

- They are also known as pre-fabricated crown as they can be found in different sizes and materials, which permits the operator to choose the crown according to the patient's need
- Moreover, they can be modified to fit the tooth preparation
- **Table 28.1** depicts various advantages and disadvantages of preformed provisional restorations.

Custom Made Provisional Restorations

- For preparing custom made provisional restoration, the impression of the tooth preparation is taken, for which a cast is poured
- The prepared tooth is then waxed up
- It is further carved to reproduce original contours of the tooth
- Its advantages and disadvantages are listed in **Table 28.2**.

Type of Material Used in Fabrication

Classification of provisional crowns on the basis of type of material used in fabrication are enumerated in **Table 28.3**.

Table 28.1: Advantages and disadvantages of preformed provisional restorations

Advantages	Disadvantages
It requires less operatory time	Mostly, insufficient to fulfil the requirements of original contours of the tooth
	Requires self-cure resin for customisation
	Can only help in restoring provisional restoration of a single tooth

Chapter 28 Provisional Restorations and Laboratory Procedures

Table 28.2: Advantages and disadvantages of custom made provisional restorations

Advantages	Disadvantages
The crown can be made from different materials through this process	The process is time consuming
Occlusal interferences are minimum	More number of laboratory procedures are required
Aid in determining accuracy of the tooth preparation	

Table 28.3: Types of provisional restorations according to the type of material used in fabrication

Metal based provisional restorations	Resin based provisional restorations
Nickel-chromium	Polycarbonate
Tin-silver	Chemically activated resin—Poly-methyl methacrylate
Aluminium	Light-cured resins—Urethane di-methylacrylate
	Resins with greater strength—Poly-R methacrylate
	Cellulose acetate

Duration of Usage

The choice of provisional restorations is also dependent upon the duration for which the restoration has to be used. Thus, on the basis of time period, it can be categorised as:
1. Long-term provisional restorations—Can be used from 2 weeks to a few months **(Table 28.4)**.
2. Short-term provisional restorations—Can be used up to 2 weeks **(Table 28.4)**.

Table 28.4: Characteristic features of long-term and short-term provisional restorations

Long-term provisional restorations	Short-term provisional restorations
Made of cast metals	Most frequently are made of aluminium or polycarbonates
Exhibit good strength	Usually available as custom-made resins or preformed crowns
Are used for treatment of longer duration	Used when the restoration is used for a maximum period of 2 weeks
Used for posterior fixed partial dentures	Used in patients after tooth preparation in fixed partial dentures
Used in patients who exerts excessive forces on the prosthesis	

SHORT ESSAYS

Question 1

What are the steps of fabrication of an anterior polycarbonate restoration with the help of direct technique?

Answer

- The procedure begins with making an alginate impression of the prepared tooth using a stock tray, followed by pouring of the plaster cast
- Then the crown size is selected with the help of a mould guide
- The crown is tried in the mouth of the patient and the excess material is marked using a pencil and reduced gingivally
- The altered shell is tried again and compared with the adjoining teeth
- Subsequently, separating medium is painted on the prepared area and adjacent portions of the plaster cast
- The crown shell is further filled with resin and is positioned onto the prepared tooth on the plaster cast
- Trimming of the gingival excess created by the expressed acrylic is done with a garnet disc upto the level of the finish line
- The occlusion is checked with articulating paper
- Burlew disc is used to smooth axial surfaces near the margins of the restorations whereas these surfaces are polished using white polishing compound on a muslin rag wheel
- The excessive cement from the gingival cervices, after crown insertion is then removed with the help of an explorer.

Question 2

What are the most frequently used materials for preformed provisional restorations?

Answer

The most frequently used materials for preformed provisional restorations are listed in **Table 28.5**.

Essential Quick Review: Prosthodontics

Table 28.5: Commercially available preformed crowns

Cellulose Acetate	Nickel-chromium	Polycarbonate	Aluminium and Tin-silver
Can be used for all types of tooth, i.e. anterior and posterior	Can be used in patients, where long-term provisional restoration has to be used	Can be used for incisor, canine, premolar teeth	Used for posterior teeth
Transparent and exhibits a thickness of 0.2–0.3 mm	Majorly used for children with severely damaged deciduous teeth	Exhibits most natural appearance among all materials	Crowns made from these materials have occlusal and axial surfaces
Available as shells which can be cemented with the help of auto-polymerising resin	Possesses very high-strength	However, can be modified in colour due to the shade of luting agent, used for cementing	The crowns are highly ductile, therefore, additional care must be provided while try-in procedure to prevent fractures
This auto-polymerising resin provides colour to the crown	Cannot be cemented by resins and requires high-strength luting agents		Swaping or stretching with the help of an instrument can aid in cervical enlargement while insertion
Can be easily removed from the tooth	Can be re-contoured using pliers		

Question 3

What are the steps in direct fabrication of preparing a metal provisional restoration on posterior tooth?

Answer

- Vernier caliper is used to determine the mesio-distal diameter of the prepared tooth
- Then, a stretching block is used to flare the gingival margins of the preformed crown for the desired size
- The crown then should be placed and checked for the discrepancy between the height of the marginal ridge and the adjacent teeth
- If the discrepancy exists, it denotes excessive length of the crown which should be trimmed gingivally
- Approximated crown length is then removed from the gingival margin
- After the removal, the gingival margin is smoothed
- Subsequently, contouring of axial surfaces with pliers is done for better fitting of the crown
- The prosthesis is finally seated over the prepared tooth surface and is checked for correct occlusion with help of articulating paper
- The crown is then cemented with the help of zinc oxide-eugenol cement
- The margins of the crown are burnished
- A dental floss is further used to remove all the excess cement from the inter-proximal region
- Excessive cement needs to be removed from the crevice with the help of an explorer.

SHORT NOTES

Question 1

Write a short note on di lock tray system.

Answer

- A special tray with orientation grooves on inner aspect is used as a special tray to pour the cast
- The chief characteristics of the tray is that it is made of multiple components which can be assembled or dismantled as needed
- The impression is poured by a two pour technique, among which first pour is up to level of impression whereas second is poured after placing the rim of di lock tray over impression
- Prior to the setting of second pour, base of di lock tray is assembled and cast is allowed to set
- After the setting, di lock tray is dismantled and formation of grooves on base of cast is done, which acts as a guide for die sectioning.

Advantages

- The tray system is simple and easy to fabricate
- Cast can be mounted on articulator.

Disadvantage
Special equipments are required for the system.

Question 2
Mention the ideal requirements of provisional restorations.

Answer
- It should be easy to contour and polish
- It should restore periodontal health with good marginal fit
- It should not react negatively with the luting agents used for cementation of the prosthesis
- It should protect the pulp from sensitivity
- It should possess sufficient working time, easy moldability and rapid setting time
- Moreover, it should be biocompatible, i.e., non-toxic, non-allergic, non-exothermic.

Chapter 29: Cementation

LONG ESSAYS

Question 1

Describe luting agents used for cementation in fixed partial denture.

Answer

- Luting agents are the agents used for bonding of fixed restoration to prepared tooth surface
- Bonding is achieved by mechanical interlocking of cement into irregularities on restoration and tooth surface
- It consists of acid combined with metal oxide base to form salt and water
- Setting mechanism is through: Binding of unreacted powder particles by matrix of salt to form a hard set mass.

Ideal Requirements

- It should be adhesive to tooth and restoration.
- It has long working time
- It is non-irritant to pulp
- It provides good seal
- It has adequate strength
- It has low viscosity
- It has low solubility in oral fluids
- It could be compressed in thin layers
- It has case of removal of excess amount.

Types

- Zinc oxide eugenol cement (ZnOE) and modified ZnOE
- Zinc phosphate cement
- Zinc silico-phosphate cement
- Glass ionomer cement
- Zinc polycarboxylate cement
- Resin cement.

Zinc Oxide Eugenol Cement

- The cement is supplied as a powder liquid system
- Powder comprises zinc oxide with accelerators like zinc acetate, zinc propionate, zinc succinate and alcohol
- Other ingredients include Glacial acetic acid and a small amount of water
- Zinc oxide of the powder reacts with water to form zinc hydroxide
- This zinc hydroxide further reacts with eugenol to form zinc eugenolate, which acts as the chief ingredient
- The setting reactions that occur during this process are as follows:

$$Zn + H_2O \rightarrow ZnO + H_2 \uparrow$$
$$ZnO + H_2O \rightarrow Zn(OH)_2$$
$$\underset{\text{(Base)}}{Zn(OH)_2} + \underset{\substack{\text{(Acid} \\ \text{containing} \\ \text{eugenol)}}}{2HE} \longrightarrow \underset{\substack{\text{(Zinc} \\ \text{eugenolate)}}}{ZnE_2} + \underset{\text{(Water)}}{2H_2O}$$

Modified ZnOE cement

- Modified ZnOE cements used for luting is classified into two types:
  1. Type I ZOE + alumina/quartz + Ethoxy Benzoic acid (EBA).
  2. Type II ZOE + polymer resin.
- The cement is indicated as a luting agent in provisional restorations
- It can be used in cast restorations to protect oversensitive teeth
- It can also aid in cementing retentive, small single tooth castings and three unit fixed partial dentures
- The cement is dispensed as liquid and powder
- Powder is incorporated in bulk as two increments and is mixed using a glass slab and stainless steel spatula.

Advantages

- Has greater compressive strength
- Biocompatibility of reinforced ZOE is high

- Prevents pulpal inflammation
- Can be used in humid environment.

Disadvantage

Exhibits high solubility

Zinc Phosphate Cement

- Zinc phosphate, a widely used cement is indicated as a luting agent in the cementation of permanent and long-term provisional restorations
- It is also found in powder and liquid systems. Among which, powder includes heavy metal oxides like zinc oxide, magnesium oxide whereas phosphoric acid and Water (28–38%) are the liquid components. Moreover, aluminium phosphate is also found in small amount
- Mixing of the cement requires cool slab technique
- The powder is mixed in rotary motion in increments with liquid in the ratio of 1.4 g :0.5 ml
- In the setting reaction, the phosphoric acid attaches to the surface of the powder particles and resultant complex formed by the dissolution of zinc oxide is zinc alumino-phosphate gel.

Advantages

- Its mechanical properties are good
- Has good compressive strength
- Has limited solubility.

Disadvantages

- Has slow setting time
- Causes pulpal inflammation due to low pH.

Zinc Silico-phosphate Cement

- Among the various categorization of this cement, type I can be used as a luting cement
- The cement is manipulated by bulk mixing of powder and liquid
- Powder, a type of glass contains silica, alumina, fluoride such as NaF, CaF_2, Na_3AlF_6 and calcium salts like $Ca(PO_4)_2 \cdot 2H_2O$ or CaO
- The components of liquid are phosphoric acid, water, buffer salts
- Setting reaction includes release of Ca^{++}, Al^{+++} and F^- ions due to the attack of acid in the liquid on the surfaces of the powder particles
- The metal ions released in conjugation with phosphoric acid in the liquid precipitate as phosphates which results in the formation of the cement matrix in which fluoride ions are dispersed.

Advantages

- Owing to the release of fluoride ions, it possesses anti-cariogenic property
- Exhibits good compressive strength.

Disadvantage

Prone to cause pulpal irritation due to high acidic pH.

Glass Ionomer Cement (GIC)

- Type I GIC is the most frequently used cement as a luting agent
- It is indicated for routine clinical use in patients which require cementation of long span bridges
- It exhibits superiority as can be used in patients with extreme caries activity
- It can also aid in post and core cementation
- Available in powder and liquid form. Powder contains acid-soluble calcium-fluoro-alumino-silicate glass with a higher silica alumina ratio, calcium fluoride, sodium fluoride, aluminium phosphate and agents used for radio-opacity such as lanthanum, strontium, barium or zinc oxide
- Liquid components contain water as vital constituent, polyacrylic acid in the form of a copolymer with itaconic, maleic or tricarboxyllic acids and tartaric acid
- The resultant mixture formed by the attack of acid in the liquid on the surface of glass particles of powder causes leaking of calcium, aluminium, sodium and fluoride ions into the aqueous medium
- Calcium polysalts are formed followed by aluminium poly salts which cross-link with the polyanion chains
- These salts in turn hydrate to form a gel matrix where unreacted glass particles are embedded.

Advantages

- Exhibits anti-cariogenic property
- Has high flow
- Prevents pulpal inflammation
- Has good adhesive property
- Has good compressive strength.

Disadvantage

Can cause dentinal sensitivity during initial setting of cementation.

Zinc Polycarboxylate Cement

- The cement is used for routine clinical use and is preferred for sensitive teeth receiving cast restorations

- Powder components include zinc oxide, magnesium oxide, bismuth and aluminium oxide, stannic oxide may be substituted for MgO and traces of stannous fluoride
- Moreover, liquid contains polyacrylic acid, or copolymer of acrylic acid and other unsaturated carboxylic acids like itaconic acid
- A glass slab is used to mix powder, which is incorporated in large quantities into liquid within 30 seconds
- The mechanism involved in setting is that the surface of the powder particles are attacked by the acid resulting in the release of zinc, magnesium and tin ions
- These ions subsequently, react with the carboxyl group of adjacent polyacrylic acid chain
- This reaction further results in the formation of a cross-linked salt leading to the setting of the cement
- This set cement, thus, comprises of an amorphous gel matrix in which residual powder particles are dispersed.

Advantages

- It is considered as the ideal luting agent
- Prevents post-operative sensitivity
- Exhibits anti-cariogenic property (lesser than GIC)
- Offers adhesion to the tooth structure
- Adequate compressive strength (less than zinc phosphate).

Disadvantages

- It has thick consistency and poses difficulty to flow (thixotropic nature)
- Setting time is shorter which makes it inadequate for the cementation of long span bridges.

Resin Cements

- Flowable, micro-filled BisGMA resins with low viscosity is used for cementing laminate veneers, all ceramic restorations, castable ceramics and maryland bridges
- The adhesion of these cements to tooth structure can be either mechanical or chemical
- The underlying mechanism of mechanical adhesion is due to the flow of resin tags in-between the etched enamel crystals
- However, chemical adhesion is done with the help of bonding agents like hydroxy ethyl meth acrylate (HEMA) or 4-methacryloxy ethyl trimellitic anhydride (META)
- The procedure of using resin cement contains acid etching with the help of 35–37% phosphoric acid on the enamel surface for 15–30 seconds
- This etched tooth surface is then applied with bonding agent, after which resin is placed on the prosthesis for final setting.

Advantages

- Has good strength
- Provides excellent choice of various shades according to the colour of the tooth
- Insoluble in oral fluids
- Easy to use
- Can be mechanical adhered to tooth surface.

Disadvantages

- Does not possess anti-cariogenic property
- Can cause periodontal problems
- Has polymerisation shrinkage leading to marginal leakage
- Has greater film thickness in contrast to other cements.

Question 2

Write in detail about try-in procedures for cast metal restorations.

Answer

Following features are checked in the cast restoration:
- Proximal contact
- Marginal integrity
- Stability
- Occlusion.

Checking for Proximal Contacts

- The proximal contact between the crown and a natural tooth should allow the passage of floss
- The operator should compare the contacts of other teeth in the dentition
- Ideally the contacts should be stable and easy to maintain
- Subjective symptoms (patients response) are sufficient to confirm a tight contact
- The most common problem seen in relation to a proximal contact is excessive tightness
- This can be corrected by:
  - Adjusting with a rubber wheel (all metal restoration)
  - Adjusting with a cylindrical mounted stone (porcelain restoration).
- Deficient proximal contacts in a gold casting can be corrected by soldering.

Checking for Marginal Integrity

- Margin adaptation with a gap around 30 μm is clinically acceptable
- Testing whether the casting binds to the tooth surface, is helpful to determine the marginal integrity. This can be done using the following materials:
  - Disclosing waxes

- Suspension of rouge in chloroform or ether (Pressure indicating paste)
- Air abrasion to form a matte finish
- Powdered sprays
- Water soluble marking agents
- Elastomeric detection paste (by far the most reliable).
▫ Marginal integrity can be assessed by moving a sharp explorer from the restoration to the tooth and from the tooth to the restoration.

Checking for Stability

▫ The restoration should not rock or rotate when a force is applied
▫ Instability produced by a small positive nodule on the fitting surface can be corrected by trimming
▫ If the instability is due to a distorted wax pattern, the casting procedure should be repeated.

Checking for Occlusion

Occlusal discrepancies are one of the most common errors that occur during the fabrication of a fixed partial denture. Hence, occlusal adjustment during eccentric movements (clinical correction) is necessary.

Occlusal discrepancies can be corrected by the following techniques:
▫ Technique 1: Colored ribbons, placed interocclusally are used to determine the occlusal contacts (red ribbon is used to record centric contacts and green ribbon is used to record eccentric: Proximal contacts are tested with dental floss contacts)
▫ Technique 2: A matte finish is given on the occlusal surface of the metal restoration and the patient is asked to occlude in centric and eccentric relations (areas of contact appear shiny). But this technique has the following disadvantages:
- It is not possible to differentiate between centric and eccentric contacts
- Time consuming
- Can be used only for cast metal restorations.

Correcting Occlusal Discrepancies

▫ Occlusal discrepancies can be checked either in the clinic or in the lab
▫ Laboratory analysis requires a remount procedure (a new inter-occlusal record is made and the casts are articulated in a semi-adjustable articulator
▫ The premature contacts are corrected in the lab using a rubber wheel
▫ After refining the occlusion, it is rechecked in the mouth.

Try-in Procedure for Ceramic Restoration

During the try-in of a porcelain restoration, the following factors should be examined.

Checking for Proximal Contact and Marginal Fit in Ceramic Restoration

▫ They are examined as explained in cast metal restorations
▫ When metal ceramic restorations are to be reduced, the metal and ceramic surfaces should be ground simultaneously in order to prevent ceramic from being stained by the metal particles
▫ Grinding at the metal ceramic junction should be done in a direction parallel to the junction.

Checking for Occlusal Discrepancies in Ceramic Restorations

▫ Occlusal discrepancies can be checked using technique 1 explained in cast metal restoration
▫ They should be corrected only after glazing because unglazed ceramic shows increased pyroplastic flow (flow at high temperatures)
▫ The reduced area should be reglazed.

Evaluation of Aesthetics in Ceramic Restorations

▫ This is unique to ceramic restorations, as metals are not used to replace missing anterior teeth
▫ The contour of the gingival embrasure space and the placement of the incisal edge are important factors to be considered during anterior try-in.

Checking for Embrasure Contour

▫ Proper contour of the gingival embrasures is essential to minimize the dark spaces formed between the prosthetic components
▫ This is more important in anterior teeth as these dark spaces produce a very unaesthetic appearance
▫ These spaces should be evaluated clinically and should be corrected by adding porcelain and recontouring the restoration.

Checking for the Location of the Incisal Edge

It can be checked by asking the patient to pronounce the letter 'F' so that the incisal edge touches the vermillion border.

Aesthetic Characterizations

Some mild discrepancies can be incorporated into the restoration to produce a natural appearance. A staining kit

can be used to replicate the following characterizations on the restorative surface.
- Enamel cracks
- Stained crack lines
- Exposed occlusal dentin
- Incisal halo.

SHORT ESSAY

Question 1

Define cementation. Discuss the procedure followed during cementation of a restoration.

Answer

According to GPT, cementation is ascribed as the process of attaching parts by means of a cement.

The various procedures followed during cementation of a restoration are as follows:
- Cleaning of tooth surface or making it contamination free is the primary goal during cementation, as it negatively impacts the activity of luting agent
- Moreover, the surface should be dried without dessicating the odontoblasts for better adhesion of luting agent
- Thereafter, cavity varnish should be applied on tooth surface, if a non-adhesive cement like zinc phosphate has to be used
- In addition, oxalate treatment of the tooth surface should be performed to prevent dentinal sensitivity
- This is followed by preparation of the casting by sandblasting with 50 μm alumina or by steam. For further cleaning, processes like ultrasonic or organic cleaning are performed
- The operatory site should be isolated with cotton rolls
- Subsequently, mixing of the cement to a luting consistency should be done which is applied on the internal surface of the casting
- The prosthesis is then, inserted with a firm, rocking dynamic seating force to prevent incomplete seating and fracture
- Clinician should check the margins of the retainers to substantiate the accurate fit of the prosthesis
- With the help of an explorer, remove the excess cement from the gingival crevice whereas floss is used to remove the excess cement in the inter-proximal surface
- After the setting of cement, occlusion is checked with Mylar shim stock or articulating paper to remove any occlusal prematurities
- The patient is then instructed to avoid loading for the first 24 hour.

SHORT NOTES

Question 1

What are the various types of soldering?

Answer

According to the technique used, soldering can be of following types:
- Soldering for Metal Ceramic Restorations
  - The soldering is done generally before ceramic application at the temperature of 1075 to 1120°C and thus, termed as pre-ceramic soldering
  - However, post-ceramic soldering which is done after ceramic application is performed at 920°C.
- Oven soldering
  - Also known as furnace soldering as it is performed under vacuum or in air
  - They generate superior joint strength.
- Torch soldering
  - It is performed under direct flame with the help of a gas air torch
  - The torch flame has two parts; the reducing part and the soft brush part, among which the reducing part is at a higher temperature in comparison to the soft brush flame.
- Infrared soldering
  - It has good accuracy and is used for low-fusing connectors
  - The strength is comparative to conventional soldering.
- Laser welding.
  - In this type of soldering, pulsed high power Neodymium lasers with very high density are used
  - It is used to join titanium components of dental crowns, bridges and partial denture frameworks.

Chapter 29 Cementation

Question 2

What are the various steps of casting procedure?

Answer

- Preparing the wax pattern for casting
- Spruing the wax pattern
- Attaching the sprue to the crucible former
- Investing the pattern in a casting ring
- Burnout of the wax pattern
- Casting
- Recovery
- Finishing and polishing.

Question 3

Write a short note on nickel-chromium crowns.

Answer

- Nickel-chromium crowns are one of the most commonly available preformed provisional restorations, used primarily in children with severely damaged deciduous teeth
- They can also be used in patients, where long-term provisional restoration are required
- These crowns exhibit very high-strength
- Therefore, cannot be cemented by resins and requires high-strength luting agents
- However, these crowns can be re-contoured or altered with the help of pliers.

Question 4

What is soldering? Also mention the properties of a solder.

Answer

Soldering involves joining two components of metal with an intermediate metal whose melting temperature is lower than the parent metal.

Properties of a Solder

- Should fuse safely below the sag or creep temperature of the parent alloy
- The joint of the solder should be strong
- Should be resistant to tarnish and corrosion
- Should be free flowing
- Should be non-pitting
- Should has similar colour as that of parent metal.

Chapter 30: Maxillofacial Prosthetics and Implants

LONG ESSAYS

Question 1

Discuss in detail the obturators used in maxillofacial prosthesis.

Answer

Obturators

It is defined as a prosthesis used to close a congenital or acquired tissue opening, primarily of the hard palate and/or contiguous alveolar structures. Prosthetic restoration of the defect often includes use of a surgical obturator, interim obturator and definitive obturator.

An obturator is used in the rehabilitation of maxillary resection. It is done in three phases namely; first, second and third phase. In the first phase, a surgical obturator is used. An interim obturator and a definitive obturator is placed in the second phase and the third or final phase, respectively.

Types

It can be categorized as follows:
- On the basis of phase of treatment
  - Surgical obturator
  - Interim obturator
  - Definitive obturator.
- On the basis of the material used
  - Metal obturator
  - Resin obturator
  - Silicone obturator.
- On the basis of the area of restoration
  - Palatal obturator
  - Meatal obturator.

Surgical obturator

- It is defined as a temporary prosthesis used to restore the continuity of the hard palate immediately after surgery or traumatic loss of a portion or all of the hard palate and/or contiguous alveolar structures (i.e., gingival tissue, teeth)
- It is further divided into two types namely; immediate and delayed surgical obturator. Immediate surgical obturator is inserted at the time of surgery whereas delayed surgical obturator is inserted 7–10 days post-surgery.

Interim obturator

- It is defined as a prosthesis that is made several weeks or months following the surgical resection of a portion of one or both maxillae
- It frequently includes replacement of teeth in the defect area
- This prosthesis, when used, replaces the surgical obturator that is placed immediately following the resection and may be subsequently replaced with a definitive obturator.

Definitive obturators

It is defined as a prosthesis that artificially replaces part or all of the maxilla and the associated teeth lost due to surgery or trauma.

Palatal obturator

- This obturator serves as a stable matrix for surgical packing
- It is advantageous as aids in decreasing oral contamination
- Post-operatively, with the help of this obturator, speech gets effective
- It allows the process of deglutition
- Moreover, it also reduces the psychological impact of the surgery
- In some cases, it can also reduce the period of hospitalisation.

Meatal obturator

- A significant type of obturator, extending upto nasal maetus is used to form the closure of nasal structures against the conchae and the roof of the nasal cavity
- The closure establishes at a level posterior and superior to the posterior border of hard palate
- This is indicated in the patients where separation of oral and nasal cavity is required
- Patients with extensive soft palate defects can also be benefitted with the use of meatal obturator
- However, it cannot control nasal air emission and causes alterations in nasal resonance.

Question 2

Write in detail about maxillary defects.

Answer

Patients with maxillary defects faces difficulties in normal physiological functions such as speech, mastication and deglutition. Therefore, maxillofacial prosthesis are used to restore these functions.

Types of Maxillary Defects

It can be categorised as follows:
- Congenital
    - Cleft lip
    - Cleft palate.
- Acquired
    - Total maxillectomy
    - Partial maxillectomy.

Congenital Maxillary Defects

- The most frequently encountered defects are cleft lip and cleft palate
- Other defects like sub-mucous cleft palate, Pierre Robin syndrome, hemifacial microsomia are also found and their management is similar to that of cleft lip/palate cases.

Types of congenital maxillary defects

- Cleft lip, a significant congenital maxillary defect results due to the inappropriate fusion between the fronto-nasal and maxillary process
- If this occurs on one side it forms a unilateral cleft and when occurs on both sides, it causes a bilateral cleft
- The aetiological factors includes infections, drugs like phenytoin, poor diet, and hormonal imbalance in the first trimester and genetic factors
- Cleft lip can be classified according to the extent of the defect, which is as follows:
    - Class I: Cleft lip involving cleft alveolus (primary palate)
    - Class II: Cleft of hard and soft palate (secondary palate)
    - Class III: Combination of class I and I.
- Cleft palate, another common congenital maxillary defect is classified according to Veau's classification, which is as follows:
    - Class I: Cleft involving the soft palate, which can also be a sub-mucous cleft with normal appearance
    - Class II: A midline cleft involving the bone, present only on the posterior part of the palate
    - Class III: A unilateral cleft extending along the mid-palatine suture and a suture between premaxilla and palatine shelf
    - Class IV: A unilateral cleft extending along the mid-palatine suture and both the sutures between pre-maxilla and palatine shelf.

Acquired Maxillary Defects

- Mostly, surgical resection of tumours causes acquired maxillary defects
- Among which, benign lesions need smaller resection while malignant tumours need extensive resection
- Therefore, restoration of resection of maxillary tumours is difficult in comparison to that of benign lesions
- Moreover, trauma can be other crucial cause for an acquired maxillary defect.

Types

- They are categorised on the basis of their extent
- The defect resulting from the ressection of both the maxillae is considered as total maxillectomy whereas the resection of one or a part of the maxilla or palate is recognised as partial maxillectomy
- According to Aramany, partial maxillary defects can be classified on the basis of their extent
    - Class I: It is a unilateral defect involving one half of the arch and the adjacent palatine shelf. The defect extends to the midline (all the teeth in that side of the arch are missing)
    - Class II: It is a unilateral defect involving one side of the arch posterior to the canine (teeth posterior to the canine are absent)
    - Class III: It is a defect involving the centre of the palatine shelves (all the teeth are present)
    - Class IV: It is a bilateral defect involving one side of the arch along with the entire pre-maxilla (all anteriors along with the posteriors of one side are missing)

- Class V: It is a bilateral posterior defect (teeth anterior to the second premolar are present)
- Class VI: It is a bilateral anterior defect (teeth anterior to the second premolar are absent).

Question 3

Define implants. What are the parts of implants?

Answer

A dental implant is defined as a substance that is placed into the jaw to support a crown or fixed or removable denture.

Parts

The parts of the implant are as follows:
- Implant body or fixture
- Healing screw
- Healing cap
- Abutment
- Impression post
- Laboratory analogues
- Waxing sleeves
- Prosthesis retaining screws
- Implant super-structures

Implant Body or Fixture

- The implant body, the constituent can be threaded or non-threaded and is positioned within the bone during first phase of surgery
- Threaded type of implant bodies are available commercially as pure Titanium (Ti) or as Ti alloys
- The Ti or Ti alloys may or may not exhibit a hydroxyapatite coating.

Healing Screw

- This screw is usually positioned in the superior surface of the body during the healing phase
- It aids in increasing the suturing of soft tissues
- In addition, it impedes the growth of the tissue over the edge of the implant.

Healing Cap

- After the second phase of surgery and prior to the insertion of the prosthesis, healing cap is placed over the sealing screw
- It is dome-shaped which may range in length from 2–10 mm
- It protudes through the soft tissue into the oral cavity
- Moreover, it help in the prevention of overgrowth of tissues around the implants during the healing phase.

Abutment

- It is similar to a prepared tooth in shape, and is designed to be screwed into the body of the implant
- It acts as the primary component and offers retention to the fixed partial denture.

Impression Post

- Impression post, a small stem, serves as to promote the transfer of the intra-oral location of the implant or abutment to a similar position on the cast
- It is positioned over the implant body during impression making.

Laboratory Analogue

- It represent the body of the implant and is a machined structure
- It is placed over prepared bone cavity in which implant body is inserted during surgery
- It helps in the fabrication of an implant-supported prosthesis
- Subsequently, the analogue is fixed over the impression post
- An impression is made and the analogue impression post complex gets attached to the impression and comes away with it
- Then the impression is poured and the impression post analogue complex gets lodged to the cast.

Waxing Sleeves

They are joined to the laboratory analogue during the fabrication of the super structure and attaches themselves to the body of the implant.

Prosthesis Retaining Screw

It penetrates the fixed prosthesis and secures it to the abutment.

Implant Super-structure

- It acts as an abutment and is fabricated over the implant after its final positioning
- It is connected to the implant through attachment
- Overdentures, fixed bridges, fixed detachable bridges and single crowns are the most frequently used super-structures.

Chapter 30 Maxillofacial Prosthetics and Implants

SHORT ESSAY

Question 1

Discuss polymers and composites in implants.

Answer

Polymers and Composites in Implants

- Polymers and composites, predominantly are used as connectors for osseointegrated implants for the distribution of internal force from implants to the tissues
- Among these, polymers are made-up both in solid and porous forms
- The solid form is used for tissue attachments whereas porous form aid in replacement augmentations
- Moreover, they require special handling techniques, and are sensitive to sterilisatiion.

Advantages

- Composites have excellent biocompatibility and are in use for a very long time
- They can be altered to suit the clinical situations
- The primary disadvantage is that they are sensitive to handling and sterilisation and cannot be sterilised using steam or ethylene oxide
- Long term experience
- Excellent biocompatibility
- Ability to control properties through composite structures.

Disadvantages

- Composites have excellent biocompatibility and are in use for a very long time. They can be altered to suit the clinical situations. The primary disadvantage is that they are sensitive to handling and sterilisation and cannot be sterilised using steam or ethylene oxide
- Porous polymers undergo elastic deformation and lead to closing or opening of regions intended for tissue ingrowth.
- Difficult to clean the contaminated, porous particles.

SHORT NOTES

Question 1

Describe meatal obturator.

Answer

- A significant type of obturator, extending upto nasal maetus is used to form the closure of nasal structures against the conchae and the roof of the nasal cavity
- The closure establishes at a level posterior and superior to the posterior border of hard palate
- This is indicated in the patients where separation of oral and nasal cavity is required
- Patients with extensive soft palate defects can also be benefitted with the use of meatal obturator.

Question 2

What are the properties of ceramics?

Answer

- Ceramics are intermediate in density between polymers and metals in the range of 2-6 gms/cm3
- Less resistance to shear and tensile stress
- They are electrical insulators under most circumstances due to the presence of hydroxyapatite crystals
- Modulus of elasticity for hydroxyapatite and bio-glass is 40 to 120 GPa and 40 to 140 GPa, respectively
- They possess high compressive strength upto 500 MPa
- Bending stress is 40 to 300 MPa (hydroxyapatite) and 20 to 350 MPa (bio-glass)
- Most ceramics are clear or transparent with some scattering or diffusion of light
- They usually have good chemical resistance to weak acids and weak bases
- They tend to be rigid and brittle and are not capable of much plastic deformation.

Question 3

What are the advantages of implants?

Answer

- The design of the implants should be such that the effect of deleterious forces can be minimized
- The effectiveness of chewing by implants is comparison to other prosthesis
- They are more comfortable in comparison to other prosthetic replacements

- They provide a natural-like appearance as if the tooth emerges directly from the soft tissues
- They also aid in stimulating the bone like a natural tooth and thus, prevent residual ridge resorption
- They possess good stability and retention due to osseo-integration.

Question 4

What are the material used in implants?

Answer

Materials used in dental implantology can be broadly studied under four groups, which are as follows:

Metals

- Stainless steel
- Cobalt-Chromium-Molybdenum alloys
- Titanium and its alloys
- Surface coated Titanium
- Gold
- Tantalum.

Ceramics

- Hydroxyapatite
- Bio-glass
- Aluminium oxide.

Polymers and Composites

Others

Carbon.

SECTION 4

RECENTLY ASKED QUESTIONS

Chapter 31: Recently Asked Questions

INTRODUCTION TO COMPLETE DENTURES

Long Essays

1. Discuss in detail how you will manage mandibular poor foundation case for complete denture fabrication. [MUHS]
2. Define physiologic rest position of mandible. Give the importance of Silverman's closest speaking space and discuss the effects of increased vertical dimension in complete dentures. [MUHS]
3. Classify denture stomatitis and write its causative factors. [MUHS]
4. What do you mean by physiological rest position? What is the importance of it in constructing the successful complete denture? [MUHS]
5. Primary stress-bearing areas in mandibular arch with reasoning. [MUHS]
6. What is the importance of patient education? What instructions you will give to a patient receiving complete denture prosthesis? [RGUHS]
7. A teacher aged 50 years wearing complete denture for last ten years visits your office for consultation. Give your method of examining treatment procedure. [RGUHS]
8. Define denture aesthetics and discuss the various factors influencing denture aesthetics. [RGUHS]
9. Enumerate the reasons for loss of teeth. What are the consequences of loss of teeth? What are the methods of prosthodontic replacements? [BUHS]

Short Essays

1. Compare residual ridge resorption of maxillary and mandibular edentulous ridge. [RGUHS]
2. Mental attitude of patients. [NTR-NR]
3. Edentulous state. [NTR-OR]
4. Metallic denture base. [NTR-OR]
5. Ridge resorption. [NTR-OR]

Short Notes

1. What are the objectives of complete denture prosthodontics? Explain them. [MUHS]
2. Fabrication of custom tray for completely edentulous arches. [TN]
3. Rougae area and its clinical application in complete denture prosthodontics. [MUHS]
4. Xerostomia. [RGUHS]
5. Advantages of metal bases. [RGUHS]
6. RRR. [RGUHS]
7. Polished surface. [NTR-NR]
8. Metallic denture base. [RGUHS]
9. Define the term geriodontology. What are the age changes occurring in geriatric patient? [MUHS]
10. Polishing surfaces of the complete denture. [GOA]
11. What are the soft tissues covering the hard palate and their relevance to complete dentures? [MUHS]
12. Draw maxillary and mandibular edentulous cast and label the anatomical landmarks of clinical importance. [MUHS]
13. Soft palate. [RGUHS]
14. What are the stress-bearing and relief areas of maxillary foundation? [MUHS]

DIAGNOSIS AND TREATMENT PLANNING

Long Essays

1. What do you understand by the term 'Examination of the patient?' Name the objectives of examination of a patient. Discuss in detail the clinical significance of anatomical landmarks of edentulous maxilla and mandible. [TN]

2. Discuss in detail the clinical significance of the following for ensuring success of complete denture treatment.
   a. Pre-extraction records.
   b. Examination, diagnosis, and treatment planning. [MUHS]
3. Diabetic patient aged 65 years with few teeth remaining comes to your dental college hospital for dental prosthesis. Discuss the treatment planning and special steps to be taken by you for the management of the patient. [NTR-OR]
4. A teacher aged 50 years' wearing complete denture for last ten years visits your office for consultation. Give your method of examining treatment procedure. [BUHS]
5. Discuss the significance of case history recording, diagnosis, and treatment planning in the fabrication of complete dentures prosthesis. [GOA]

Short Essays

1. Importance of preprosthetic evaluation of the edentulous area before making impression. [MUHS]
2. Why should complete radiograph examination be made of an edentulous mouth? [MUHS]
3. Influence of saliva on retention and stability. [RGUHS (OS)]
4. Discuss the diagnosis and treatment planning in complete denture patients. [GOA]

Short Notes

1. Importance of full mouth intraoral radiographs in edentulous patients. [RGUHS (RS2)]
2. Mental attitudes of patients. [TN]
3. Significance of retromolar pad. [NTRUHS]
5. Undercuts in complete denture. [RGUHS (RS)]
6. Preprosthetic surgery. [GOA]
7. House classification of mental attitudes. [GOA]

DIAGNOSTIC IMPRESSIONS IN CD AND MOUTH PREPARATION FOR CD

Long Essays

1. Define impression. Discuss the biological considerations for a maxillary impression. [RGUHS (RS)]
2. Define complete denture retention. Enumerate the various factors of retention. [RGUHS (RS2)]
3. Define impressions in prosthodontics. Why is it called as biological? Discuss the principles and objectives of impression making in complete denture prosthesis. [GOA]
4. Discuss the mouth preparation of compete dentures. [TN]

Short Essays

1. Importance of preprosthetic evaluation of the edentulous area before making impression. [MUHS]
2. Diagnostic cast and its uses. [RGUHS (OS)]
3. Preprosthetic surgery. [RGUHS; NTR-NR]
4. Vestibuloplasty. [NTR-NR]
5. Preprosthetic surgical managements in complete denture. [NTR-OR]

Short Notes

1. Mandibular stress-bearing areas. [RGUHS (RS)]
2. Retromolar pad. [NTRUGHS]
3. Preprosthetic surgery. [RGUHS (RS)]
4. Buccal shelf area. [RGUHS (RS2); TN]
5. Anterior reference points. [NTRUGHS]
6. Incisive papilla. [RGUHS (OS)]
7. Muscles of mastication and facial expression. [TN]
8. Muscles of the soft palate. [TN]
9. Alveolingual sulcus. [TN]
10. Balanced occlusion. [TN]

PRIMARY IMPRESSION IN COMPLETE DENTURES AND LAB PROCEDURES PRIOR TO MASTER IMPRESSION MAKING

Long Essays

1. Define stability and support in complete dentures. Describe the methods to obtain stability and support. [RGUHS (RS)]
2. Write in detail the supporting and limiting structures of maxillary and mandibular edentulous arch. [RGUHS (RS2)]
3. Write in detail about the anatomical landmarks of maxillary and mandibular edentulous arches in relation to complete denture construction. [TN]
4. Define the term 'impression' in complete denture prosthodontics. Classify impression techniques and explain the objectives and theories of impression making. [TN NTR-OR]

Chapter 31 Recently Asked Questions

5. Define and discuss retention in complete denture. [RGUHS (OS)]
6. Define stability and discuss the various factors affecting stability in complete denture. [NTRUHS]
7. Mention the objects of impression making and discuss the procedure of merits and demerits of different impression techniques for a complete denture. [TN]
8. Give the importance of impression techniques used for different patient treatment planning and post-insertion instruction to the patient. [MUHS]
9. Define retention. Write briefly about the various factors involved in the retention of complete denture. [RGUHS]
10. Describe any one method of making the primary impression for a maxillary complete denture, stating step by step precautions and causes of errors in the impression. [MUHS]
11. Mention the importance of posterior palate seal in complete denture. Describe in detail the anatomic location and the methods of recording the same. [TN]
12. Define complete denture impression. Discuss in detail the aims and objectives of impression making. [RGUHS]
13. Describe in brief the principles and objectives of making maxillary final impression for complete edentulous patient and write the concepts incorporated in your impression procedure. [MUHS]
14. Define 'retention' in complete dentures. Enumerate and discuss the various factors responsible for the retention of complete dentures. [TN]
15. Neutral zone. [NTR-NR]
16. Define impression. Discuss the various theories of impression making and describe your method of making a definitive impression. [GOA]
17. Define impression making in complete denture. Name the objectives of impression making. Discuss the factors affecting the retention. [TN]
18. Discuss the aims and objectives of impression making in complete denture treatment. [GOA]
19. Define retention, stability, and support. Explain how you will achieve these factors in complete denture prosthesis. [GOA]
20. Define retention, stability, and support in complete denture. Write in detail about the factors influencing retention. [NTR-OR]
21. Discuss the anatomical landmarks in case of a completely edentulous patient. [NTR-OR]
22. What do you understand by term 'stability' of complete denture? Write the factors which influence stability in CD. [RGUHS]
23. Discuss the factors affecting retention and stability in complete dentures. [MUHS]
24. Discuss posterior palatal seal in detail. [MUHS]
25. Define retention, stability, and support. Discuss the importance of stress and non-stress-bearing areas in complete denture patient. [RGUHS]
26. Define the term 'retention'. Describe the factors of retention in complete denture. [NTR-OR]
27. Define impression. Discuss the aims and objectives of impression for a complete denture patient. [BUHS]
28. What is 'Posterior palatal seal? Describe how it is obtained? [MUHS]
29. What are the various causes for inadequate retention in complete denture? What precautions would you take to achieve good retention in complete denture? [MUHS]
30. What are the objectives of impression making and how will you achieve them during impression making? [NTR-OR]
31. What do you understand by the terms retention, stability, and support? What factors affect stability of the complete denture? [MUHS]
32. What is mucostatic impression? Give in detail the mucostatic impression procedure with special reference to its underlying principle. Describe its merits. [RGUHS]
33. What is posterior palatal seal and give its significance? Describe one of the methods of projecting posterior palatal seal in complete denture patient. [BUHS]
34. With the help of a diagram, discuss the denturebearing area of edentulous mouth. Give the clinical importance of anterior palatal seal and retromolar pad. [RGUHS]
35. With the help of a diagram, discuss the denturebearing area of edentulous mouth. Give the clinical importance of anterior palatal seal and retromolar pad. [BUHS]
36. Discuss the various factors related to retention and stability in complete dentures. [MUHS]
37. What do you understand by the terms, retention and stability in complete denture prosthesis? Discuss the various doctrines incorporated in prosthesis for guessing good retention in conversional complete denture prosthesis. [RGUHS]
38. Explain how different groups of muscles cause dislodgement of maxillary and mandibular complete denture and how muscular power can be harnessed for further retention of complete denture? [BUHS]
39. What do you understand by the terms, retention and stability in complete denture prosthesis? Discuss the various doctrines incorporated in prosthesis for guessing good retention in conversional complete denture prosthesis. [BUHS]
40. Describe in detail the various anatomical landmarks in an edentulous mouth to be considered for construction of complete denture. [RGUHS]

41. What do you understand by the term 'stability' of complete denture? Write the factors which influence stability in CD. [TN]

Short Essays

1. Physical factors of retention of dentures. [RGUHS (RS2)]
2. Factors affecting stability of complete dentures. [NTRUHS (NR)]
3. Alginate impression material. [NTRUHS (NR)]
4. Objectives of impression making. [MUHS NTRUHS]
5. Impression compound. [NTRUHS (OR)]
6. Pressure theory of impression making. [RGUHS (OS)]
7. Relief areas. [NTRUHS]
8. Factors affecting stability of complete dentures. [NTRUHS]
9. Write about the significance of posterior palatal seal in maxillary prosthesis. [RGUHS]
10. Alveolingual sulcus. [RGUHS (RS)]
11. Retromolar pad. [RGUHS (OS)]
12. Discuss the materials and methods for recording complete denture impressions. [GOA]
13. Posterior palatal seal. [NTR-NR NTR-OR]
14. Maxillary anatomic landmarks. [NTR-NR]
15. Impression technique for a flabby ridge. [TN]
16. Microscopic anatomy of supporting and limiting structures of maxilla. [TN]
17. Factors for retention and stability of complete denture. [TN]
18. Retention in complete dentures. [NTR-NR ; NTR-OR]
19. Define retention, stability, and support. Discuss the various causes for inadequate retention in complete dentures. [GOA]
20. Define and explain the significance of posterior palatal seal with diagram. [RGUHS]
21. Incisive papilla. [NTR-NR NTR-OR]
22. Buccal sheet area. [NTR-OR]
23. Factors affecting retention in complete dentures. [NTR-OR]
24. Role of saliva in edentulous patients. [MUHS]
25. Enumerate the various objectives of impression making in complete denture. Discuss the various philosophies of impression making in complete denture. [MUSH]
26. Enumerate the various objectives of impression making in complete denture. Discuss the various philosophies of impression making in complete denture. [MUHS]
27. Role of saliva in edentulous patients. [MUHS]
28. Significance of retromolar pad. [NTR-OR]
29. Primary stress-bearing areas. [NTR-OR]
30. Classify the various methods of impression making in complete denture. [MUHS]
31. Write a note on surverying. [GOA]
32. Saliva and its role in complete dentures. [NTR-OR]
33. Retromolar pad. [NTR-OR]
34. Mylohyoid ridge. [NTR-OR]

Short Notes

1. Retromolar pad. [RGUHS; TN]
2. Disinfection of impression. [NTRUGHS]
3. Dual arch impression. [NTRUGHS]
4. Neutral zone. [RGUHS TN]
5. Primary stress-bearing area. [RGUHS(RS2)]
6. Buccal shelf. [NTRUHS (NR)]
7. Ring form. [RGUHS (OS)]
8. Stress-bearing areas. [NTRUHS (NR); RGUHS (RS); TN]
9. Anterior and posterior vibrating lines. [RGUHS (RS2)]
10. Rugae. [RGUHS(RS2)]
11. Retention. [NTRUHS]
12. Stability. [NTRUHS]
13. Selective pressure impression technique in complete denture patients. [TN]
14. Vibrating line of palate. [RGUHS (RS)]
15. Retention in complete denture. [RGUHS; TN]
16. Classify impression materials. [NTRUHS]
17. Tissue conditioners. [NTRUHS]
18. What is the significance of a posterior palatal seal? Enumerate the techniques used to develop the same. [MUHS]
19. Posterior palatal seal area. [MUHS]
20. Significance of centric relation. [RGUHS (RS)]
21. Enumerate the functions of posterior palatal seal. [MUHS]
22. Syneresis and imbibition. [RGUHS (RS)]
23. Disadvantages of condensation silicones. [RGUHS (RS)]
24. Labial frenum. [RGUHS (RS)]
25. Significance of incisive papilla? [NTR-NR]
26. How you will record buccal frenum in maxillary impression? Name the muscles associated with it. [MUHS]
27. Objectives of final impression making in complete denture prosthodontics. [MUHS]
28. Ruguae support. [RGUHS]
29. Torus palatines. [RGUHS]
30. Saliva's influence on denture retention and stability. [RGUHS]
31. Factors affecting complete denture retention. [NTR- NR]
32. House's palate classification. [NTR-NR]
33. How would you locate the posterior palatal seal area? Describe any one method of incorporating the effect in the maxillary complete denture. [MUHS]
34. What are the advantages of zinc oxide eugenol impression paste? State its composition. [MUHS]

35. Define retention as applicable to complete dentures and list five possible causes for failure in achieving it. [MUHS]
36. Anterior and posterior vibrating lines. [RGUHS]
37. Retention and stability. [TN]
38. Selective pressure impression. [RGUHS]
39. Mechanism of complete denture support. [TN]
40. Objectives of impression making in complete dentures. [MUHS]
41. Materials which can be used fof wash impressions in final impression for complete dentures. [MUHS]
42. Define posterior palatal seal and give conventional method to record it. [MUHS]
43. What is a functional impression and write the technique for making the same? [MUHS]
44. Posterior palatal seal area [NTR-NR]
45. Masseteric notch. [RGUHS]
46. Mention the physical factors which aid in retention of complete dentures. [MUHS]
47. Marking of vibrating line. [RGUHS]
48. What is the purpose of border moulding? [MUHS]
49. Marking of vibrating line. [RGUHS]
50. Factors of retention in complete denture. [MUHS]
51. Atmospheric pressure. [NTR-NR]
52. Stability in complete dentures. [NTR-OR GOA]
53. Mucocompressive impression theory. [RGUHS]
54. Stress-bearing areas of the edentulous arches. [GOA]
55. Soft palate. [BUHS]

SECONDARY IMPRESSION IN COMPLETE DENTURES AND LAB PROCEDURES PRIOR TO JAW RELATION

Long Essays

1. Define articulators. Give classification, and discuss the uses of articulators. [GOA]
2. Define articulators. Give classification, uses of articulators, and discuss in detail about a semi-adjustable articulator. [NTRUHS]
3. Define impression for complete denture and discuss in detail the anatomic structures influencing the impression of edentulous mandible. [NTR-NR]
4. Define complete denture impression. Discuss the various theories of impression making. [NTR-OR]
5. What is posterior palatal seal? Describe how it is obtained. [GOA]
6. Write in detail about the need for balanced articulation and explain in detail the factors governing balanced articulation. [TN]
7. Define impression. Discuss in detail about the most widely accepted technique of making impression in complete denture treatment. [NTR-NR]
8. Define the term impression' in complete denture prosthodontics. Classify impression techniques and explain the objectives of impression making. [NTR-OR]
9. Define articulators. Give any two classifications of articulators. Write the advantages and disadvantages of mean value articulators. [GOA]
10. Describe the theories of impression making in complete dentures prosthodontics. Describe the impression procedure you will follow for a patient with upper anterior movable flabby tissue. [NTR-OR]
11. What is posterior palatal seal and give its significance? Describe one of the methods of projecting posterior palatal seal in complete denture patient. [RGUHS]
12. What are the objectives of impression making and how you will achieve them during impression making? [NTR-OR]
13. What is mucostatic impression? Give in detail the mucostatic impression procedure with special reference to its underlying principle and describe its merits. [BUHS]

Short Essays

1. Selective pressure impression theory [RGUHS (RS)]
2. Posterior palatal seal. [NTRUHS (OR), RGUHS (RS); TN]
3. Semi-adjustable articulator. [RGUHS (RS2)]
4. Draw a neat labelled diagram of mean value articulator. [RGUHS (RS)]
5. Selective pressure impression technique. [NTR-NR; NTRUHS]
6. Articulators. [NTRUHS; TN]
7. Rubber base impression materials. [TN]
8. Various theories of impression making of edentulous arches. [NTR-NR]
9. Discuss the materials and methods for recording complete denture impressions. [GOA]
10. Trial denture. [NTR-NR]
11. Selective compression theory. [NTR-OR]
12. Define and explain the significance of posterior palatal seal with diagram. [RGUHS]
13. Pascal's law. [NTR-OR]

14. Controlled pressure theory of impression making. [NTR-OR]
15. Define articulator. Classify and discuss the importance of articulators in prosthodontics. [GOA]
16. Selective pressure theory of impression. [NTR-OR]
17. Border moulding in mandible. [NTR-OR]

Short Notes

1. Articulators-classification. [NTRUHS (OR)]
2. Primary stress-bearing area. [NTRUGHS]
3. Disinfection of impressions. [NTRUHS (NR)]
4. Mean value articulator. [RGUHS (RS)]
5. Significance of posterior palatal seal. [RGUHS (RS)]
6. Define articulator. Classify them. [NTRUHS]
7. Hinge axis. [NTRUHS]
8. Vibrating line. [RGUHS (OS)]
9. Border moulding. [RGUHS (RS)]
10. Hinge axis. [RGUHS (OS)]
11. Disinfecting the impression. [NTRUHS]
12. Significance of peripheral seal in complete denture. [TN]
13. Posterior palatal seal area. [RGUHS; TN]
14. Bennett angle. [BUHS NTRUHS]
15. Functions of posterior palatal seal. [TN]
16. Materials used for master impression. [RGUHS]
17. Final impression materials for complete denture. [NTR-NR]
18. Articulators and their uses. [TN]
19. Occlusion rims for construction of complete denture. [TN]
20. Average movement articulators. [TN]
21. Posterior palatal seal area. [GOA; TN]
22. Maxillary tuberosity. [TN]
23. Mucocompressive impression theory. [RGUHS]
24. Selective pressure impression. [BUHS]
25. Bennett movement. [BUHS]

MAXILLOMANDIBULAR RELATIONS

Long Essays

1. Write the importance of centric relation in complete denture treatment. Write in brief the methods to record centric relation in complete dentures. [TN]
2. Define face-bow. Give classification and utility of face-bow in complete denture prosthodontics. [NTRUGHS]
3. What are jaw relations? Discuss the biological significance of following during complete denture preparation? [TN]
4. Define centric jaw relation. Classify different methods and explain any one method for recording jaw elation. [RGUHS (RS2)]
5. Define centric relation. Explain its significance. Discuss the various methods of recording centric relation in edentulous patients. [NTRUHS]
6. Define centric jaw relation. Mention in brief the various methods of recording it. [NTRUHS]
7. Describe and classify face-bow. Mention the parts of face-bow. Discuss the uses of face-bow. [RGUHS (OS)]
8. Define centric relation and write its significance. List the methods of recording centric relation in complete dentures. Write in detail any one of them. [RGUHS (OS)]
9. Define centric relation. Explain its significance and methods of recording the centric relation. [TN]
10. Mention recordable jaw relation for complete dentures. Describe in detail the vertical jaw relation. [RGUHS (OS)]
11. Define centric relation. Name the different methods of recording centric relation of an edentulous patient. Describe in detail one of the methods you choose for recording centric relation in your clinic. [RGUHS; TN]
12. What is balanced articulation and mention its importance? Describe the factors responsible for balanced articulation in complete dentures. [NTRUHS]
13. What is orientation relation? Write in detail about recording of orientation relation in complete denture patient. [MUHS]
14. Define balanced occlusion. Write in detail about the various factors that contribute to balanced occlusion? [RGUHS]
15. Define and classify jaw relation. Discuss the methods of establishing vertical relations. [GOA]
16. Shade selection. [NTR-NR]
17. Define balanced occlusion. Explain its significance. What are the factors affecting it? Explain each in detail. [NTR-NR]
18. Signification of centric relation. [RGUHS]
19. What is articulator? Classify articulator. Write the uses and requirements of an articulator? [RGUHS]
20. Define jaw relations. Enumerate the various jaw relations. Mention the significance of physiologic rest position. Discuss the effects of increased andreased vertical jaw relation. [NTR-OR; TN]

Chapter 31 Recently Asked Questions

21. Classify jaw relation. Define centric relation. Explain its clinical significance. What are the methods for recording centric relation? Explain one in detail. [NTR-NR]
22. Write in detail the procedures involved in selection of anterior teeth in complete denture patients. [RGUHS]
23. What is an articulator? Write the uses and requirements of an articulator. Classify articulator. [RGUHS]
24. Define centric relation. Discuss the methods of recording centric relation. [GOA]
25. What is face-bow? Discuss the importance of same in complete dentures in removable partial prosthesis. [GOA]
26. Dentogenic concept. [NTR-NR]
27. Define physiologic rest position of mandible. Give the importance of Silverman's closest speaking space and discuss the effects of increased vertical dimension in complete dentures. [M]
28. Define balanced occlusion. Describe in brief the factors to be considered to obtain balanced occlusion in a complete denture. [BUHS RGUHS]
29. Define .centric relation. Classify the different methods of recording the same and discuss the significance of centric relation in complete denture prosthodontics. [MUHS]
30. Define centric relation. Explain the different methods of recording the same. [RGUHS]
31. Describe the principles of selection of teeth for complete denture patient. [NTR-NR]
32. What is jaw relation? Classify jaw relation. Enumerate the various methods of recording different jaw relations. Discuss in detail any one method of recording vertical jaw relation. [TN]
33. Define balanced occlusion. Explain the rationale of balanced occlusion. Discuss the factors controlling the balanced occlusion. [NTR-OR]
34. Describe the principles of selection of teeth for complete denture patient. [NTR-NR]
35. Define centric relation. List the various methods to record it and explain one of them in detail. Add a note on the difficulties encountered while recording centric relation. [TN]
36. Define jaw relations. Classify and write briefly about the methods of recording vertical jaw relation. [TN]
37. Define articulator. Mention the different types of articulators and discuss a semi-adjustable articulator. [NTR-NR]
38. Define centric relation. Write in detail one method of recording centric relation in a complete denture patient. [NTR-OR]
39. What are the types of jaw relation? Write in detail about the definition and different methods or recording vertical jaw relation. [NTR-OR]
40. What is an articulator? Give the classifications, functions, and requirements of an articulator. [NTR-OR]
41. What are the different maxillomandibular relationships? Discuss their importance and different methods of recording horizontal jaw relation in complete denture patient. [MUHS]
42. Define the term 'centric relation'. Mention the significance of centric jaw relation. Enumerate the methods of recording centric relation. Describe in detail your method of recording centric jaw relation. [NTR-OR]
43. What are the vertical jaw relations? Why is it important to record the correct vertical jaw relation? What is the method followed in your clinic to record vertical jaw relation? [GOA]
44. Describe the technique of establishing and verifying vertical jaw relationship in completely edentulous patient, who has no pre-extraction records. [MUHS]
45. Define vertical dimension of occlusion. Give briefly any one method that you know of registering the same. [RGUHS BUHS]
46. Anterior teeth for an edentulous patient. [NTR-OR]
47. Define centric relation. Describe a method for record centric relation for complete denture construction. [NTR-OR]
48. Discuss aesthetics in complete denture and discuss the factors which favour the selection of anterior teeth. Write the uses and requirements of an articulator selection of anterior teeth. [BUHS]
49. Describe the methods of selecting anterior teeth for an edentulous patient. [NTR-OR]
50. Squint test. [BUHS]
51. Describe the methods of selecting anterior teeth in edentulous patients. [NTR-OR]
52. Discuss the physical and biological factors for the selection of teeth for complete denture construction in edentulous patient. [BUHS]
53. What are centric and eccentric jaw relations? Enumerate the methods of recording centric jaw relation and describe your method for recording the same. [RGUHS]
54. What are centric and eccentric jaw relations? Enumerate the methods of recording centric jaw relation and describe your method for recording the same. [BUHS]
55. What is a face-bow? Discuss the importance of face-bow transfer for an edentulous patient. [MUHS]
56. Define physiological rest position of mandible. Describe the method of establishing and verifying vertical jaw relation for edentulous patient. [BUHS]
57. What are the consequences of incorrect vertical dimension record in complete denture construction? Describe your methods of obtaining vertical dimension records. [MUHS]

58. Define denture aesthetics and discuss the various factors influencing denture aesthetics. [BUHS]
59. What is balanced occlusion and articulation? What are the laws of articulation of developing balanced occlusion in complete denture prosthesis? [BUHS]

Short Essays

1. Plane of orientation. [RGUHS (OS)]
2. Vertical jaw relationship. [RGUHS (RS)]
3. Methods of recording vertical jaw relation. [RGUHS (RS2)]
4. Gothic arch tracing. [RGUHS (RS2)]
5. Alveolingual sulcus. [NTRUHS (OR)]
6. Physiologic rest position. [NTR-NR NTRUHS]
7. Method of training the patient to retrude the mandible. [NTRUHS]
8. Centric relation. [RGUHS (RS)]
9. Significance of recording centric relation. [NTR-OR, RGUHS (RS2)]
10. Face-bow. [NRT-NR NTR- OR; NTRUHS RGUHS (OS)]
11. Classification of jaw relations. [RGUHS (RS)]
12. Articulators. [NTR-OR; NTR-NR]
13. Physiologic rest position and its significance. [NTR-NR]
14. Colour selection of teeth. [RGUHS]
15. Write about orientation relation in complete denture. [RGUHS]
16. Method of recording centric jaw relation. [NTRUHS]
17. Effect of incorrect vertical dimensions. [NTRUHS]
18. Write about Arcon articulators. [RGUHS]
19. Enumerate the factors affecting balanced occlusion. [NTR-NR]
20. Increased vertical dimension. [RGUHS]
21. Shade selection. [NTR-NR, NTR-OR]
22. Dentogenic concept. [NTR-NR]
23. Pre-extraction guides for complete denture. [NTR-NR]
24. Increased vertical relation. [NTR-OR]
25. Laws of balanced occlusion? [RGUHS]
26. Requirements of an articulator. [NTR-NR , NTR-OR]
27. Neutral zone. [NTR-NR]
28. Needles chew-in technique. [TN]
29. Discuss the various jaw relation recording procedures in complete denture patients. [GOA]
30. Principles of arrangement of teeth in complete denture. [NTR-NR]
31. Rationale of balanced occlusion. [NTR-OR]
32. Condylar guidance. [NTR-OR]
33. Non-anatomic teeth. [NTR-OR]
34. Vertical dimension. [NTR-OR]
35. Anatomical articulators. [NTR-OR]
36. Non-anatomic tooth. [NTR-OR]
37. Anatomical articulators? [NTR-OR]
38. Classify jaw relation. Discuss in detail the significance of horizontal jaw relations in complete denture construction. [GOA]
39. Define orientation relation and give its importance in complete dentures. [MUHS]
40. Define centric relation and give its significance. [MUHS]
41. Orientation jaw relation. [NTR-OR]
42. Balanced occlusion. [NTR-OR]
43. Significance of centric relation. [NTR-OR]
44. Reased vertical dimension. [NTR-OR]
45. Physiologic rest position of mandible. [NTR-OR]
46. Freeway space (interocclusal distance). [NTR-OR]
47. Gothic arch tracing. [NTR-ORNTR-OR]
48. Bennet movement and Bennet angle. [NTR-OR]
59. Condylar and incisal guidance. [BUHS]
50. Compensating curves. [NTR-OR]
51. Physiologic rest position of mandible. [BUHS]
52. Importance of pre-extraction records. [BUHS]

Short Notes

1. Selective grinding in complete denture. [NTRUGHS]
2. Chamfer finish line. [RGUHS (RS)]
3. Gothic arch tracing. [RGUHS,TN; NTRUHS]
4. Merits of face-bow. [NTRUHS (OR)]
5. Vertical dimension at rest. [NTRUHS (OR)]
6. Overjet and overbite. [RGUHS (RS)]
7. Hazards of increased vertical dimension. [RGUHS (RS2)]
8. Parts of face-bow. [RGUHS (RS)]
9. Origination jaw relation. [RGUHS (OS)]
10. Bennett movement. [RGUHS (RS2)]
11. Altered vertical dimension. [RGUHS(OS)]
12. Freeway space. [BUHS RGUHS(OS); NTRUHS]
13. Face-bow. [TN]
14. Vertical jaw relations. [TN]
15. Needle-House chewing technique. [TN]
16. Define face-bow. Enumerate its types. [NTRUHS]
17. Rest position of mandible. [RGUHS (OS)]
18. Freeway space. [NTR-NR; TN]
19. Oveijet and overbite. [NTRUHS]
20. Closest speaking space. [RGUHS (RS,OS)]
21. Describe the importance of marking the midline, the canine line, and the high lip line during jaw relation. [MUHS]
22. Physiologic rest position. [NTRUHS]
23. State the consequence of increased vertical relation recording in complete denture case. [MUHS]
24. Enumerate the various methods of determining vertical relation of occlusion. [MUHS]
25. Define centric relation. Write in brief about the different methods to record it. [MUHS]

26. Altered VD. [RGUHS]
27. Group function. [RGUHS]
28. Interocclusal clearance. [RGUHS]
29. Significance of centric relation. [TN]
30. Centric jaw relation record. [RGUHS]
31. Lingualized occlusion. [NTR-NR]
32. Compensating curves. [TN]
33. Silverman speaking space. [TN]
34. Increased vertical relation. [RGUHS]
35. Posterior tooth forms. [NTR-NR]
36. Give any one definition of centric relation of mandible. Describe any two important consequences of failure to record it correctly for complete dentures. [MUHS]
37. Write the various methods for assisting the patient to retrude the mandible during centric relation registration. [MUHS]
38. Hinge axis. [NTR-NR]
39. Beyron's point. [RGUHS]
40. Effect of increased vertical dimension. [TN]
41. Perleche. [RGUHS]
42. Canine-guided occlusion. [RGUHS]
43. Difference between natural and artificial dentition. [RGUHS]
44. Niswonger's method of establishing vertical examples. [MUHS]
45. Closest speaking space. [RGUHS]
46. Problems with reduced vertical dimension in complete dentures. [MUHS]
47. Vibrating line of palate and its importance in complete denture. [TN]
48. Retruding the mandibular to centric relation. [TN]
49. Define centric relation and give its significance. [MUHS]
50. Relief factor. [GOA]
51. Cuspless teeth. [NTR-NR]
52. Significance of rest position of the mandible. [TN]
53. Freeway space and its importance. [MUHS]
54. Write the differences between arbitrary and kinematic face-bow. [MUHS]
55. Enumerate the characteristics of increase of vertical relation in complete denture patient. [MUHS]
56. Define centric relation. [MUHS]
57. Methods of recording centric relations. [RGUHS]
58. Methods of recording centric relations. [BUHS]
59. Face-bow transfer. [RGUHS]
60. Neutrocentric occlusion. [BUHS]
61. Physiologic rest position of mandible. [RGUHS GOA]
62. Anatomical articulator? [BUHS]
63. Face-bow. [RGUHS]
64. Importance of pre-extraction records. [RGUHS]
65. Articulator. [BUHS]
66. Christianson phenomenon. [RGUHS]

LAB PROCEDURES PRIOR TO TRY-IN

Long Essays

1. Define balanced occlusion. Enumerate the advantages of a balanced occulsion. Describe any two factors that jg affect a protrusive balance. [MUHS]
2. Define articulators. Give the classifications and uses of articulators and discuss in detail about semi-adjustable 1, articulator. [NTRUGHS]
3. Discuss occlusion in complete denture. [RGUHS (OS)]
4. What is balanced occlusion? Write in brief the factors jy governing balanced occlusion. [RGUHS (RS)]
5. Selection of anterior and posterior teeth in complete 20. denture. [RGUHS (RS2)]
6. Discuss the various factors to be considered in selec- 21. tion of teeth for complete denture patient. [MUHS TN]
7. What is articulator? Classify articulator. Write the uses and requirements of an articulator [RGUHS]
8. Define articulator? Discuss the advantages, disadvan- 22. tages, and classifications of articulators. [TN]
9. What is an articulator? Write the uses and requirements of an articulator. Classify articulator [RGUHS]
10. Write in detail the procedures involved in selection of anterior teeth in complete denture patients. [RGUHS]
11. Discuss the importance of try-in stage in complete denture prosthodontics. [MUHS]
12. Mention the importance of occlusion in complete dentures. Write in brief about the factors governing balanced articulation. [TN]
13. Define denture aesthetics. Discuss selection of artificial teeth for a complete denture. [GOA]
14. Describe in brief the various posterior tooth forms for dentures. [TN]
15. Describe in detail about tooth selection for treating a fully edentulous patient. [TN]
16. Define balanced occlusion. Describe in brief the factors to be considered to obtain balanced occlusion in a complete denture. [RGUHS]

17. Discuss the factors which help in the selection of artificial teeth in complete denture prosthodontics. [GOA]
18. What are the factors for selection of anterior teeth for a complete denture patient? [MUHS]
19. Discuss the various factors to be considered in the selection of teeth for complete denture patient. [GOA MUHS]
20. What is balanced occlusion? How do you establish it while fabricating a complete denture? [TN]
21. Write the aims, objectives, and scope of prosthodontics. Discuss the role of arrangement of artificial teeth in the success of complete denture. [GOA]
22. Define balanced occlusion and articulation? Discuss in brief determination of balanced occlusion. [GOA]
23. Discuss the principles in arrangement of artificial teeth in complete denture prosthesis. [GOA]
24. Requirements of articulator. [MUHS]
25. Discuss physical and biological factors for the selection of teeth for complete denture construction in edentulous patient. [RGUHS]
26. Define denture aesthetics. Write in detail about the aesthetic requirements of complete denture prosthesis. [GOA]
27. Discuss aesthetics in complete denture and discuss the factors which favour the selection of anterior teeth. [RGUHS]
28. What is balanced occlusion and articulation? What are the laws of articulation of developing balanced occlusion in complete denture prosthesis? [RGUHS]

Short Essays

1. Hinge axis. [NTRUGHS]
2. Anterior tooth selection for complete denture. [NTRUHS]
3. Dentogenic concept. [NTRUHS, NTRUHS (NR)]
4. Types of posterior teeth. [RGUHS (RS2)]
5. Anterior teeth selection. [NTRUHS]
6. Factors affecting balanced occlusion. [RGUHS (RS2)]
7. Posterior selection of teeth. [RGUHS (OS)]
8. Principles in teeth arrangement for completely edentulous patients. [RGUHS (RS2)]
9. Discuss the selection of posterior teeth in complete denture. [MUHS]
10. Rationale of balanced occlusion. [RGUHS]
11. Laws of balanced occlusion. [RGUHS]
12. Try-in procedure. [NTR-OR]

Short Notes

1. Neutral zone. [NTRUHS, RGUHS (RS)]
2. Balanced occlusion. [GOA; TN; NTRUGHS]
3. Hanau's quint. [TN]
4. Arcon articulators. [TN]
5. Non-anatomic teeth. [RGUHS (RS), (RS), (OS), (OS)]
6. SPA factor. [RGUHS (RS2)]
7. Semi-adjustable articulators. [TN]
8. Bilabial sounds. [RGUHS (RS)]
9. Compensating curve. [NTRUHS]
10. Porcelain denture teeth. [NTRUHS]
11. Dentogenic concept. [GOA; TN]
12. SPA factor. [GOA, RGUHS (OS)]
13. Classify articulators. Give two examples for each type. [MUHS]
14. Define centric relation and give its significance. [MUHS]
15. Discuss in short, neutral zone. [MUHS]
16. Define retention and stability. [NTRUHS]
17. Describe the various dimensions of colour. [MUHS]
18. Occlusal refining. [RGUHS]
19. Finishing and polishing agents for acrylic dentures. [RGUHS]
20. Classify articulators. [MUHS]
21. Define guiding planes. [MUHS]
22. Canine-guided occlusion. [RGUHS]
23. Selection of anterior teeth. [GOA]
24. Laws of articulation in complete denture. [MUHS]
25. Write the methods of selecting the colour/shade of artificial teeth. [MUHS]
26. Differences between natural and artificial dentition. [RGUHS, GOA]
27. ASP factor in complete denture. [TN]
28. Define articulator and name the different types of articulators. [MUHS]
29. Selection of posterior teeth. [GOA; TN]
30. Posterior teeth selection for complete denture. [TN]
31. Post-insertion problems of complete denture. [TN]
32. Differences between natural and artificial occlusion. [GOA]
33. Importance of try-in complete dentures. [MUHS]
34. Factors on which dentogenic concept of selection of teeth is based. [MUHS]
35. Define terminal hinge axis and give its importance. [MUHS]
36. Selection of teeth for geriatric patients. [TN]
37. Selection of anterior teeth. [RGUHSil]
38. What are the criteria for selection of anterior teeth for a complete denture patient? [MUHS]
39. Importance of age factor in selection of teeth. [MUHS]
40. Indications of non-anatomic teeth in complete denture. [MUHS]
41. Try-in complete dentures. [GOA]

42. Importance of compensatory curve. [MUHS]
43. Concept of mutually protected occlusion. [MUHS]
44. Squint test. [RGUHS]
45. Factors determining neutrocentric occlusion. [MUHS]
46. Neutrocentric occlusion. [RGUHS]
47. Anatomical articulator. [RGUHS]
48. Condylar and incisal guidance. [RGUHS]
49. Articulator. [RGUHS]
50. Bennett angle. [RGUHS]
51. Bennett movement. [RGUHS]

LAB PROCEDURES PRIOR TO INSERTION AND COMPLETE DENTURE INSERTION

Long Essays

1. Write an essay on sequelae of complete denture wearing. [NTRUHS (OR)]
2. What are the various post-insertion problems and their management? [NTR-NR]
3. Discuss in detail the various post-insertion problems in edentulous patients using complete dentures. [NTR- NR]
4. Discuss in detail about the insertional instructions and aftercare of the complete denture. [NTR-NR]
5. Give your method of fitting complete denture prosthesis and instructions and aftercare to patients. [GOA]
6. What is the importance of patient education? What instructions you will give to a patient receiving complete denture prosthesis? [BUHS]
7. What are the post-insertion problems in complete dentures? Discuss the methods of rectifying the same. [MUHS]
8. Give your method of fitting/insertion of complete denture and aftercare for complete denture prosthesis. [BUHS]
9. Discuss in brief the post-insertion management in complete denture prosthodontics. [NTR-OR]

Short Essays

1. Denture stomatitis. [RGUHS; NTRUHS, NTRUGHS]
2. Burning mouth syndrome. [RGUHS (RS)]
3. Denture resins. [NTRUHS (OR)]
4. Denture stomatitis. [NTRUHS]
5. Instructions to complete denture patients. [RGUHS(RS2)]
6. Neutral zone. [NTRUHS; TN]
7. Describe the steps in delivering complete denture. [GOA]
8. Importance of finishing and polishing of complete dentine. [MUHS]
9. Write about the instructions to complete denture patient at the time of denture delivery. [MUHS]
10. Problems associated with complete denture use. [TN]
11. Write the instructions given to the patient during insertion of new complete dentures. [MUHS]
12. Compare residual ridge resorption of maxilary and mandibular edentulous ridge. [RGUHS]
13. Denture cleansing agents. [NTR-OR]
14. Instructions to be given to patient receiving complete denture. [NTR-OR]
15. What are the post-insertion problems in complete dentures? Discuss the methods of rectifying the same. [MUHS]
16. Mechanism of action of denture cleansers. [MUHS]
17. Give your method of fitting/insertion and aftercare for complete denture prosthesis. [RGUHS]
18. Importance of patient education. [NTR-OR]

Short Notes

1. Tissue conditioners. [RGUHS; GOA; TN]
2. Injection-moulded glass ceramic. [RGUHS (OS)]
3. Role of tissue conditioners. [TN]
4. Denture adhesives. [NTRUHS (OR), NTRUHS, NTRUHS]
5. Tissue conditioner. [RGUHS (RS), RGUHS (OS)]
6. Need for periodic recall of complete denture patients. [NTRUHS]
7. Denture stomatitis. [RGUHS (RS2), GOA; TN]
8. Denture cleaning agents. [RGUHS (RS); TN]
9. Diet in complete denture. [RGUHS (OS)]
10. Residual ridge resorption. [TN]
11. Articulating paper. [RGUHS (OS)]
12. Denture hyperplasia. [TN]
13. Denture irritation hyperplasia. [RGUHS (RS)]
14. Denture irritation hyperplasia. [RGUHS (RS)]
15. Epulis fissuratum. [RGUHS; NTR-NR]
16. Perleche. [RGUHS]
17. Treatment of abused tissues. [TTN]
18. Gag reflex. [GOA]
19. Denture allergy. [RGUHS]

RELINING AND REBASING IN COMPLETE DENTURES

Long Essays

1. Patient aged 55 years, who is wearing complete prosthesis for last 15 years complains of skidding of prosthesis on examination, both maxillary and mandibular ridges being hyperplastics. Give your method of treatment for the patient. [GOA]
2. Tissue conditioner. [NTR-NR, NTR-OR]
3. Conditioning of abused and irritated tissues. [RGUHS]
4. What is relining and rebasing of complete dentures? How would you proceed to reline the maxillary complete denture? [MUHS]
5. What are the post-insertion problems in complete dentures? Discuss the methods of rectifying the same. [MUHS]
6. State the clinical indications for relining and rebasing of complete denture and discuss the hazards of relining procedures. [RGUHS]

Short Essays

1. Age change in edentulous patients. [RGUHS (OS)]
2. Repair of complete denture. [NTRUHS]
3. Post-insertion problems in complete denture patients. [RGUHS (OS)]
4. Repair and relining of complete denture. [RGUHS (RS2)]
5. Open mouth relining technique. [RGUHS (RS2)]
6. Importance of counselling for a complete denture wearer. [TN]
7. Indications, diagnosis, and contraindications for relining and rebasing of complete denture. [NTR-NR]
8. Dentures relining. [RGUHS]
9. Midline fracture of complete denture. [RGUHS]
10. Complete denture repair. [RGUHS]
11. Relining and rebasing. [NTR-OR]
12. Relining and rebasing of complete denture. [NTR-OR]
13. Closed-mouth technique for relining of denture. [MUHS]
14. Causes for midline fractures of maxillary complete denture. [BUHS]

Short Notes

1. Relining and rebasing. [GOA, NTRUHS (OR); TN]
2. Tissue conditioners. [NTRUGHS]
3. Rebasing. [GOA, RGUHS(OS)]
4. Tissue preparation for relining. [RGUHS (OS)]
5. Relining. [RGUHS (OS)]
6. Dentures relining. [RGUHS, RGUHS (RS2)]
7. Resilient liners. [TN]
8. Soft reliners. [TN]
9. Steps in rebasing of complete dentures. [NTR-NR]
10. Rebasing and relining of denture. [TN]
11. Complete denture repair. [RGUHS]

SPECIAL COMPLETE DENTURES AND MISCELLANEOUS

Long Essays

1. What are overdentures? Describe their indications, contraindications, and advantages. [MUHS]
2. Enumerate the advantages and disadvantages of overdentures. [MUHS]
3. Define overdenture. Discuss in detail the following in treatment planning of an overdenture.
   a. Selection and preparation of abutment teeth.
   b. Objectives or goals of overdenture treatment. [MUHS]
4. What are overdentures? State the indications, advantages, and disadvantages of overdentures. [MUHS]
5. What are the indications and contraindications for an immediate complete denture? [RGUHS]
6. What is 'Preventive prosthodontics'? Give the principle, advantages, and disadvantages of overdentures. [MUHS]
7. Define interim removable dentures and give indications for use. [MUHS]
8. What are the advantages and disadvantages of immediate denture service? [MUHS]
9. Discuss why are dentures necessary for semi-edentulous and completely edentulous patients. [RGUHS]
10. Enumerate the reasons for loss of teeth. What are the consequences of loss of teeth? What are the methods of prosthodontic replacements? [RGUHS]

Short Essays

1. Advantages of immediate denture. [MUHS, RGUHS (RS2)]

2. Single complete denture. [RGUHS (RS), RGUHS(RS2); NTRUGHS]
3. Immediate dentures. [NTR-OR; NTRUGHS]
4. Advantages of overdenture. [NTR-ORRGUHS (RS)]
5. Immediate complete denture. [NTR-OR, NTRUHS]
6. Infection control in prosthodontics. [RGUHS]
7. Requirements of an overdenture. [RGUHS (RS2)]
8. What is immediate denture? Write about indications and contraindications. [MUHS]
9. What are overdentures? Write the advantages and disadvantages. [RGUHS]
10. Write the disadvantages of immediate complete denture. [MUHS]
11. What is a refractory cast? Write its fabrication. [MUHS]
12. Pre-extraction guides for complete denture fabrication. [NTR-NR]
13. Overdenture. [NTR-NR, NTR-OR]
14. Types of implant denture. [NTR-NR]
15. Methods of training the patient to retrude the mandible. [NTR-NR]
16. Rationale and advantages of immediate complete denture. [NTR-NR]
17. Die spacers. [NTR-NR]
18. Laboratory remounting. [NTR-NR]
19. Altered cast. [NTR-NR]
20. Interocclusal recording media. [NTR-NR]
21. Drawbacks of single complete denture. [NTR-NR]
22. Indication of immediate denture. [NTR-NR]
23. Problems encountered in single denture construction. [NTR-OR]
24. Clinical remount procedure? [NTR-OR]
25. Indications for immediate denture. [MUHS]
26. Pascal's law. [NTR-OR]
27. Altered cast technique. [NTR-OR]
28. Immediate dentures, their advantages and disadvantages. [NTR-OR]
29. Implant dentures. [NTR-OR]
30. Single dentures. [NTR-OR]
31. Importance of study cast. [BUHS]
32. Split cast technique. [NTR-OR]
33. Granular porosity in dentures. [BUHS]

Short Notes

1. Pindex system. [NTRUGHS]
2. Tooth-supported overdentures. [TN]
3. Obturators. [NTR-OR, NTR-NR; NTRUGHS]
4. Disinfecting dentures. [NTRUGHS]
5. Endosseous implant. [NTRUGHS]
6. Advantages of partial denture. [NTRUHS (OR)]
7. Screw-retained prosthesis. [NTRUHS (OR)]
8. Combination syndrome. [TN]
9. Immediate denture. [GOA; NTRUHS; TN]
10. Immediate overdenture. [NTRUHS (OR)]
11. Muscles producing protrusive and retrusive mandibular movements. [RGUHS (RS2)]
12. Disadvantages of immediate denture. [RGUHS(RS2)]
13. Abutment considerations of overdentures. [NTRUHS]
14. Advantages of metal denture implants. [RGUHS (RS)]
15. Enumerate the different types of obturators, their functions, and the materials used for making them. [MUHS]
16. Overdenture advantages. [MUHS]
17. Temporary prosthesis. [RGUHS]
18. Types of bar-retained overdentures. [NTR-NR]
19. What are the causes of gagging? [RGUHS]
20. Write in brief, the treatment planning for maxillary obturator prosthesis. [RGUHS]
21. Group function. [RGUHS]
22. Advantages of immediate complete dentures. [RGUHS]
23. Occlusal refining. [RGUHS]
24. Kelly's combination syndrome. [TN]
25. Remounting procedures in complete dentures. [RGUHS]
26. Name the different maxillary prostheses and facial prostheses and the materials used. [MUHS]
27. Write the concept and the advantages of overdenture. [MUHS]
28. Edentulous state. [RGUHS]
29. Describe the components of a sub-periosteal dental-implant-supported complete denture. [MUHS]
30. Advantages of immediate dentures. [RGUHS]
31. Write in brief the concept of osseointegration. [MUHS]
32. Overdenture. [NTR-NR, GOA, GOA; TN]
33. Define and mention the factors of dentogenics. [NTR- NR]
34. Realeff effect. [NTR-NR]
35. Define tooth-supported CD and give its advantages. [MUHS]
36. Rationale of overdentures. [TN]
37. Immediate denture. [RGUHS; TN]
38. Midline fracture of complete denture. [RGUHS ; TN]
39. Occlusal pivots. [NTR-NR]
40. Appliance versus prosthesis. [RGUHS]
41. How will you make a treatment plan for a cleft palate patient? [MUHS]
42. Define implants. Enumerate the various materials used for implants. [MUHS]
43. Clinical remounting. [NTR-NR]
44. Transitional denture. [NTR-NR]

45. Immediate complete denture. [TN]
46. Appliance versus prosthesis. [RGUHS]
47. Advantages of overdentures. [MUHS]
48. Temporary prosthesis. [RGUHS]
49. Transitional denture. [NTR-OR]
50. Processing errors in complete denture prosthesis. [GOA]
51. Immediate obturator. [NTR-OR]
52. Advantages and disadvantages of immediate denture. [RGUHS]
53. Split cast techniques. [RGUHS]
54. Obturator. [RGUHS]
55. Hybrid dentures. [NTR-OR]
56. Interim denture. [BUHS]
57. Interim denture. [RGUHS]
58. Implant denture. [NTR-OR]
59. Importance of study cast. [RGUHS]
60. Gunning splint. [BUHS; RGUHS]
61. Causes for midline fractures of maxillary complete denture. [RGUHS]
62. Granular porosity in dentures. [RGUHS]

INTRODUCTION TO FIXED PARTIAL DENTURES

Long Essays

1. Discuss in detail about the advantages, disadvantages, indications, and contraindications of FPD. [TN]
2. Importance of radiograph in fixed partial denture treatment. [MUHS]
3. Abutment. [MUHS]
4. Discuss the indications and contraindications for a fixed partial denture. Describe components of a fixed partial denture in detail. [GOA]
5. Indications and contraindications for fixed partial dentures. [MUHS]
6. Abutments for fixed partial prosthesis. [MUHS]
7. Discuss the importance of diagnosis and treatment planning in fixed partial prosthodontics. [GOA]
8. What are questionable abutments? Give the management of such abutment successfully in a fixed partial denture. [MUHS]
9. Describe the advantages and disadvantages of fixed partial prosthodontics. [NTR-OR]

Short Essays

1. Fibre-reinforced bridges. [NTRUGHS]
2. Resin-bonding bridges. [NTRUGHS]
3. Indications for fixed partial denture. [MUHS]
4. Importance of radiographs in fixed partial dentures. [MUHS]
5. Criteria for ideal abutment. [MUHS]
6. Write four uses of radiographs in FPD. [MUHS]

Short Notes

1. Contraindications of fixed partial denture. [TN]
2. Cantilever restoration. [NTRUGHS]
3. Splints and stents. [NTRUGHS]
4. Indications for FPD. [RGUHS]
5. Significance of radiographs in fixed partial denture. [NTR-OR]
6. Indications and contraindications for fixed partial denture. [TN]
7. Importance of radiographs in crown and bridge. [NTR-OR]

PARTS AND DESIGN OF FIXED PARTIAL DENTURES

Long Essays

1. Define pontic. Discuss in detail about pontic designs. [NTRUHS]
2. Classify pontic. Discuss in detail the various pontics used in FPD. [RGUHS (RS2)]
3. Discuss the various components of partial denture and the functional role played by, them individually. [RGUHS (RS2)]
4. Describe the component parts of fixed partial denture. [RGUHS (RS); TN]
5. Define and classify pontics. Write in detail indications, design, and advantages of different types of pontics. [NTRUHS]
6. Name the component parts of a bridge. Define and classify pontics and add a note on selection of pontic design and requirements of pontic. [NTRUHS (OR)]
7. Define and classify pontic. Discuss the indications and contraindications of various types of pontics. [GOA]
8. Classify bridge pontics. Discuss in detail regarding the principles of designing pontic. [TN]

9. What is fixed partial denture prosthesis? How do you classify them? Discuss with reasons in your choice of materials for construction of 3-unit bridge for missing. [RGUHS]
10. Discuss the indications and contraindications for a fixed partial denture. Describe the components of a fixed partial denture in detail. [GOA]
11. Define pontics. Classify them and discuss the principles for designing pontics. [MUHS]
12. Define and classify pontics of fixed partial denture. Explain the indications, design, and advantages of any three types. [RGUHS]
13. Define pontics in fixed partial denture. Classify and discuss the selection and fabrication of pontics. [TN]
14. Define fixed partial denture. Mention the different types of retainers and the criteria for the selection of the retainers. Add a note on care for the prosthesis. [NTR-OR]
15. Define bridge retainer. Requirements in selection of retainer. Mention cast restoration which can be used as retainer. [RGUHS]
16. Discuss the management of endodontically treated abutment tooth in fixed dental prosthesis. [NTRUGHS]
17. Discuss in detail the factors affecting retention in fixed partial prosthesis. [MUHS]
18. Discuss the connectors used in fixed partial prosthesis. [MUHS]
19. Define an abutment and enumerate the criteria involved in abutment selection. [RGUHS]
20. Describe the concept, design, and placement of margins of crown and retainers in fixed partial dentures. [RGUHS]
21. Define and classify pontics of fixed partial denture. Explain the indications, design, and advantages of any three types. [RGUHS]
22. Define pontic and classify the pontics. [NTR-OR]
23. Describe the concept, design, and placement of margins of crown and retainers in fixed partial dentures. [NTR-OR]
24. Classify bridge pontics. Discuss in detail regarding the principles of designing pontics. [BUHS]
25. Define abutment. Describe the factors to be considered in selection of a bridge abutment. [RGUHS]
26. What is fixed partial denture prosthesis? How do you classify them? Discuss with reasons in your choice of materials for construction of 3-unit bridge for missing [NTR-OR]

Short Essays

1. Rigid and non-rigid connectors in FPD. [RGUHS (OS)]
2. Sanitary pontic. [RGUHS (RS)]
3. Types of connectors used in FPDs. [RGUHS]
4. Ridge lap and modified ridge lap pontic. [RGUHS (RS2)]
5. Selection of retainers for a fixed partial denture. [RGUHS (RS); TN]
6. Connectors in fixed partial dentures. [NTR-NR]
7. Pontic. [MUHS]
8. Define pontic. Describe the various types with indication. [RGUHS]
9. Define and classify pontic. Describe the various types of pontic with indication. [GOA]
10. Define and classify connectors in FPD. [RGUHS]
11. Classify connectors in FPD. [MUHS]
12. Types of bridges. [MUHS]
13. Adhesive bridge. [NTR-OR; MUHS]
14. Define and classify retainers in fixed partial prosthesis. Describe in detail the principles of tooth preparation for the mandibular first molar to receive a fill cast metal crown. [GOA]
15. Connectors in FPD. [NTR-OR; MUHS]
16. Define components of fixed partial prosthesis and classify the same. Give your design of pontics with necessary indications. [GOA]
17. Achieving retention in FPD. [MUHS]
18. Maryland bridges. [NTR-OR]
19. Non-rigid connectors in crown and bridge. [NTR-OR]
20. Bridge retainer. [NTR-OR]
21. Soft tissue management in FPD. [RGUHS (RS)]
22. Hygienic pontic. [NTR-NR]
23. Ante's law. [NTRUHS (OR)]
24. Define pontic. Write about the different types of pontic designs and their indications in case of posterior fixed prosthesis. [RGUHS]
25. Sanitary pontic. [RGUHS]
26. Define pontic. Describe its types with indications. [RGUHS]
27. Modified ridge lap pontic. [NTR-NR]
28. Pontic. [NTR-NR, NTR-OR]
29. Requirements of pontics. [RGUHS]
30. Hygienic pontic. [NTR-OR]
31. Root extension pontic. [NTR-OR]
32. Disadvantages of ridge lap type pontic. [NTR-OR]
33. Discuss biomechanical principles used in the preparation of vital teeth to receive a fixed partial denture. [GOA]

Short Notes

1. Hygienic pontic. [TN]
2. Ovate pontic. [RGUHS (OS); TN]
3. Mesial half crown. [RGUHS (RS)]
4. Sanitary (Hygienic) pontic. [NTRUHS (OS); TN]
5. Altered vertical dimension. [RGUHS (OS)]

6. Modified ridge lap pontics. [RGUHS (OS)]
7. Spheroidal pontic. [RGUHS (RS2)]
8. Connectors in FPD. [NTR-NR, MUHS, RGUHS, TN]
9. Define pontic. Enumerate the types of pontic. [NTRUHS]
10. Bullet-shaped pontic. [RGUHS (RS2)]
11. Enumerate the factors affecting retention form for a fixed partial denture. [MUHS]
12. Ridge lap pontics. [TN]
13. Sanitary pontic. [RGUHS]
14. Pontics. [GOA TN]
15. Choice of pontic as related to tissue contacts. [MUHS]
16. What is pontic? Give its classification. [MUHS,]
17. Components of FPD. [RGUHS TN]
18. Requirements of pontics. [RGUHS]
19. Pontic design. [TN]
20. Radiographic evaluation of prospective abutment teeth for fixed partial denture. [TN]
21. Classify bridges and give their types. [MUHS]
22. What are the ideal requirements of pontic design? [MUHS]
23. Extracoronal retainers in fixed partial prosthodontics. [TN]
24. Write the ideal requirements for retainers in FPD. [MUHS]
25. Classify retainers in FPD. [MUHS]
26. Non-precision fixed bridges. [BUHS]
27. Non-rigid connectors in FPD. [MUHS]
28. Radicular bridge retainers. [BUHS]
29. Sanitary pontic. [NTRUGHS]
30. Pier abutments. [NTRUGHS]
31. Abutment evaluation in fixed partial denture. [TN]
32. Crown-root ratio. [RGUHS(RS2)]
33. Treatment protection to prepared abutment. [RGUHS]
34. Ante's law. [RGUHS, GOA]
35. Factors in selection of abutment in FPD. [RGUHS]

OCCLUSION IN FIXED PARTIAL DENTURES

Long Essays

1. What is balanced occlusion? Write in brief about the factors governing balanced occlusion. Write in detail about the principles of tooth preparation for fixed partial denture. [RGUHS (RS)]

Short Essays

1. Achieving retention in fixed partial denture. [GOA]
2. Recording of jaw relation records for crown and bridge. [RGUHS (OS)]
2. Achieving retention in fixed partial denture. [GOA]
4. Clinical remounting. [GOA]

Short Notes

1. Types of occlusion in FPD. [NTR-NR]
2. Selective grinding. [RGUHS (RS2), (OS) TN]
3. Selective grinding procedure. [RGUHS]

TYPES OF ABUTMENTS

Long Essays

1. Define abutment. Explain the criteria for selection of teeth for a fixed partial denture abutment. [RGUHS (RS); TN]
2. Define an abutment and enumerate the criteria involved in abutment selection. [RGUHS]
3. Selection of abutment for FPD. [RGUHS (RS)]
4. Define an abutment and discuss the biomechanical principles involved in abutment preparations. [GOA]
5. Define the term 'Abutment' in fixed partial dentures. Describe the factors responsible for selection of an abutment. [NTR-OR]
6. Define an abutment and a pier. How will you manage abutment with compromised periodontal conditions? [MUHS]
7. Define abutment. Describe the factors to be considered in selection of a bridge abutment. [BUHS]

Short Essays

1. Pier abutment. [RGUHS (RS)]
2. Ideal abutments. [RGUHS (RS2)]
3. Abutment selection. [NTR-NR]
4. Abutment selection for FPD. [RGUHS (RS2)]
5. Post and core. [RGUHS (RS2)]

6. Factors affecting selection of abutment tooth. [NTR- NR]
7. Factors in selection of abutment in FPD. [RGUHS]
8. What is an ideal abutment? Discuss selection of abutment teeth for a fixed partial prosthesis. [GOA]
9. Bridge abutment. [NTR-OR]
10. Ante's law. [NTR-NR]
11. Selection of bridge abutment. [NTR-OR]

Short Notes
1. Parapost. [RGUHS (OS)]
2. Ideal abutments. [NTRUHS (OR)]
3. Pier abutment. [NTR-NR; NTRUHS (NR); NTRUHS; NTRUHS]
4. Cantilever fixed partial denture. [RGUHS(OS)]
5. Osseointegration. [RGUHS (RS)]
6. Ante's law. [NTR-NR]

TOOTH PREPARATION

Long Essays

1. Give in detail the step by step procedure for preparing metal-ceramic crowns for a maxillary central incisor. [RGUHS (OS)]
2. Define retention and resistance in fixed partial dentures. What are the factors affecting retention and resistance in posterior tooth preparation? [NTRUHS (OR)]
3. Discuss, the principles of tooth preparation in detail. [NTRUHS]
4. What is balanced occlusion? Write in brief about the factors governing balanced occlusion. Write in detail about the principles of tooth preparation for fixed partial denture. [RGUHS (RS)]
5. Discuss in detail the principles of tooth preparation to receive artificial crown. [NTRUHS]
6. What is crown? How do you prepare a maxillary centre incisor to receive a complete ceramic crown? [RGUHS (OS)]
7. Enumerate the principles of tooth preparation in fixed prosthesis. Write the factors affecting retention and resistance. [BUHS; TN]
8. What are the biomechanical principles of tooth preparation? Discuss the biologic principles in detail. [MUHS]
9. Describe in detail about the steps in preparation of tooth for receiving full metal crown. [NTR-OR]
10. Write in detail about the biomechanical considerations for preparation of a tooth for fixed prosthesis? [RGUHS]
11. Enumerate and discuss the principles of preparation of tooth to receive artificial crown. [RGUHS]
12. Give a step by step description of preparation of a mandibular first molar for receiving a ceramic-metal crown with reasons for amount of reduction and from to the tooth. [MUHS]
13. Define an abutment and discuss the biomechanical principles involved in abutment preparations. [GOA]
14. List the principles of tooth preparation. Describe each with examples and instructions. [NTR-OR; TN]
15. Describe tooth preparation of a maxillary central incisor to receive porcelain jacket with justification. Illustrate with diagram. [MUHS]
16. Describe the principles of tooth preparation and write about mechanical considerations in detail. [RGUHS]
17. Write about biomechanical principles of tooth preparation. [TN]
18. What are the biomechanical principles in tooth preparation? Discuss. [TN]
19. Describe the principles of abutment preparation for fixed partial denture. [NTR-OR]
20. What is FPD prosthesis? Give its classification with reasons in your choice of materials for 3-unit bridge for missing 26? [RGUHS]
21. Steps in the preparation of upper central incisor to receive a jacket crown. [RGUHS]
22. Discuss the recent advances in materials used for fixed partial dentures. [MUHS]
23. Discuss the recent advances in materials used for fixed partial dentures. [MUHS]
24. Enumerate the principles of tooth preparation aside in detail the mode of preparation of 36 to receive a ¾ crown. [RGUHS]
25. Discuss the mechanical, biological, and aesthetics involved in tooth preparation in fixed bridge prosthesis. [MUHS]
26. Discuss the biological and mechanical considerations in tooth preparation to receive a fixed partial denture. [GOA]
27. Discuss the mouth preparation of a patient for fixed partial denture. [NTR-OR]
28. What are the principles in tooth preparation? Explain each in detail. [NTR-OR]
29. Discuss the principles of tooth preparation to receive artificial crown. [NTR-NR]

30. Discuss the principles and design of a tooth preparation for receiving a cast complete veneer restoration. [GOA]
31. Discuss the principles of preparation of abutment teeth for partial veneer crown. [NTR-ORI]
32. Define retainer in FPD. Classify the retainers in FPD and describe the step by step preparation of posterior tooth to receive a complete veneer crown. [NTR-OR]
33. What are the principles of tooth preparation? Describe the various steps in the preparation of maxillary central incisor to receive a ceramic-metal restoration. [MUHS]
34. Define and classify retainers in FPD. Describe in detail the principles of tooth preparation for first maxillary molar. [RGUHS, BUHS]
35. Enumerate the principles of tooth preparation in fixed prosthesis. Write the factors affecting retention and resistance. [RGUHS]
36. Describe the biomechanical principles of tooth preparation in fixed partial denture. [BUHS]
37. Discuss the biomechanical principles of tooth reduction in fixed partial denture prosthodontics. [NTR-OR]
38. Describe the clinical and laboratory steps in the preparation of a porcelain jacket crown. [BUHS]

Short Essays

1. Finish lines in FPD. [NTR-NR; MUHS NTR-OR; NTRUHS (OR)]
2. Principles of tooth preparation. [RGUHS(OS); TN]
3. Supragingival finish line. [RGUHS (RS2)]
4. Step-wise tooth preparation of a molar tooth for crown and prosthesis. [RGUHS (OS)]
5. Describe the indications, contraindications, advantages, and disadvantages of partial veneer crowns. [RGUHS]
6. Indications, advantages, and disadvantages of ¾th partial veneer crown. [NTR-NR]
7. Briefly write on the principles of tooth preparation. [TN]
8. Proximal groves in partial veneer crown. [NTR-OR; TN]
9. Describe the indications, advantages, and disadvantages of subgingival finish line. [RGUHS]
10. Give the advantages and disadvantages of porcelain jacket crown. [RGUHS]
11. Gingival finishing lines. [MUHS NTR-OR]
12. Axioproximal grooves. [NTR-NR, NTR-OR TN]
13. Marginal finish lines. [NTR-NR]
14. What are the advantages of porcelain jacket crown? [MUHS]
15. Indications and contraindications of porcelain jacket crown. [RGUHS]
16. PFM (porcelain fused to metal restoration). [NTR-NR]
17. Define and classify retainers in fixed partial prosthesis. Describe in detail the principles of tooth preparation for the mandibular first molar to receive a fill cast metal crown. [GOA]
18. Partial veneer crown. [NTR-OR]
19. Advantages of porcelain jacket crown. [NTR-OR]
20. Dowel crown. [NTR-OR]
21. Metal crown. [NTR-OR]
22. Discuss the biomechanical principles used in the preparation of vital teeth to receive a fixed partial denture. [GOA]
23. Etch cast restorations. [MUHS]
24. Principles of tooth preparation. [NTR-OR]
25. Full veneer crown. [NTR-OR]
26. Retention grooves in anterior and posterior partial veneer crowns. [MUHS]
27. Post and crown. [NTR-OR]
28. Finish line - location and types. [NTR-OR]
29. Porcelain jacket crown. [NTR-OR]
30. Post core crown. [BUHS]
31. Shoulder. [NTR-OR]
32. Types of gingival finish lines in crown preparation. [NTR-OR]
33. Comparison of acrylic and porcelain crown. [MUHS]

Short Notes

1. Advantage of partial denture. [NTRUHS (OR)]
2. Functional cusp bevel. [NTRUHS (NR)]
3. Chamfer finish line. [NTRUHS (NR), RGUHS (RS), (RS2)]
4. Shoulder finish line. [RGUHS(OS)]
5. Gingival finish lines. [GOA, TN]
6. Ante's law. [RGUHS (RS)]
7. Chamfer. [RGUHS (RS)]
8. Resistance and retention form in tooth preparation. [TN]
9. Cervical finish lines in tooth preparation. [TN]
10. Shoulder with bevel. [RGUHS (OS)]
11. Tensofrictional resistance. [RGUHS (OS), TN]
12. Dowel post. [NTRUHS]
13. Maintenance of air rotor hand pieces. [RGUHS (OS)]
14. What are the requirements of an ideal abutment? [MUHS]
15. Discuss in short, the validity of Ante's law as applicable to fixed prosthodontics. [MUHS]
16. Maryland bridges and their limitations. [MUHS]
17. Importance of functional cusp bevel. [MUHS]
18. What are the different types of finish lines? Write about heavy chamfer type of finish line. [MUHS]

19. Types of cervical finish fines in fixed prosthesis. [RGUHS]
20. Disadvantages of subgingival finishing fines. [NTR-NR]
21. All ceramic systems. [RGUHS]
22. Disadvantages of partial veneer crown. [NTR-NR]
23. What are the purposes for establishing a clear gingival finishing fine in tooth preparations for crowns? What are the possible location of the finishing fine and their reason? [MUHS]
24. Name and draw different finish fines with one indication of each. [MUHS]
25. Finishing fines in fixed partial dentures. [GOA]
26. Depth orientation groove. [TN]
27. Biological considerations in tooth preparation for crown and bridge. [TN]
28. Enumerate the various margins design in fixed partial denture giving examples. [MUHS]
29. Indications and contraindications of partial veneer crown. [RGUHS]
30. Jacket crown. [NTR-NR]
31. Give the benefits of supragingival margins in fixed prosthodontics. [MUHS]
32. What are the different types of finish fines? What finish fine is used for metal-ceramic restoration and why? [MUHS]
33. Advantages of porcelain jacket crown. [NTR-NR]
34. Chamfer. [NTR-NR]
35. Different margin designs with indications. [MUHS]
36. Supragingival finish fine. [BUHS]
37. Proximal grooves in anterior PVC. [BUHS]
38. Indications and contraindications for acrylic jacket crown. [BUHS]
39. Chamfers. [RGUHS]

TYPES OF FIXED PARTIAL DENTURES

Long Essays

1. Name the component parts of a bridge. Define and classify pontics and add a note on selection of pontic design and requirements of pontic. [NTRUHS (OR)]
2. What is partial veneer crown? Mention about its indications and contraindications. Describe about the steps of preparation for a three-quarter crown preparation on maxillary cuspid with diagram. [MUHS]
3. Describe tooth preparation of a maxillary central incisor to receive porcelain jacket with justification. Illustrate with diagram. [MUHS]
4. Discuss the tooth preparation for a metal-ceramic restoration in maxillary central incisors. [TN]
5. Mention the indications and contraindications for a metal-ceramic crown. Describe the step by step procedure in the preparation of molar tooth for a metal-ceramic crown. [TN]
6. Discuss the recent advances in materials used for fixed partial dentures. [MUHS]
7. Name the various types of bridges. Diagrammatically name the parts of a bridge. Classify the retainers. Discuss in detail about radicular retainers. [TN]
8. Briefly enumerate the step by step preparation of a maxillary premolar to receive a complete ceramic-metal restoration. [MUHS]
9. Describe the clinical and laboratory steps in the preparation of a porcelain jacket crown. [RGUHS]
10. Enumerate the principles of tooth preparation aside in detail the mode of preparation of 36 to receive a ¾ crown. [NTRUHS (OR)]
11. What is FPD prosthesis and give its classification with reasons in your choice of materials for C 3-unit bridge for missing 26. [NTRUHS (OR)]
12. Steps in the preparation of upper central incisor to receive a jacket crown. [NTRUHS (OR)]

Short Essays

1. All-ceramic crown. [NTRUGHS]
2. Dental ceramics. [NTRUGHS]
3. Cantilever fixed partial denture. [NTRUHS (OR)]
4. Rochette bridge. [NTRUHS (OR)]
5. Types of fixed partial denture. [RGUHS (RS2)]
6. Full veneer crown. [RGUHS (RS2)]
7. Resin-bonded fixed partial dentures. [NTRUHS]
8. Indications for jacket crown. [RGUHS (RS)]
9. Enumerate the various failures in fixed partial denture. [RGUHS (RS2)]
10. Comparative merits of complete veneer and partial veneer, crowns. [RGUHS (RS2)]
11. Describe the indications, contraindications, advantages, and disadvantages of partial veneer crowns. [RGUHS]
12. Give the advantages and disadvantages of porcelain jacket crown. [RGUHS]
13. Failure effect in post and core restorations [MUHS]
14. Alloys used in FPD. [MUHS]

15. What are the different types of finish lines? What finish line is used for metal-ceramic restoration and why? [MUHS]
16. Define and classify retainers in fixed partial prosthesis. Describe in detail principles of tooth preparation for the mandibular first molar to receive a fill cast metal crown. [GOA]
17. Indications and contr indications of porcelain jacket crown. [RGUHS]
18. Comparison of acrylic and porcelain crown. [MUHS]
19. Retention grooves in anterior and posterior partial veneer crowns. [MUHS]

Short Notes

1. Pier abutment. [NTRUHS (NR)]
2. Tooth preparation for anterior all-ceramic crown. [TN]
3. Porcelain jacket crown. [RGUHS (OS)]
4. Resin-retained bridges. [RGUHS (RS2)]
5. Anterior partial veneer crown [NTRUHS]
6. Resin-bonded fixed partial denture. [TN]
7. Indications and contraindications of partial veneer crown. [RGUHS, (OS)]
8. Advantages of porcelain veneer. [RGUHS (RS)]
9. Advantages of partial veneer crown. [RGUHS (RS), (OS)]
10. Maryland bridge. [RGUHS (OS) TN]
11. Partial veneer crown. [GOA TN]
12. Indications of anterior jacket crown. [TN]
13. Compound bridge. [RGUHS (RS2)]
14. Resin-bonded bridges. [NTRUHS]
15. Indications and contraindications for porcelain jacket crown. [NTRUHS]
16. Adhesive bridges. [TN]
17. What is ceramic laminate? Write about its indications. [MUHS]
18. Advantages of partial veneer crowns over full veneer crowns. [MUHS]
19. Post core crown. [RGUHS, TN]
20. Metal-free ceramics. [TN]
21. Acid-etched bridges. [TN]
22. Telescopic crowns. [TN]
23. Polycarbonate crowns. [RGUHS]
24. Cantilever fixed partial dentures. [RGUHS]
25. Metal-ceramic crown. [TN]
26. What are the advantages of porcelain jacket crown? [MUHS]
27. Richmond crown. [TN]
28. Complete veneer crown. [GOA]
29. Cast porcelain crowns. [RGUHS]
30. Radicular bridge retainers. [RGUHS]
31. Non-precision fixed bridges. [RGUHS]
32. Indications and contraindications for acrylic jacket crown. [RGUHS]
33. Cast core.

IMPRESSION MAKING IN FIXED PARTIAL DENTURES

Long Essays

1. What is impression? Enumerate the impression theories. Explain the selective pressure impression theory and classify fixed partial denture. Explain the selection of abutment for a fixed partial denture. Advantages of porcelain veneer crown. [RGUHS (OS)]
2. Describe the technique of impression making in fixed partial denture treatment. [NTR-NR]
3. Describe the methods to control saliva and soft tissue management for fixed partial denture procedure. [TN]
4. What are the objectives of an impression and explain your techniques in recording the impressions of a FPD? [TN]
5. Describe the gingival tissue management in fixed prosthesis. [MUHS]
6. What do you understand by the term 'tissue dilatation' and what are the different methods to obtain it? [MUHS]

Short Essays

1. Various retraction methods in FPD. [RGUHS (RS2)]
2. Gingival retraction. [NTR-NR, NTR-OR TN NTRUHS, (OR), RGUHS (RS)]
3. Indications and advantages of all-ceramic crown. [NTRUHS]
4. Gingival retraction techniques. [RGUHS (RS)]
5. Write in detail the impression procedures in crown and bridge prosthesis. [RGUHS (OS)]
6. Write about the different methods of gingival retraction. [MUHS]
7. Role of special trays in fixed partial denture impression making. [RGUHS]
8. Impression materials in FPD. [NTR-NR]
9. What do you understand by the term 'tissue dilatation' and what are the different methods to obtain the same? [GOA]
10. Methods of gingival dilatation. [MUHS]

11. Rubber base impression materials. [NTR-NR]
12. Double impression technique in FPD? [NTR-OR]
13. Impression procedures in fixed partial denture. [NTR- OR]
14. Methods of gingival retraction. [MUHS]
15. Gingival management. [MUHS]
16. Describe the various methods of gingival retractions in fixed prosthodontics. [BUHS]
17. Gingival dilation. [MUHS]
18. Elastomeric impression materials. [MUHS]

Short Notes

1. Selective pressure impressions technique. [GOA TN]
2. Functions of saliva. [NTRUHS (OR)]
3. Gingival retraction techniques. [TN]
4. Gingival retraction [NTRUHS; TN, GOA,TN]
5. Triple tray impression. [NTRUHS]
6. Fluid wax impression. [TN]
7. Enumerate the various impression materials used for crown and bridge work. [RGUHS (RS2)]
8. Reversible colloid. [NTR-NR]
9. Gingival tissue retraction. [RGUHS (RS2)]
10. Recent advances in FPD. [RGUHS]
11. Write the various types of gingival retraction cords. [MUHS]
12. Tissue management in FPD. [TN]
13. Retraction cord. [NTR-NR]
14. Purpose of gingival retraction. [NTR-NR]
15. Cantilever fixed partial dentures. [RGUHS]
16. Ante's law. [GOA]
17. McLean's physiologic impression. [TN]
18. Impression materials in fixed partial dentures. [MUHS; TN]
19. Selective pressure technique. [TN]
20. Write the four advantages of subgingival margin. [MUHS]
21. Maryland bridges. [NTR-OR]
22. Double impression technique in fixed partial prosthodontics. [GOA]
23. Impressions. [RGUHS, BUHS]

TEMPORISATION OR PROVISIONAL RESTORATIONS AND LAB PROCEDURES INVOLVED IN FABRICATION OF FPD

Long Essays

1. What is provisional restoration? What are the requirements of a provisional restoration? Write an account of the various types of provisional restorations. [TN]
2. Discuss in detail the fixed partial denture failures. [TN]
3. Discuss temporization in fixed partial denture. [NTRUHS (NR)]
4. What is the need for temporization after tooth preparation? Discuss the various methods to achieve it. [MUHS]
5. What are provisional restorations? Justify their need and discuss their limitations. [MUHS]
6. Discuss the role of provisional restorations in FPD and describe the different types used. [MUHS]
7. Dies and die materials. [MUHS]
8. Describe the clinical and laboratory steps in the preparation of a porcelain jacket crown. [NTR-OR]

Short Essays

1. Failures in FPD. [RGUHS (RS)]
2. Temporization in fixed partial prosthesis [RGUHS (RS2)]
3. Provisional restoration. [NTR-NR; RGUHS (RS)]
4. Enumerate the various failures in fixed partial denture. [RGUHS (RS2)]
5. Enumerate the die materials and die systems. Write in brief on divestment technique. [MUHS]
6. Role of special trays in fixed partial denture impression making. [RGUHS]
7. Describe the die systems used in FPD and describe any one of them. [RGUHS]
8. Treatment protection to prepared abutment. [RGUHS]
9. Define die and name the various die materials. [MUHS]
10. Requirements of provisional restoration. [RGUHS]
11. Indirect procedure of fabricating provisional restoration. [RGUHS]
12. List temporary tooth protection materials. Explain anyone technique of temporary tooth preparation. [RGUHS]
13. Advantages of porcelain jacket crown. [NTR-NR]
14. Temporary protection of prepared tooth. [TN]
15. Write about try-in of FPD. [MUHS]
16. Provisional restorations. [MUHS]

17. Write the requirements of provisional restoration. [MUHS]
18. Give your method of cementing 3-unit fixed partial prosthesis and instructions and aftercare to patients. [GOA]
19. Temporization. [MUHS; NTR-OR]
20. Porcelain jacket crown. [NTR-OR]
21. Temporary tooth protection. [NTR-OR]
22. Temporary crowns. [MUHS]
23. Metal-ceramic crown. [TN]
24. PFM (Porcelain-fused metal restoration). [TN]

Short Notes

1. Provisional restorations. [GOA; NTRUHS (OR); TN]
2. Temporization. [GOA, RGUHS (RS2); TN]
3. Requirement of provisional restoration. [RGUHS (OS)]
4. Need for temporization. [NTRUHS]
5. Abrasives and polishing agents. [RGUHS(OS)]
6. Polycarbonate crowns. [RGUHS, RGUHS (RS2)]
7. Cements used in fixed prosthesis. [RGUHS (RS2)]
8. Enumerate the requirements of a provisional restoration. [MUHS]
9. Temporary protection of prepared abutment. [TN]
10. Different polishing agents used in dentistry. [RGUHS (OS)]
11. Temporization in fixed partial denture. [MUHS]
12. Provisional crowns. [TN]
13. Temporary crown. [RGUHS]
14. Suck back porosity. [NTR-NR]
15. Types of fixed partial dentures. [GOA]
16. Management of endodontically treated teeth [GOA]
17. Casting defects. [NTR-NR]
18. What is temporization? Give its importance and the technique. [MUHS]
19. Importance of provisional restorations in fixed partial denture. [MUHS]
20. Give the biologic requirements of provisional restorations. [MUHS]
21. Cementation of a fixed partial denture. [GOA]
22. Difference between natural and artificial occlusion. [GOA]
23. Luting agents. [GOA]
24. Jacket crown. [NTR-NR]
25. Metal-ceramic restoration. [BUHS]
26. Cast porcelain crowns. [BUHS]

CEMENTATION OF FIXED PARTIAL DENTURES AND MISCELLANEOUS

Long Essays

1. Explain in detail cementation of FPD. [MUHS]
2. Soldering. [NTRUHS (OR)]
3. Luting agents used in fixed prosthesis. [MUHS]

Short Essays

1. Castable ceramics. [RGUHS (RS)]
2. Compare and contrast acrylic partial denture with cast partial dentures. [RGUHS (RS)]
3. Casting defects. [NTRUHS, RGUHS (RS)]
4. Porosities in casting. [RGUHS (OS)]
5. Die materials. [NTRUHS]
6. Sprue former. [RGUHS (OS)]
7. Working cast and die preparation. [RGUHS (OS)]
8. Factors affecting colour of ceramics. [RGUHS (RS2)]
9. Porosities in noble metal castings. [RGUHS (RS2)]
10. Cements used in fixed partial dentures. [RGUHS; NTRUHS]
11. Veneering materials. [NTR-NR]
12. Luting agents in FPD. [NTR-NR]
13. Diagnostic aids for FPD evaluation. [RGUHS]
14. Ceramics. [NTR-NR]
15. Luting cements for FPD. [NTR-NR]
16. List temporary tooth protection materials. Explain anyone technique of temporary tooth preparation. [RGUHS]
17. Porcelain teeth. [NTR-OR]
18. Splints. [NTR-OR]

Short Notes

1. Removable dies. [RGUHS (RS2)]
2. Welding and soldering. [RGUHS (OS)]
3. Porcelain fused to metal crown. [RGUHS(OS)]
4. Metal-free ceramics. [RGUHS (RS2)]
5. Titanium alloy. [RGUHS (OS)]
6. Die spacer. [RGUHS (OS)]
7. Cements used in fixed partial dentures. [RGUHS]
8. Prothero's cone theory. [NTR-NR]
9. Solders for dental cast units assembly. [NTR-NR]
10. Tooth coloured cements for all-porcelain crowns [NTR-NR]
11. Casting failure. [TN]

12. Phosphate-bonded investment. [TN]
13. Enumerate the tooth coloured veneering material. [NTR-NR]
14. Dicor. [NTR-NR]
15. Cerestore. [NTR-NR]
16. Nickel-chromium alloy. [NTR-NR]
17. Dental ceramics. [GOA]

MAXILLOFACIAL PROSTHETICS AND IMPLANT DENTISTRY

Short Essays

1. Dental solder. [NTRUGHS]
2. Die materials. [NTRUGHS]
3. Casting defects. [NTRUGHS]
4. Biomaterials used in implants. [RGUHS (OS)]
5. Permanent obturator. [RGUHS (RS)]
6. Obturators. [NTRUHS (OR)]
7. Ear prosthesis. [NTRUHS (OR)]
8. Armani's classification. [NTRUHS (OR)]
9. Implant materials. [NTR-NR; RGUHS(RS2)]
10. Osseointegration. [RGUHS (RS)]
11. Role of occlusal equilibration in the treatment of MPD syndrome. [RGUHS (OS)]
12. Endosseous implants. [NTRUHS]
13. Requirements for successful osseointegration. [RGUHS (RS2)]
14. Arrangement for segregation and disposal of clinical waste of all kinds. [RGUHS (RS2)]
15. Types of obturator. [RGUHS (RS)]
16. Advantages of implant prosthodontics over conventional complete denture. [RGUHS (RS)]
17. Osseointegration. [NTR-NR]
18. Osseointegration of dental implants. [RGUHS]
19. Retention in maxillofacial prosthesis. [NTR-NR]
20. Materials used for maxillofacial prosthesis. [NTR-NR]
21. Implant denture. [NTR-OR, RGUHS]
22. Implant. [RGUHS]
23. Indication for dental implant. [RGUHS]

Short Notes

1. Endosseous implants. [NTRUHS]
2. Post and core crowns. [NTRUHS]
3. CAD/CAM restoration. [NTRUGHS]
4. Osseointegration. [RGUHS (RS) TN, NTR-NR]
5. Sub-periosteal implants. [RGUHS (RS)]
6. Dowel post. [NTRUHS (NR)]
7. Osseointegration of dental implants. [RGUHS(OS); TN]
8. Management of mutilated tooth. [TN]
9. Obturators. [GOA, TN]
10. Implant. [BUHS, NTRUHS, (OR) TN]
11. Surgical obturator. [RGUHS (OS)]
12. Classification of dental implants. [RGUHS (RS)]
13. Subperiosteal implants. [RGUHS (RS2)]
14. Endosseous implants. [RGUHS (RS)]
15. Write in brief the treatment planning for maxillary obturator prosthesis. [TN]
16. Splints. [NTRUHS]
17. Speech-aid prosthesis. [RGUHS (RS)]
18. Dowel pin. [TN]
19. Types of implants. [NTR-NR]
20. Parts of implant. [NTR-NR]
21. Mention the materials used for fabrication of maxillofacial prosthesis. [NTR-NR]
22. Dowel core. [RGUHS (RS)]
23. Classify obturators. [RGUHS (OS)]
24. Types of obturator. [RGUHS (RS)]
25. Advantages of implant prosthodontics over conventional complete denture. [RGUHS (RS)]
26. Hallow bulb obturator. [TN]
27. Implant biomaterials. [TN]
28. Retention form for a post-retained crown. [TN]
29. Implant denture. [BUHS TN]
30. Dental implants. [GOA]
31. Implants in prosthodontics. [GOA]
32. Indication for dental implant. [BUHS]

INTRODUCTION TO REMOVABLE PARTIAL DENTURES

Long Essays

1. Classify partially edentulous areas according to Applegate-Kennedy's classification and mention Applegate's rules for Kennedy's classification. [RGUHS(RS2)]
2. Present the entire Applegate-Kennedy's classification of partially edentulous situation with the latest nomenclature and modification. [RGUHS (OS)]

3. What is removable partial denture prosthesis? How do you classify the partially edentulous situations? Discuss the principles in designing of tooth-tissue-supported and tooth-supported removal partial denture prosthesis. [RGUHS (OS) BUHS]
4. Describe the Kennedy's classification of partially edentulous arches along with the rules governing the classification. Draw diagrams. [NTR-OR]
5. What are the requirements of classifying partially edentulous arch? Explain Kennedy's classification of partially edentulous arch with diagram. List Applegate's rules applied for classification of partially edentulous arch. [RGUHS]
6. Explain the mode of classification of removable partial denture with a diagram. Give the importance of such a classification. [TN]
7. Describe in detail about Kennedy's classification of partial dentures. [RGUHS]
8. Classify semi-edentulous arches as per Kennedy's classification and give Applegate rules for Kennedy's classification. [RGUHS]
9. Discuss the importance of diagnostic and treatment planning in removable partial denture prosthodontics. Enumerate the Applegate's rule for applying the Kennedy' classification. [NTR-OR]

Short Essays

1. Kennedy-Applegate's classification for partially edentulous arches. [NTRUHS]
2. Kennedy's classification of partially edentulous arches. [RGUHS (RS)]
3. Kennedy's classification. [NTRUHS, RGUHS]
4. RPD design options for Kennedy's class II situation in maxillary arch. [RGUHS (OS)]
5. State Kennedy's classification and state Applegate's rules. [MUHS]
6. Swing-lock dentures. [NTRUHS (OR)]
7. Kennedy's classification in removable partial denture. [MUHS]
8. Give the requirements of acceptable classification system in partially edentulous arches. [MUHS]
9. Kennedy's classification of partially edentulous conditions. [TN]
10. Ideal classification system in RPD. [MUHS]
11. Describe Applegate-Kennedy's classification. [MUHS]
12. Discuss the requirements of acceptable classification system. [MUHS]
13. Need for bilateral design in Kennedy's Cl II partial denture. [MUHS]
14. Classify partial edentulous jaw. Give in detail about the Kennedy's classification of partial edentulous jaws with Applegate's rules. [GOA]

Short Notes

1. End of reversible partial denture. [RGUHS]
2. Kennedy's classification. [NTR-OR, NTRUGHS]
3. Define immediate partial denture. [RGUHS]
4. Applegate rules for Kennedy's classification of partially edentulous arches. [NTR-NR]
5. Kennedy-Applegate's classification. [RGUHS, TN]
6. Advantages of tooth-supported prosthesis [RGUHS]
7. Immediate partial denture. [NTR-OR]
8. Classification of partially edentulous arches. [NTR-NR]
9. Fulcrum line. [NTR-NR]
10. What points should be checked when a partial denture is placed in the mouth? [MUHS]
11. Describe the sequelae to loss of teeth. [MUHS]
12. Limitations of Kennedy's classification of partially edentulous spaces. [NTR-OR]
13. Swing-lock partial denture prosthesis. [BUHS]
14. Denture base. [BUHS]

TREATMENT PLANNING AND MOUTH PREPARATION

Long Essays

1. Discuss the mouth preparation in removable partial dentures. [TN]
2. Define removable partial denture prosthesis. Describe in detail mouth preparation for removable partial denture. [RGUHS]
3. Describe in brief the various types of mouth preparation procedures undertaken in a case of removable partial denture service. [RGUHS]
4. Discuss the importance of diagnostic and treatment planning in removable partial denture prosthodontics. Enumerate the Applegate's rule for applying the Kennedy's classification.

Short Essays

1. Treatment partial dentures. [RGUHS (RS)]
2. Splints. [RGUHS (RS2)]

3. Diagnostic cast and its uses. [RGUHS (RS2)]
4. Mouth preparation for removable partial denture. [RGUHS(OS)]
5. Uses of diagnostic casts in removable partial dentures. [RGUHS (OS)]
6. Pre-prosthetic surgery. [GOA]

Short Notes

1. Refractory cast. [NTRUGHS]
2. Disinfection of impressions. [NTRUHS (NR)]
3. Importance of mouth preparation in partial denture treatment. [TN]
4. Mouth preparation prior to RPD services. [TN]

MAJOR AND MINOR CONNECTORS

Long Essays

1. Define major connectors in removable partial denture. Discuss with diagrams different mandibular major connectors. [TN]
2. Write briefly on the requirements of major connectors. Add notes on the advantages and disadvantages of maxillary major connectors. [NTRUGHS]
3. Explain in detail the various types of minor connectors. Add a note on the function of minor connector. [RGUHS (RS)]
4. Discuss the diagnostic choice of major connectors in the treatment of mandibular partial edentulous condition. [RGUHS]
5. Maxillary major connectors. [RGUHS(OS)]
6. What is major connector? Describe the different types of maxillary and mandibular major connectors. [TN]
7. What is the major connector? Describe in detail the mandibular major connectors. [MUHS]
8. Enumerate the various components of a removable partial denture and discuss major connectors. [TN]
9. Enumerate the parts of removable partial denture. Define major connector. Give their ideal requirements and describe maxillary major connectors. [NTRUHS]
10. Mention the parts of a cast partial denture and describe the different maxillary major connectors. [TN]
11. Classify major connectors and discuss the role of major connector in removable partial dentures prosthodontics. [NTR-OR]
12. Write the components of cast partial denture and write in detail about direct retainers. [TN]
13. Discuss the requirements of major connectors. Explain the indications, contraindications, advantages, disadvantages, and design features of mandibular major connectors. [TN]
14. Draw a design for a partially edentulous patient, mentioning each component. [MUHS]
15. Define a major connector in removable partial denture. Discuss with diagram the various types of maxillary major connector. [TN]
16. Write an essay on 'Minor Connector. [TN]
17. Define major connector. Write in detail about the requirements and types of mandibular major connectors. [NTR-NR]
18. Describe mandibular major connectors and write in detail about lingual bar. [RGUHS]
19. Discuss in detail the principles of designing a cast partial denture. [TN]
20. Classify the major connections. Write briefly on the principles and indications in major connector designing. [TN]
21. What are major and minor connectors? Describe their different types and discuss the requirements. [MUHS]
22. Define major corrector. What are the design requirements for major connector? Discuss in detail the mandibular major connector. [NTR-OR]
23. Name the different components of cast removable partial denture. Describe in detail the different types of major connectors used in mandibular removable partial denture. [RGUHS]

Short Essays

1. Maxillary major connectors. [RGUHS (RS)]
2. Non-rigid connectors. [NTRUHS (OR)]
3. Mandibular major connectors. [MUHS, NTRUHS (NR)]
4. Mandibular major connectors. [RGUHS (RS2)]
5. Occlusal rest. [RGUHS (RS2), (OS)]
6. Bar clasp. [RGUHS (OS)]
7. Neutral zone. [NTRUHS; TN]
8. Function of major connector. [RGUHS (RS2)]
9. Lingual bar. [RGUHS (RS)]
10. Maxillary major connectors. [NTR-NR, MUHS, RGUHS (OS)]
11. Define major connector. Enumerate the indications for use of linguoplate major connector. [MUHS]
12. Functions of reciprocal arm. [RGUHS (RS)]
13. Minor connectors. [NTRUHS]
14. Occlusal rest. [NTRUHS]

15. Define rest. Describe the functions and design of occlusal rests. [NTRUHS]
16. Stress breakers. [RGUHS (RS)]
17. Abutment preparation for removable partial denture. [RGUHS (OS)]
18. Advantages of lingual plate major connecto. [MUHS]
19. Selection of major connectors in various Kennedy's classifications of mandibular arch. [MUHS]
20. Write in brief about the different types of mandibular major connector. [MUHS]
21. Major connector in maxilla. [NTR-NR, NTR-OR]
22. Minor connectors. [NTR-NR, NTR-OR, MUHS]
23. What will be the Kennedy's classification for a maxillary arch with both first molars missing? Name the components of a removal cast partial denture for such a situation with reason. [MUHS]
24. Describe designing a lingual bar with diagrams. Name two indications of the same. [RGUHS]
25. Define major connectors and mandibular major connectors. [MUHS]
26. Define and classify major connectors. Discuss their indications and contraindications. [GOA]
27. Requirement of major connectors in removable partial dentures. [RGUHS]
28. U-shaped or horseshoe-shaped major connector. [NTR-NR]
29. Minor connectors - definition and types. [MUHS]
30. Give the advantages and disadvantages of lingual plate major connector. [MUHS]
31. Describe designing a lingual bar with diagrams. Name two indications of the same. [RGUHS]
32. Define and explain the various types of minor connectors. [RGUHS]
33. Enumerate the major connectors. [MUHS]
34. U-shaped maxillary major connector. [RGUHS]
35. Define major and minor connectors. Describe the different types of major connectors. [GOA]
36. Write the various major connectors used in RPD and discuss mandibular major connectors. [MUHS]
37. Name the different components of removable partial denture. Discuss the various maxillary major connectors. [GOA]
38. Posterior palatal bar. [NTR-NR]
39. Lingual bar. [NTR-NR]
40. Define direct retainers in removable partial prosthesis. Classify and give different designs. [GOA]
41. Mirror connectors used with denture bases. [MUHS]
42. Mandibular major connector used with high lingual frenum. [MUHS]
43. Different types of minor connectors. [MUHS]
44. Minor connector in partial denture. [NTR-OR]
45. Major connector. [NTR-OR, RGUHS]
46. Swing-lock partial denture prosthesis. [NTR-NR]

Short Notes

1. Precision attachments. [NTRUGHS]
2. Bar clasp. [TN]
3. Ring clasp. [RGUHS (OS)]
4. I-bar clasps. [TN]
5. Canine rest. [RGUHS (RS)]
6. Combination clasp. [NTRUHS (NR); TN]
7. Non-rigid connectors. [RGUHS (RS2)]
8. Circumferential clasp. [RGUHS (RS2)]
9. Stress breakers. [RGUHS (RS2); TN]
10. Reciprocal arm. [RGUHS(RS2)]
11. Stress equalizers. [TN]
12. Maxillary major connectors. [NTRUHS]
13. Splints. [NTRUHS]
14. RPI concept. [NTRUHS (OR); TN]
15. Compare retentive and reciprocal arm in removable partial dentures. [TN]
16. Gingivally approaching clasp. [TN]
17. Selection of mandibular major connector. [TN]
18. Lingual bar. [RGUHS (OS)]
19. Indirect retainers. [GOA; TN]
20. RPI clasp. [TN]
21. Principles of indirect retention. [TN]
22. Functions of occlusal rest. [TN]
23. Advantages of metallic denture bases. [TN]
24. Cingulum rest. [NTRUHS]
25. Part of surveyor. [NTRUHS]
26. Advantages of vertical projection clasps [NTRUHS]
27. Major connectors. [GOA, TN]
28. Role of stress breakers. [RGUHS (RS2)]
29. Internal occlusal rests. [RGUHS (RS2)]
30. Indirect retention. [TN]
31. Aker's clasp. [RGUHS (OS); TN]
32. Clasp assembly. [TN]
33. Factors affecting support in distal extension. [TN]
34. Define path of insertion and path of removal in partial denture. [NTRUHS]
35. RPI system. [NTRUHS]
36. Minor connectors. [GOA, TN]
37. Circumferential clasp. [RGUHS (RS)]
38. Fulcrum axis and its importance in RPD design. [TN]
39. Requirement of a clasp design. [TN]
40. Occlusal rest seat. [GOA, TN]
41. Radicular retainers. [GOA]
42. Internal attachment prosthesis. [GOA]

Chapter 31 Recently Asked Questions

RESTS AND REST SEATS

Long Essays

1. Classify 'Rests' in removable partial denture. Describe the function and topography of occlusal rest, illustrating with diagram the occlusal rest seat. [TN]

Short Essays

1. Indirect retainers. [MUHS]
2. Occlusal rest. [RGUHS,TN]
3. Define occlusal rest and rest seat and describe the preparation of occlusal rest. [RGUHS]
4. Rest seat preparation [TN]
5. Write the characteristics of occlusal res,t seat. [MUHS]
6. Rests and rest seats. [MUHS]
7. Define occlusal rest and explain the designing of occlusal rest seat.

Short Notes

1. What are the requirements of an occlusal rest seat preparation for a premolar? [MUHS]
2. Rest seat. [RGUHS]
3. Occlusal rest and rest seat. [MUHS]
4. What are the different components of cast partial denture? Give details about the rest and rest seat preparation. [MUHS]
5. Write the procedure of occlusal rest seat preparation in enamel. [MUHS]
6. Occlusal rest seat preparation. [RGUHS, NTR-OR]
7. Rests in RPD. [NTR-NR]
8. Define occlusal rest and rest seat and describe the preparation of occlusal rest. [RGUHS]
9. Occlusal rest seat. [RGUHS, NTR-OR, TN]
10. Give the functions of rest in removable partial dentures. [MUHS]
11. Rests and rest seats. [GOA]
12. Occlusal rest. [GOA, TN]
13. Functions of occlusal rest. [NTR-OR]
14. Occlusal rest-functions, diagnosis and rest seat preparation. [NTR-OR]
15. Function of rest in RPD. [MUHS]
16. Define occlusal rest and explain the designing of occlusal rest seat. [BUHS]

DIRECT AND INDIRECT RETAINERS

Long Essays

1. Define direct retainer. Discuss in detail the extracoronal direct retainer. [MUHS]
2. Define direct retainers. Classify extracoronal direct retainers. Discuss the application and design of RH clasp. [MUHS]
3. Define direct retainer. Write the various principles of designing a clasp. Add a note on the various types of clasp. [RGUHS]
4. Classify extracoronal retainers in removable partial dentures. Discuss the factors which influence the quality and efficiency of clasp. [MUHS]
5. Define direct retainers. Classify them and discuss the principles of designing them for a successful remov-able partial denture. [MUHS]
6. Define a removable partial denture. How do you choose a direct retainer for a removable partial denture case? [NTR-NR]
7. Write in detail about the various modifications of circumferential clasps and add a note on intracoronal direct retainers. [TN]
8. Define direct retainers in removable partial dentures. Classify them and discuss their indications. [MUHS IS]
9. Draw a design for a partially edentulous patient mentioning each component. [MUHS]
10. What is direct retainer? Describe the parts of direct retainer. What are the requirements of an ideal clasp design? [NTR-OR]
11. Discuss the RPI system and describe the design. [MUHS]
12. Define indirect retainer. Describe the indications and reasons for the use of indirect retainer and its requirements. [NTR-OR]
13. Discuss the indirect retention in removable partial prosthodontics. [GOA]
14. Discuss the factors which determine the choice of direct retainer. [MUHS]
15. What is direct retainer? Describe the parts of a direct retainer and mention its function [RGUHS, BUHS]
16. Discuss the role of indirect retainers in a distal extension partial denture. Name the various types of indirect retainers and discuss the principles for correct location of indirect retainers. [MUHS]

17. What are the internal attachments in removable partial dentures? [RGUHS]
18. Define retainer, connector, and stress breakers. Describe in brief the various types of maxillary direct retainers used in removable prosthodontics. [RGUHS]
19. Classify 'rests' in removable partial denture. Describe the function and topography of occlusal rest, illustrating with diagram the occlusal rest seat. [TN]
20. Define direct retainer. Write the various principles of designing a clasp. [TN]
21. Classify direct retainers in removable partial denture. Explain the different occlusally approaching clasps. [RGUHS (OS)]
22. Define a clasp. Describe the parts of clasps. Illustrate with diagram about the various configurations of clasps and their relevance to survey lines. [TN]
23. Write the components of cast partial denture and write in detail about direct retainers.
24. Define a clasp. Describe the parts of clasps. Illustrate with diagram about the various configurations of clasps and their relevance to survey lines.

Short Essays

1. Radicular retainer. [RGUHS (RS2)]
2. RPI concept. [NTRUGHS]
3. Indirect retainer. [NTR-OR, MUHS, NTRUHS (OR)]
4. Circumferential clasp. [RGUHS (RS)]
5. Indirect retainers in RPD. [RGUHS (RS2)]
6. Bar clasp. [RGUHS (RS2)]
7. Gingivally approaching clasp. [RGUHS, NTR-NR]
8. Retentive and reciprocal arms. [RGUHS (RS2)]
9. Compare between direct and indirect retention in removable partial dentures. [RGUHS]
10. What are direct retainers? Discuss the different types of direct retainers in removable partial prosthesis. [GOA]
11. Direct and indirect retention. [NTR-NR]
12. Direct retainers in RPD. [NTR-NR, NTR-OR]
13. Aker's clasp. [NTR-NR]
14. Define direct retainers. Discuss in detail an ideal circumferential clasp direct retainer. [GOA]
15. Classification of clasp. [NTR-OR]
16. Define direct retainers. Enumerate and discuss the different types of direct retainers in removable partial denture prosthesis. [GOA]
17. Ring clasp. [NTR-OR]
18. Define direct retainers in removable partial prosthesis. Classify and give the different designs. [GOA]
19. Combination clasp. [NTR-OR]
20. Direct retainers (clasp). [NTR-OR]
21. Factors governing the clasp design. [NTR-OR]
22. Requirements of clasp design. [MUHS]

Short Notes

1. Direct retainers. [GOA, NTRUHS (OR), TN]
2. Reciprocation. [NTRUHS]
3. Porosities in casting. [RGUHS (OS)]
4. Roach clasp. [RGUHS (OS)]
5. Reciprocal arm. [RGUHS (OS)]
6. Enumerate the factors influencing effectiveness of indirect retainers. [MUHS]
7. Reciprocation. [NTRUHS]
8. Guiding planes. [NTRUHS]
9. Indirect retention. Add a note oniding the location of the same. [MUHS]
10. Ring clasp. [NTRUHS]
11. What is indirect retainer? And what are the different forms of indirect retainer? [MUHS]
12. Indirect retainers. [RGUHS]
13. Extracoronal retainers. [RGUHS]
14. Aker's clasps with diagram. [TN]
15. Parts of clasp. [RGUHS]
16. Indications of embrasure clasp. [NTR-NR]
17. Precession attachment. [RGUHS]
18. Requirements of extracoronal direct retainers. [MUHS]
19. Infrabulge. [RGUHS]
20. Parts of clasp. [RGUHS]
21. Types of bar clasps. [TN]
22. Indirect retainers. [GOA]
23. Ring clasp. [NTR-NR]
24. Classify extracoronal direct retainers by giving examples. [MUHS]
25. Circumferential clasp. [GOA]
26. Functions of indirect retainer. [MUHS]
27. Clasp assembly. [NTR-NR; TN]
28. Half and half claps. [NTR-NR]
29. Occlusally approaching clasps. [TN]
30. Radicular retainers. [GOA]
31. Clasp units. [GOA]
32. Gingivally approaching clasp. [RGUHS]
33. Bar clasp. [RGUHS]
34. Intracoronal retainers. [BUHS, RGUHS]
35. RPI clasp. [RGUHS]
36. Combination clasp. [RGUHS]
37. RPI clasp. [BUHS]

Chapter 31 Recently Asked Questions

DENTURE BASE CONSIDERATIONS

Long Essays

1. Discuss how you will minimize the stress on abutment in case of distal extension partial denture. [MUHS]

Short Essays

1. Stress breakers. [MUHS, NTRUHS (OR)]

Short Notes

1. Denture bases for cast RPD. [TN]
2. What is the concept of stress breakers? Write the different types of stress breakers. [MUHS]

PRINCIPLES OF RPD DESIGN

Long Essays

1. Enumerate the components of removable partial denture. Discuss the principles of partial denture design. [NTR-OR]
2. Describe the principles involved in RPD designing. [NTRUHS (OR)]
3. Discuss the various components of removable partial denture designed for Kennedy's class II situation. [NTR-NR]
4. Discuss the principles in removable partial denture design. [RGUHS, BUHS]

Short Essays

1. Factors influencing design of RPD. [RGUHS (RS)]
2. Stress breakers. [NTR-OR, RGUHS RGUHS (RS2)]
3. Disadvantages of stress breakers. [NTR-OR]
4. Problems encountered in distal extension partial denture. [NTR-NR]
5. Stress breaking principle. [NTR-NR]
6. Stress breakers in partial denture. [NTR-OR]
7. Denture base. [RGUHS]

Short Notes

1. Stress breakers. [NTR-NR, GOA]
2. Precision attachment. [RGUHS]
3. Fulcrum line. [NTR-NR]

SURVEYING AND PREPARATION OF MOUTH FOR RPD

Long Essays

1. Define a surveyor. What is the purpose of surveying and explain in detail about the step by step procedure in surveying diagnostic and master cast? [RGUHS]
2. Discuss the role of surveyor in removable partial denture treatment. [NTRUHS (NR)]
3. Describe in detail the denture surveyor. [RGUHS (OS)]
4. Define dental cast surveyor. Enumerate the functions. Describe the surveying procedure. [RGUHS (RS2)]
5. What is a surveyor? Mention its uses and describe step by step procedure of surveying a diagnostic cast. [TN]
6. Define a surveyor. Mention its parts. Explain in detail step by step procedure in surveying. [NTR-NR]
7. Define a surveyor. Describe the parts of a surveyor and the importance of surveying. [GOA]
8. Write in brief the importance of dental cast surveyor in designing biologically acceptable removable partial denture. [TN]
9. Define path of insertion and path of removal in a removable cast partial denture. Discuss the factors affecting the same and the role played by the surveyor. [TN]
10. Mouth preparation in removable partial dentures. [MUHS]
11. Describe a dental cast surveyor. Describe the factors responsible for the path of insertion of a removable partial denture. [NTR-OR]
12. Selection of teeth for distal extension partial dentures. [MUHS]
13. Anterior teeth replacement in removable partial denture. [MUHS]

14. Discuss how you will minimize the stress on abutment in case of distal extension partial denture. [MUHS]
15. Define removable partial, denture prosthesis. Describe in detail mouth preparation for removable partial denture. [RGUHS BUHS]
16. Describe a dental cast surveyor. Describe the factors responsible for the path of insertion of a removable partial denture. [NTR-OR]
17. Describe in brief the various types of mouth preparation procedures undertaken in case of removable partial denture service. [RGUHS]

Short Essays

1. Survey line. [RGUHS (RS)]
2. Survey lines. [RGUHS NTRUHS (OR)]
3. Guiding plane. [RGUHS (RS)]
4. Define surveyor. What are the objectives of surveying? [NTRUHS]
5. Uses of surveyor. [RGUHS (RS)]
6. Undercut gauge. [RGUHS (RS)]
7. Surveyor. [RGUHS (OS)]
8. Axioproximal grooves. [RGUHS (RS)]
9. Factors influencing design of removable partial denture. [RGUHS (RS)]
10. Define dental surveyor. Discuss the factors affecting path of insertion and removal. [GOA]
11. Dental model surveyor. [NTR-NR]
12. Surveying line. [NTR-NR]
13. Infrabulge. [RGUHS]
14. Surveying tools. [RGUHS; NTR-NR]
15. Preparation of mouth for impressions. [RGUHS]
16. Define surveyor. Give the classification and discuss the uses of an articulator. [GOA]
17. Discuss the importance of surveying and the various steps in removable partial denture fabrication. [GOA]
18. Refractory cast for removable partial denture. [TN]
19. List the types of surveyors and explain the various uses of surveyors. [RGUHS]
20. Surveyor. [NTR-NR NTR-OR]
21. Guide planes. [RGUHS]
22. Mouth preparation in RPD. [NTR-OR]
23. Dental cast surveyor. [RGUHS TN]
24. Surveying. [NTR-OR]
25. Define surveying. Describe dental surveyor and its uses in designing of a removable partial prosthodontics. [GOA]
26. Write a note on surveying. [GOA]
27. Dental cast surveyor. [NTR-OR]
28. Dental surveyor. [NTR-OR]
29. Stress breakers. [MUHS]

Short Notes

1. Factors influencing the path of insertion on removable prosthesis. [TN]
2. Surveyors [RGUHS (OS); TN]
3. Surveying tools. [RGUHS(OS)]
4. Provisional restoration. [NTRUHS (OR)]
5. Uses of surveyors. [RGUHS (OS); NTR-NR]
6. Undercut gauges and their application in surveying. [TN]
7. Height of contour. [RGUHS]
8. Tripoding. [NTR-NR TN]
9. Dental surveyor. [GOA TN]
10. Remounting procedure. [TN]
11. Surveyor - draw the diagram and label the parts. [TN]
12. Tripoding the cast. [RGUHS]
13. Surveyor and its uses. [TN]
14. What is the concept of stress breakers? Write the different types of stress breakers. [MUHS]
15. Factors determining path of insertion of removable partial denture. [GOA]
16. Factors affecting path of placement. [GOA]

IMPRESSION MATERIALS AND PROCEDURES FOR RPD

Long Essays

1. What is functional impression in removable partial denture? How will you obtain such an impression? [RGUHS BUHS]

Short Essays

1. Surgical obturators. [RGUHS(RS2)]
2. Impression techniques in removable partial dentures. [RGUHS (RS)]
3. Impression procedures in removable partial denture. [RGUHS,(RS2), (RS2)]
4. Functional form of impression in removable partial denture. [RGUHS (RS)]
5. Enumerate the methods of making a functional impression for removable partial dentures. What is the significance of such functional impressions? [MUHS]

Chapter 31 Recently Asked Questions

Short Notes

1. Physiological impression in RPD. [NTR-NR]
2. Altered cast technique. [RGUHS (RS2); TN]
3. Altered impression technique. [NTRUHS (OR)]
4. Impression in distal extension partial denture. [TN]
5. Impression procedure for distal extension PD. [NTR-OR]

SUPPORT FOR THE DISTAL EXTENSION DENTURE BASE, OCCLUSAL RELATIONSHIP FOR RPD, LABORATORY PROCEDURES AND WORK AUTHORIZATION FOR RPD

Long Essays

1. State how indirect retainer helps in distal extension base partial denture. Explain the effective method of recording impression for the same. [MUHS]
2. Methods of establishing occlusal relationships in RPD. [RGUHS]
3. Working model. [MUHS]
4. Discuss the need for special impression procedures in removable partial dentures and describe the various methods in detail. [MUHS]
5. Discuss stress optimization in bilateral long-span extension partial denture. [MUHS]
6. Explain altered cast technique. [MUHS]
7. Dentures base material in RPD. [MUHS]

Short Essays

1. Factors influencing the support of the distal extension base. [RGUHS (OS)]
2. Functional impressions for distal extension partial dentures. [MUHS, NTRUHS]
3. Distal extension denture base in removable partial denture construction. [RGUHS (RS)]

Short Notes

1. Lingualized occlusion. [TN]
2. Define stress breaker (stress equalizer) and discuss in short its role in distal extension partial denture. [MUHS]
3. Ring clasp. [NTRUHS]
4. Distal extension denture base in removable partial denture construction. [TN]
5. Support for the removable partial denture. [RGUHS (RS2)]
6. Methods of special impression procedure in removable partial denture which is already' in use with drawbacks. [MUHS]
7. Occlusal registration in removable partial denture. [TN]

CORRECTION OF RPDS, REPAIRS AND ADDITIONS TO RPD, RELINING AND REBASING TNE RPD AND MISCELLANEOUS

Long Essays

1. Discuss why are dentures necessary for a semi-edentulous and completely edentulous patients. [BUHS]

Short Essays

1. Kelly's combination syndrome. [NTR-NR]
2. Block out procedure in cast partial denture. [NTR-NR]
3. Pain control in tooth preparation for retained prosthesis. [NTR-OR]
4. Path of insertion of removable partial dentures. [NTR- OR]
5. Splints. [NTR-OR]
6. Surgical splints. [NTR-OR]
7. Soldering and its implications and procedures. [NTR-OR]
8. Soldering and its applications and procedures. [NTR-OR]
9. Guide planes. [NTR-OR]
10. Key and key way attachment. [NTR-OR]
11. Path-of insertion. [NTR-OR]

Short Notes

1. Tensofriction. [NTR-NR]
2. Combination syndrome. [TN]
3. Guiding planes in RPD. [RGUHS]
4. Pressure indicating paste. [RGUHS]
5. Refractory cast. [NTR-NR]
6. Reciprocation in RPD. [NTR-NR]
7. Enameloplasty in RPD. [NTR-NR]